Philosophy of Science for Nursing Practice:
Concepts and Application

Michael D. Dahnke, PhD, is assistant teaching professor, Department of Health Sciences & Health Administration and Doctoral Nursing Department, Drexel University, Philadelphia. Dr. Dahnke's PhD is in Philosophy from Temple University (2002) and his BA is in Liberal Studies from Bowling Green State University (1990). His dissertation was *Film and the Aesthetic Construction of Self/Sex/Gender* under the supervision of Dr. Charles Dyke. His areas of specialty include Philosophy of Science, Ethics, Aesthetics, Philosophy of Film, and Contemporary Continental Philosophy. He has taught a wide range of philosophy and ethics courses to BSN, MSN, DrNP, and other health professions students, including: Health Care Ethics, Advanced Ethical Decision Making in Health Care, Moral Philosophy, and Health & Vulnerable Populations. Dr. Dahnke has taught NURS 700: *Philosophy of Natural & Social Science: Foundations for Inquiry into the Discipline of Nursing* in Drexel University's DrNP program for 6 years, since the inception of the course. He has developed and revised this course and has a great appreciation for the kinds of concepts and principles that are particularly germane to the critical thinking development of a doctoral nursing student. He is the author of *Film, Art, and Filmart: An Introduction to Aesthetics through Film* (University Press of America, 2007), a chapter in Lachman's, *Applied Ethics in Nursing* (LWW, 2005), and "The Role of the ANA Code of Ethics in Ethical Decision Making" in the journal *Holistic Nursing Practice* (2009). He recently presented at the 2008 International Nursing Ethics Conference at Yale University and at the 2009 DNP Conference at Hilton Head Island, SC on *How Much Does Philosophy of Science Belongs in a Doctor of Nursing Practice Curriculum?* His work is becoming increasingly visible in scholarly nursing circles.

H. Michael Dreher, PhD, RN, is associate professor with Tenure and Chair, Doctoral Nursing Department, Drexel University, Philadelphia (appointed 2004). His PhD is in Nursing Science from Widener University (2000) and AS (1984), BSN (1988), and MN (1991) from the University of South Carolina, Columbia. His dissertation was *The Effect of Caffeine Reduction on Sleep and Well-being in Persons with HIV* (published in the *Journal of Psychosomatic Research*, 2003) under the supervision of the deceased Dr. Susan Kun Leddy (author of six editions of *Leddy and Pepper's Conceptual Bases of Professional Nursing* (LWW, 2009). Dreher is a dynamic leader, innovator, and educator. He has led Drexel to the forefront of doctoral nursing education and spear-headed the Drexel DNP Conferences on DNP Education in Annapolis in 2007 and in Hilton Head Island, SC in 2009 (the 3rd conference is scheduled for Fall 2011). In 2007, he established the first mandatory doctoral study abroad program in nursing (London/Dublin). His clinical nursing experience (1984–2000) has focused primarily on Adult Health/Coronary Care/Home Care of Cardiac Patients, and he completed a postdoctorate in sleep and respiratory neurobiology at the University of Pennsylvania (2001–2003). He has participated in the Harvard Macy Institute Program for Leading Innovation in Healthcare & Education (Harvard Business School/Medical School—2007) and established the first MSN in Innovation (2007). Dr. Dreher has published more than 70 journal articles and has been PI or Co-PI on more than 20 funded projects. His current scholarship has focused on innovation, "boomer health," professional/practice doctorate issues, and in expanding his Model of Practice Knowledge Development. He recently presented two papers at the first International Conference on Professional Doctorates in London (11/2009) and was the invited endnote speaker at the Southern Universities Alliance for Doctoral Education's Professional Doctorate Conference at the University of Brighton, UK (4/2009). Dr. Dreher conceived and has taught NURS 716: *The Structure of Scientific Knowledge in Nursing* to Doctor of Nursing Practice students for several years and is coauthor on another forthcoming text from Springer (12/2010) on *Role Development for Doctoral Advanced Nursing Practice* with Dr. Mary Ellen Smith Glasgow.

Philosophy of Science for Nursing Practice: Concepts and Application

Michael D. Dahnke, PhD
H. Michael Dreher, PhD, RN

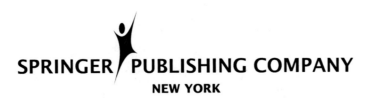

SPRINGER PUBLISHING COMPANY
NEW YORK

Springer Publishing Company, LLC
11 West 42nd Street
New York, NY 10036
www.springerpub.com

Acquisitions Editor: Margaret Zuccarini
Senior Editor: Rose Mary Piscitelli
Cover design: Steven Pisano
Project Manager: Nick Barber
Composition: Techset Composition India Pvt Ltd

ISBN: 978-0-8261-0554-7
E-book ISBN: 978-0-8261-0555-4

12 13/ 5 4

The author and the publisher of this Work have made every effort to use sources believed to be reliable to provide information that is accurate and compatible with the standards generally accepted at the time of publication. Because medical science is continually advancing, our knowledge base continues to expand. Therefore, as new information becomes available, changes in procedures become necessary. We recommend that the reader always consult current research and specific institutional policies before performing any clinical procedure. The author and publisher shall not be liable for any special, consequential, or exemplary damages resulting, in whole or in part, from the readers' use of, or reliance on, the information contained in this book. The publisher has no responsibility for the persistence or accuracy of URLs for external or third-party Internet Web sites referred to in this publication and does not guarantee that any content on such Web sites is, or will remain, accurate or appropriate.

CIP data is on file at the Library of Congress

Printed in the United States of America by Gasch Printing.

To
My parents William and Raymonde Dahnke
and
HMD

Michael David Dahnke

and

To
My parents Larry Dreher and Hazel Evenich
and
MDD
and
to the memory of Lavinia Lloyd Dock (1858–1956), a feminist, author,
pioneer in nursing education, social activist, and one helluva radical nurse,
born in the town of my dad's birth

Heyward Michael Dreher

Contents

Reviewers

Ann H. Cary, PhD, MPH, RN, A-CCC   Professor, Director, School of Nursing, Loyola University of New Orleans, Robert Wood Johnson Foundation Executive Nurse Fellow 2008–2011, New Orleans, Louisiana

Eileen Chasens, DSN, RN   Assistant Professor, Health and Community Systems, School of Nursing University of Pittsburgh, Pittsburgh, Pennsylvania

Veronica A. Clarke-Tasker, PhD, RN, MBA, MPH   Professor, Division of Nursing, College of Pharmacy, Nursing & Allied Health Sciences, Howard University, Washington, DC

Barbara Granger, PhD, CPRP, LLC   Granger Consultation Services, Philadelphia, Pennsylvania

Cheryl Holly, EdD, RN   Associate Professor and Co-Director of the NJ Center for Evidence-Based Practice, Chair, Doctor of Nursing Practice Program, School of Nursing, University of Medicine and Dentistry New Jersey

Alice Marie S. Poyss, PhD, MSN, CS, APRN-BC   Clinical Associate Professor, College of Nursing and Health Professions, Drexel University, Philadelphia, Pennsylvania

Foreword

The rapid emergence of the Doctor of Nursing Practice (DNP) degree in the United States during the past five years has been remarkable. Also remarkable is the significant debate about knowledge generation and whether knowledge generation belongs within the competencies of the nurse holding a DNP degree. The "knowledge" debate has largely been an "either/or" phenomenon about who generates and who applies knowledge. The debate has focused less on what knowledge development and implementation looks like when contextually driven in real-world practice environments. There is a linear tendency to compartmentalize research and practice as separate entities rather than view these as intricately intertwined and rooted in the same foundations of philosophies of science and epistemologies.

One argument for the separation of nursing theory development from nursing practice reflects long-standing ideologies stemming from nursing's quest for academic disciplinary status. While academe is the traditional bastion of knowledge discovery, the academy has also been criticized as sometimes being removed from the realities practitioners encounter everyday, and that science does not always address the questions driven through practice. The traditional theory–practice gap may reflect the location of scientists and practitioners as well—the former more likely being housed in traditional academic environments and the latter found in service.

As the debate about knowledge development and the DNP continues to unfold, envisioning what constitutes an inclusive knowledge development environment, who engages science, and what competencies doctorally prepared clinicians need in the current health care sector are imperative. It is unlikely that nurse scientists can effectively answer all the questions posed by practice. Moreover, the numbers of advanced practice nurses prepared to conduct research under conditions posed by real-world practice conditions are limited. From a practical standpoint research findings often tell clinicians more about efficacy than effectiveness. Yet, clinicians must make treatment decisions without the evidence of how a treatment works under ordinary and variable conditions, prescribed by clinicians with varying degrees of expertise, and practicing across the spectrum of healthcare settings, to treat a heterogeneity of eligible patients. Showing that an intervention is efficacious under homogeneous (e.g., randomized clinical trials) conditions *and* effective under real-world heterogeneity does not ensure that it will be adopted in the broader population, public health, or clinical practice settings.

Challenges associated with getting research findings into practice are long standing, yet evidence alone may not influence practice. An assumption of the evidence-based practice movement is that research evidence and best practice guidelines are crucial for treatment decisions. Yet, treatment decisions largely remain at the level of the individual clinician, and in the current health-care environment it can be argued that treatment decisions have a wide degree of variability. For advanced practice nurses, who are currently the largest constituents of the DNP degree, the greater body of evidence for advanced nursing practice is also likely to come from non-nursing disciplinary research (e.g., pharmacotherapeutics and medical science). What changes are necessary to transform *nursing* into the discipline that is leading knowledge development for practice?

In *Philosophy of Science for Nursing Practice: Concepts and Application*, Dahnke and Dreher argue that we can no longer ignore the need for clinicians to be educated in the principal concepts of philosophy of science. Debate, again largely fueled by the expansion of the practice doctorate, provides a compelling opportunity to examine philosophy of science as a necessary foundation for nurses prepared at the doctoral level—whether prepared through the Doctor of Philosophy (PhD) or Doctor of Nursing Practice (DNP) degree. The text is organized into three sections. Section I focuses on practice and the practice disciplines. Section II focuses on philosophy, science, and the philosophy of science, and argues that philosophy of science is fundamental for all scientific work. Section III traces the history of nursing science and the book culminates by presenting practice knowledge development as an emerging epistemology in nursing. An intriguing discussion is presented about what kind of nursing knowledge DNP graduates should produce. Is it "practice inquiry" or "actionable knowledge" or "mode 2 knowledge" or perhaps simply "practice knowledge"? Those who have been engaged in the debates will recognize these terms. Further, given the complexity of nursing phenomena, are traditional methods of inquiry sufficient to explore the breadth of these phenomena? Additionally, should nursing limit inquiry to nurses holding the PhD? Clearly, this textbook raises stimulating questions that hopefully will be embraced within the nursing knowledge debate.

As the DNP movement marches forward, one risk is settling the debates too soon. Some schools are moving toward dual preparation through the DNP/PhD degree. Just as in other disciplines that promote dual preparation, there clearly is both need and place for the DNP/PhD dual preparation. It can be argued, however, that dual preparation will not sufficiently meet the demands for practice knowledge development. Greater numbers of graduates will be in the practice domain—at the points where the dots between theory and practice are connected and play out. Thus, as the practice knowledge epistemology grows, the theory and methods for conducting practice-led research must also evolve.

While the past five years have seen significant debate about what the DNP does or does not do, less attention has been given to knowledge generation as a process that all nurses engage in at all levels of educational development and across the career spectrum. Defining knowledge development as a competency to be developed across the spectrum of nursing education deserves greater attention. Educational strategies might more fully consider how theory and practice are mutually interdependent instead of mutually independent processes, particularly since all too often it takes years before research findings are implemented in practice or translated into meaningful patient outcomes.

Historically, strategies to get nursing knowledge better utilized largely concentrated on improving nurses' knowledge about research, and more recently on improving implementation of the evidence into practice. Is it really sufficient to strive for active collaboration between researchers and practitioners in the sense that the former does research and the latter applies research? If it can be accepted that this approach is not sufficient, then traditional values and boundaries must change—an argument inherent within *Philosophy of Science for Nursing Practice: Concepts and Application.* Core to the argument that traditional values and boundaries must change is the notion that *before* clinicians can evaluate the evidence they must understand something about knowledge and evidence (e.g., philosophy of science) as well as understand how evidence is generated (e.g., methodology), and this is the chief rationale for this important text.

A challenge ahead for nursing is to take the path of *most resistance* rather than the easier road of *least resistance.* The debate needs to continue and move beyond teaching our students that there is "research" and there is "practice" and that the choice of degree should reflect what one wants to do (e.g., research or practice), to debating whether nursing is teaching an appropriate level of inquiry including philosophy and methodologies specific to those real-world, rapidly changing conditions that characterize today's practice environment. Most today embrace that practice should be evidence based, yet struggle lingers with respect to the notion that doctoral level practice includes knowing the principles of philosophy and competencies to conduct research and generate practice knowledge (including what must be new and emerging theories and methodologies).

The debate also needs to grapple with the concomitant notion that *theory generation is practice* and debate whether *the nurse who is conducting research is engaging in nursing practice?* All too often theory generation is not equated with nursing practice. The comfort zone seems more aligned with the premise that nurse scientists have the skills to conduct research and practitioners have the skills to examine the evidence. The ability to generate knowledge that can be rapidly translated into practice and the determination of who is qualified to do this are arguably on the path of most resistance—a road not to be feared, but to be embraced as part of the knowledge frontier.

Dahnke and Dreher's *Philosophy of Science for Nursing Practice: Concepts and Application* is thought-provoking. The text raises questions about whether it is time to examine nursing's deeply seated values about knowledge generation, who does it, and the definitions of research versus practice, as well as timeliness for the discipline to grapple with emerging epistemologies and embrace teaching philosophy of science and research as a competency that begins with the fundamentals of nursing and is developed across practice and research settings. As such a text, it has utility for both the DNP and PhD student, as doctoral preparation, regardless of the degree, is enhanced by grappling with what it means for nursing to be a practice discipline. Dahnke and Dreher portend that critical inquiry is essential to any practice discipline that seeks the best evidence, the best interventions, and the best practices. Further, they posit that knowledge cannot be properly evaluated or advanced without an understanding of the principles of philosophy of science, which ultimately supports all types of practice-oriented decision making. From the perspective of teaching students fundamental philosophy of science content—such as "What is evidence?" "What is explanation?" or "What is inductive/deductive reasoning?"—inclusion of content on philosophy of science seems formative knowledge for the basis of critical inquiry—again, a central component of Dahnke and Dreher's perspective.

Perhaps, as Dahnke and Dreher portend, some of the struggle continues to rest with the concept of whether DNP graduates are mere users of knowledge or active

participants in the generation of practice knowledge—knowledge driven by interaction, experience, and *a priori* knowledge. The last is more than the end user and is
possibly the least defined type of (emerging) epistemology. A few years ago Gary
Rolfe suggested that nursing practice is a series of unique encounters, each of which
is different from all others. For clinicians, a practice challenge from a methods perspective is that generalizability applies to the average of large groups rather than to specific
individuals within those groups. Clinicians make treatment decisions at the individual, unique level of application. Rolfe went so far as to suggest that clinicians
should not simply engage with researchers, but that clinicians should become
researchers. He suggested that:

> ... rather than practice being informed by science, nursing practice should reformulate
> itself as science if it is to address the problem of the theory–practice gap. What is required
> is not a science of large numbers, but a science of the unique. While the social sciences
> are concerned with theorizing about people, nursing science requires theories about
> individual persons[1]
>
> —*Rolfe, 2006, p. 40*

The notion of nursing practice being reformulated as a science is intriguing as the
care of the unique individual is the domain of the clinician. Dahnke and Dreher's text
also triggers a thought that perhaps part of nursing's struggle is a need to recognize
that epistemologies are changing and revolutionary science is at play. As a consequence, our deep-seated (and hard-won) values are competing against emerging
epistemologies further driving current debate (and to some degree discord). The
path of least resistance will maintain status quo—that is, dominant paradigms will
push to maintain the division of practice and research. The debates are not surprising
and are critical to moving knowledge forward. As Thomas Kuhn pointed out, when
paradigm shifts occur, maintaining *status quo* is a response of the established scientific
community to maintain their beliefs. Scientists, especially young, unknown scientists,
are expected to conform to the dominant paradigm. New thought, theory, or scientific
findings outside of the dominant paradigm may be ridiculed and dismissed as bad
science. Kuhn also reminds us that change takes time, and often occurs away from
the mainstream, and occurs in the fringes.[2] Is the notion of practice knowledge,
practice-led or practitioner-led research an example of bad science? If one argues
that practice is the center of the design, the context of where research is conducted,
and ultimately where findings are reported and implemented, it seems nursing may
be moving toward the leading edge rather than the fringes. Perhaps a better question
is "why not pursue doctoral education that places our clinicians at the forefront of
practice-led investigative models?" It is unlikely that a linear approach to practice
knowledge development (e.g., theory-to-practice) argument can be sustained.

Finally, while the DNP has sparked significant knowledge debates that have not
always been easy, impersonal, or are even necessarily resolved, let alone have arrived
at a level enough playing field that nursing can build new practice epistemologies and

---

[1]Rolfe, G. (2006). Nursing praxis and the science of the unique. *Nursing Science Quarterly, 19*, 39–43.

[2]Kuhn, T. (1962). *The structure of scientific revolutions*. Chicago, IL: University of Chicago Press.

methodologies (with courage and a smile), I am reminded of the King of Swamp Castle from the film *Monty Python and the Holy Grail.*

> When I first came here, this was all swamp. Everyone said I was daft to build a castle on a swamp, but I built in all the same, just to show them. It sank into the swamp. So I built a second one. That sank into the swamp. So I built a third. That burned down, fell over, then sank into the swamp. But the fourth one stayed up. And that's what you're going to get, Lad, the strongest castle in all of England.[3]

Thus it goes that in the larger scheme of nursing's quest for knowledge it is likely that practice knowledge will be built in the evolutionary swamp, over and over again, brick by brick, until our practice understanding is fortified and our castle the strongest of all. Along the way, hopefully, nursing will gain strong understanding of the processes needed to educate the DNP, will assure a reasonable measure of standardization and rigor across programs, and will embrace the practice knowledge frontier as the domain of doctoral level practice—whether from the traditional perspectives of research, or clinical practice, and hopefully again as an interwoven process. That said, failure to give all of our doctoral graduates a solid understanding of where evidence comes from and skills to pursue practice knowledge presents the risk of having them sink into the practice swamp and that (arguably again!) seems daft (said with a sincere laugh!).

Sally J. Reel, PhD, RN, FNP, BC, FAAN, FAANP

Clinical Professor & Associate Dean
Academic Practice
University of Arizona College of Nursing
Tucson, Arizona

---

[3]*Monty Python and the Holy Grail.* Retrieved from http://www.imdb.com/title/tt0071853/quotes.

Preface

As more doctor of nursing practice programs embrace the concept of *practice inquiry*, we decided to write a text that we thought would be essential to its development. Any doctoral nursing program, no matter the type, must address the fundamental principles underlying "inquiry" if its graduates are going to become stewards of the discipline and advance the profession. This is a text on the philosophy of science, but one directed toward nursing, especially doctoral nursing practice. We also believe that PhD programs that have a strong connection to practice will find this text very useful too. In a unique way, we think we have embedded the philosophy of science content into the context of practice, nursing's evolution as a discipline, and philosophy's essential underpinning to what we call *practice knowledge development*.

The nature of doctoral nursing education is presently in flux and a matter of debate. What type and degree of education regarding theory and research that practice doctorates in nursing need is presently an unsettled question. Whereas many nursing PhD programs include coursework on the philosophy of science, very few doctor of nursing practice (DNP) programs have a stand-alone course devoted to the subject. However, most DNP programs do include some formal content on philosophy of science (usually embedded in other related courses) and we of course see this as essential to practice inquiry. A philosophical study like this one provides a further, deeper step into the basis of what students are learning, the essence and justification for what they are studying. There is obvious disagreement as to whether this further step is necessary or desirable. However, our review of the strongest DNP programs in the country indicate to us that coursework focusing on improving the critical inquiry of practitioners and other types of DNP students is increasing as the drive for more evidence-based practice knowledge and practice-based evidence knowledge drives DNP curricula (and PhD curricula too).

This is not a text about nursing epistemology, although the concluding chapter breaks the ice on this topic by opening a discussion surrounding a practice epistemology for nursing and we think this is particularly relevant for doctor of nursing practice programs. This text is both a contribution to this ongoing debate and a reader-friendly text on the philosophy of science. We assume minimal to no background in the formal study of philosophy for students and faculty who will use this book. Toward that end, we have included introductory materials on the essence, history and practice of philosophy in general, as well as on the philosophy of science in particular. The introductory chapters are essentially essays on the nature of practice disciplines with a nursing focus, including an essay on nursing as a practice discipline. We have emphasized issues that have been important in the evolution of nursing as a discipline, its struggle to fully embrace its identity as a practice discipline, and how the nature of doctoral nursing education, especially the practice doctorate, has now challenged the profession to revisit its disciplinary future anew and with fresh eyes. The philosophy of science chapters are written informally, in a conversational style with a minimum amount of esoteric terminology, and terminology that is included is defined in straightforward language which does not require advanced study in philosophy. The goal is to further and deepen the understanding of science for practice-doctorate nurses in a relevant and meaningful manner. The text ends with first, a chapter that traces the evolution of nursing science through the social, political, and historical prism through which nursing has evolved. The concluding chapter is a discussion of practice knowledge as an emerging epistemology for nursing and discourse on the future trajectory of the DNP as it challenges the discipline to revisit discussion on the future of nursing, disputed concepts of nursing knowledge, and the education of contemporary advance practice nurses.

In our experience of teaching doctoral nursing practice students since 2005, students are very receptive to this level of study. This has been one of the first two courses taken by our students and inevitably connections are made by them to their later studies in nursing practice and in their investigation of an important clinical problem they choose to study. From our observation, the theory–practice gap seems to collapse of its own weight through mere study, curiosity and academic rigor. Philosophy becomes a part of our nurses' knowledge-base and not simply an academic, esoteric study. At present, there appears to be no other text that addresses these issues in this manner. This is understandable, given the debate mentioned. But we offer this book not only to those nursing practice doctorate programs that currently include philosophy of science in their curriculum, but also to those that may not do so explicitly and patently, yet may include investigation into such issues more implicitly in their general curriculum. We also offer this book to those programs that are considering moving in the direction of including philosophy of science in an explicit manner in their curriculum. We think this text will also be particularly adept as a secondary text for courses in research methods, nursing epistemology, and professional DNP issues. And finally, we offer this book to those programs, faculty, and students interested and engaged in the ongoing debate regarding doctoral nursing education. Doctoral education is about debate and discourse and not merely acquiescence to another scholar's ideas, even to all of the ideas written about in this text. One of our dissertation chairs once said, "If you aren't tussling in the doctoral classroom, then what are you doing here?" We do not presume to have the final word on this debate, but hope merely to provide a thoughtful, helpful, meaningful contribution to it.

Michael D. Dahnke, PhD
H. Michael Dreher, PhD, RN

Introduction

Nursing, as a practice, as a discipline, as a science, is continually evolving and is arguably at present at a crossroad in its development. As the profession is now confronted with a new doctorate that is surging in both in enrollment and number of programs, the scope, specialties, and turf of the various forms of advance practice nurses and nurse scholars, are currently a matter of debate. Along with being a textbook, this book is a contribution to that discourse and debate. In particular, the status, purpose, and function of practice doctorate nurses (mostly DNP but DrNP too) are matters of uncertainty in the nursing discipline, its scholarship, and education today. Discussion of "evidence," however, cannot take place in a vacuum and thus the formal inquiry provided by a grounding in philosophy of science is fundamental to the discussion, conduct, and translation of evidence-based practice and practice-based evidence. We approach this work with a normative attitude toward the furtherance of education for practice doctorate nurses that advanced, fundamental knowledge, such as the philosophy of science, is not only a benefit but also a necessity for nurses at this level of education and preparation. The practice doctorate must not be a watered-down PhD. It needs to be a rigorous degree on its own merit with its own standards of academic excellence. We contend that not much has changed since Caplan (1979) observed that the two communities—one of researchers and the other of practitioners—remained apart. We hope this text can contribute to this discussion and help bridge this chasm.

Section I focuses on the nature of practice and practice disciplines, particularly nursing. Chapter 1 first introduces the concept of "practice" with an emphasis on its general use in the health professions. The nature of practice and its practice boundaries is discussed, along with a discussion of how a discipline is different from a "field" and how disciplinary membership is bestowed, and its knowledge producers legitimized. The chapter promotes the idea that it is the nature of the interpersonal and the ethical that gives rise to the status of the professional discipline. Chapter 2 takes on the challenge of providing both a historical and sociological context in which to define nursing as a practice discipline and to characterize its rise from merely work, to a field, to a fully fledged discipline. Section I concludes with Chapter 3, a discussion of the importance of philosophy of science in a practice discipline, particularly for DNP programs, and our argument is presented from both the authors' perspective as a philosopher professor and nurse professor (both doctor of nursing practice educators).

Section II focuses on philosophy, science and the philosophy of science. We find this focus valuable in preparing students to be active members in an arena of interdisciplinary advanced studies and sciences. This study is the study of the bases of all scientific work. It underlies and brings them together at their fundament. Chapters 4 through 6 are stage-setting. They provide introductory material necessary for the study to be developed through the rest of this section. Chapter 4 presents an introduction to philosophy and what it means to *do* philosophy or think philosophically. Common misconceptions of philosophy are addressed and a classic example of philosophical thinking is presented and analyzed. In addition, an introduction to basic logic is provided. This chapter will be especially helpful to students who may have never studied philosophy in a formal setting before. Chapter 5 presents a brief history of science since the Scientific Revolution. The changes—intellectual, cultural, historical, political—that occurred to bring about this revolution are addressed and the states of science pre- and post-revolution are compared. Chapter 6 is a history of the philosophy of science. By providing a historical context to this branch of philosophy, we hope to present a more holistic view of the changes, the arguments, the various schools of philosophy that comprise this study. Presenting the chapters that follow without this context runs the risk of fragmenting what is a cohesive, discursive narrative.

Chapters 7 through 12 present specific classic and contemporary questions and problems that have been raised by philosophers regarding the nature, function and practice of science. Chapter 7 presents the most fundamental of questions, "What is science?" The nature and essence of science as a means of studying the world of human experience and acquiring knowledge and justifying knowledge claims is investigated. Several classic answers are presented and critiqued. Chapter 8 investigates the scientific method with a special emphasis on the questions and problems regarding inductive logic as central to scientific investigation. Chapter 9 looks at the concept of observation. The simple notion of merely observing and reporting on phenomena is discovered to be much more complex, indefinite, and opaque than usually assumed. Chapter 10 investigates the concept of "theory" as it applies to science. The meanings and uses of theory in science are presented and critiqued. Also, the metaphysics of science are investigated as part of the study of theoretical entities. In Chapter 11, the nature of scientific explanation is explored. Explanation takes us beyond the questions of what and how to the question, why? And Chapter 12 surveys feminist critiques of both science and the philosophy of science that began during the last few decades of the 20th century.

Chapters 13 and 14 change focus to the social sciences. Since much of what is recognized as nursing science may qualify more as social science than as natural science, these chapters may be quite valuable. The dispute in nursing science between quantitative and qualitative research can be found in a much broader context within this study as well. Chapter 13 presents some of the classic problems of social science, many of which reflect problems previously studied regarding natural science but may have distinct answers due to the nature of the social sciences, while some problems may be more specific to the social sciences themselves.

Section III builds on Sections I and II. In Chapter 15, the rise of nursing science is traced through a 100 year journey of nursing's trek through time through its maturing scholarship and educational advancement. A creative use of history, sociology, and cultural commentary is used to examine how nursing rose through a century of world events and evolved to the present state of doctoral nursing education. Chapter 16 is likely the most provocative and it describes a proposed practice epistemology for the practice doctorate, practice knowledge development. Critique of the current state of the DNP degree is offered with suggestions to formalize the DNP graduate's responsibility for both disciplinary knowledge (practice knowledge) and disciplinary stewardship.

REFERENCE

Caplan, N. (1979). The two communities theory and knowledge utilization. *American Behavioural Scientist, 23,* 4.

Philosophy of Science for Nursing Practice:
Concepts and Application

1

What Is a Practice Discipline?

In responding to the challenge of relating theory to practice, it is not enough simply to argue for an "enlightenment model" which sees theoretical work as influencing practitioners and policy makers indirectly through the way in which new concepts and interpretations of social processes percolate into society at large shaping the thinking of lay and professionals alike. We must struggle to achieve a better integration of theoretical understanding and practical concerns.

NORMAN LONG[1]

INTRODUCTION

There is little doubt, at least among nursing scholars, that nursing *is* a practice discipline. However, there remains a certain amount of ambiguity surrounding the precise meaning of the word *practice*. What exactly is practice? Do all nurses[2] practice? Conversely, can a nurse *not practice*?[3] Is perhaps nursing somewhat similar to the discipline of physics where there is applied physics and also theoretical physics,[4] which is not applied but more abstract? Is the nursing scientist conducting a research study actually engaging in [applied] nursing practice or perhaps theoretical nursing? We pose this question since we are not alone in acknowledging there is real tension in nursing education and in the discipline between the acquisition of practical and theoretical knowledge and between the forces of practice and theory (Baynham, 2002; Conway, 1994; Ousey & Gallagher, 2007; Reed, 2006). As one scholar has recently

---

[1]Long, N. (1992). Introduction. In N. Long, & A. Long (Eds.), Battlefields of knowledge: The interlocking of theory and practice in social research and development (pp. 3–15). Abingdon, Oxon, UK: Routledge. Reprinted with permission of author.

[2]In this text the use of the word *nurse* will generally be defined as a registered nurse. Where the term *professional* is used, the assumption is that the nurse has at least a baccalaureate degree.

[3]That is, can a nurse who is *actively working* in nursing not be engaged in practice?

[4]*The Journal of Applied Physics* (American Institute of Physics [AIP]) web site states: they "emphasize understanding of the physics underlying modern technology, but distinguished from technology on the one side and pure physics on the other" (2010). "Theoretical physics attempts to understand the world by making a model of reality, used for rationalizing, explaining, predicting physical phenomena through a 'physical theory'." (www.wordig.com/definition/theoretical_physics, 2010, p. 1).

written, "Nursing has struggled for more than 100 years with the practice/theory dichotomy" (Apold, 2008, p. 104).

There are also skeptics who question whether nursing is a discipline, or more specifically, an *academic discipline* (Cronin & Rawlings-Anderson, 2004; Smith, 2007). The incredulous comment "You can get a doctorate in *nursing*?" continues to be expressed sometimes even from college-educated individuals. Unfortunately, this author has been asked this question multiple times and even from such persons. The issue of whether nursing is an academic discipline is even more tenuous outside of the United States where the education of nurses is usually less academically rigorous, and where the status of nurses and nursing has diminished (Hamrin, 1997). More commonly, however, is the perspective of nursing scholars who consider nursing as a relatively young and still maturing discipline (Lobo, 2005; Parse, 2005).

This first chapter will explore such questions as: What constitutes practice? What are the characteristics of a discipline? What then is a *practice discipline*? We will then address whether a practice discipline is necessarily a *profession*. Finally, we will explore some of the early practice disciplines that have parallels to nursing, and then examine the state of the contemporary health professions practice discipline. Our discussion is particularly germane to doctoral nursing students pursuing a practice doctorate, but any graduate student in nursing who deeply believes nursing scholarship must be rooted, grounded, and connected intensely to nursing practice should find this chapter and text helpful. In the next chapter we will explore these concepts as they relate specifically to nursing as a practice discipline.

WHAT IS *PRACTICE*?

Certainly the bedside registered nurse engages in practice or *nursing practice*. Similarly, the masters-prepared certified registered nurse practitioner (CRNP), certified nurse midwife (CNM), certified registered nurse anesthetist (CRNA), and clinical nurse specialist (CNS) all engage in advanced nursing practice. Recently, Dreher and Montgomery (2009) have defined the practice of the doctor of nursing practice (DNP or DrNP)[5] graduate as doctoral *advanced practice nursing* and describe how it is (or should be) different from the practice of the advanced practice registered nurse with the masters degree. But before we explore these concepts in Chapter 2, we need to first explore the origins of the word *practice* and evaluate how it is defined and operationalized among various health professions.

Elementally, the word "practice" is both a noun and a verb. The earliest English derivation of the word is from the 14th century with the word's etymology from the Middle English *practisen*, from Middle French *practiser*, from Medieval Latin *practizare*, alteration of *practicare*, from *practica* practice, noun, from Late Latin *practice*, and from Greek *praktikē*, from feminine of *praktikos* (*Merriam-Webster Online Dictionary*, 2010). As

---

[5]Both initials DNP and DrNP stand for *doctor of nursing practice*. While two of the first nine doctors of nursing practice programs in the United States were DrNP programs (Drexel University and Columbia University); now only Drexel uses those initials. In this book, when DNP is specified, for clarity both degree types are thus referenced, except where the DrNP is specifically differentiated.

a <u>noun</u> the *Oxford American Dictionary* (1980) defines it as (1) action as opposed to theory; (2) a habitual action, custom; (3) repeated exercise to improve the skill one has; and (4) professional work, the business carried on by a doctor or lawyer, the patients or clients regularly consulting these.[6] As a <u>verb</u> it is defined as (1) to do something in order to be skillful; (2) to carry out in action, to do something habitually; (3) to do something actively; and (4) to be actively engaged in professional work.[7] From these definitions, it is clear that the term *practice* indicates it is action, habitual and repeated, and professional work. *Nursing practice* is also done to be skillful, is carried out actively, and constitutes in engaging in professional work. Our view of these various definitions is that the word *practice* often has a strong connection to professional work and thus to professional disciplines.[8]

Practice Boundaries

It is incumbent upon any professional discipline, particularly health profession disciplines, to define specifically what their disciplinary practice is and to establish boundaries within the domains of these definitions. Without such defined boundaries of practice, advanced practice nurses may find themselves accused of "practicing medicine" for instance. One of the earliest cases of a nurse being accused of practicing medicine occurred in 1917 in *Frank v. South*, 175 Ky. 416 (Kentucky, 1917), Margaret Hatfield, a nurse anesthetist, was accused of practicing medicine. However, the court ruled that:

> ...the mere giving of medicines which are prescribed by a physician in charge, who has made a diagnosis and determined the disease, and determined the remedy and directs the manner and the time and the character of the medicines to be administered, has never been considered engaging in the practice of medicine.
>
> —*p. 2*

The court went on to further note:

> It is however, contended that the trained nurse, who administers an anesthetic, must, at some time, exercise her own judgment and thus bring her within the definition of 'to practice medicine' in this, that the surgeon is engaged with his duties in performing the operation and it may become necessary to apply another anesthetic, instead of the one being used .... If a physician makes a diagnosis and discovers the ailment of the patient, who is attended by a nurse, and prescribes certain medicines to be given, when the medicine already given shall affect the patient in a certain way, to determine when the medicine should be given requires the exercise of some degree of judgment by a nurse; ... in all these contingencies, the nurse would have to exercise some degree of judgment, but to hold that such would constitute her a practitioner of medicine and

---

[6] These definitions have been slightly modified for clarity (p. 700).

[7] See footnote 6.

[8] Whether all nursing practices are indeed *professional* will be discussed later in this text.

prohibit her from the rendition of such services, it would have the effect ... 'to deprive the people of all services in sickness other than those which are gratuitous, except when rendered by a licensed physician.'

—p. 7

In a more current case of the boundaries of professional practice, the Attorney General of Illinois in 2009 ruled that physician assistants or advanced practice nurses (referred to as advanced practice clinicians) were legally able to dispense RU-486 under the supervision of a physician (Olsen, 2009). This practice by non-physicians, according to the Illinois Abortion Law of 1975 (the Abortion Law—720ICLS 510/), would not constitute the practice of medicine. Another contemporary controversy over the boundaries of disciplinary practice includes, for example, whether nurse practitioners (NPs) can administer cosmetic services such as Botox independently (Buppert, 2006). Or similarly, whether dentists, who can legally use Botox to treat temporomandibular disorders (TMD) or other dental problems in the dental office, can use it for cosmetic procedures too (Bouck, 2008).[9] Complicating the complex question of the precise boundaries or domains of a professional practice is the issue of regulation and malpractice insurance. For any practitioner, while a respective state practice act may indeed indicate that the health professional is legally authorized to perform a specific procedure, it is perhaps equally important for the individual health professional to be certain their malpractice insurance offers coverage for the procedure. Ultimately, with 50 different Nurse Practice Acts, the autonomy and authority of the advanced practice nurse to practice independently varies from state to state.

Obviously, over time and with the evolution of any discipline, countless numbers of questions arise as to what actions and skills constitute the practice or professional work of the practitioner. It is not surprising that competing health professions may also dispute the legitimacy or legal authority of one health professional to perform an act they believe is in *their* domain of practice. At the beginning of the 20th century, prior to the advances in technology that have changed the landscape of health care, taking a blood pressure and pulse was the domain of medicine. Today, these still important assessments are done by nonlicensed assistive personnel. Controversy over the boundaries of a domain even happens *within* disciplines. With the invention of emergency ultrasound procedures for rapid use in the emergency room, a very large battle began over who was qualified to administer emergency radiography (Kendall, Blaivas, Hoffenberg, & Fox, 2004). Traditionally, this was the strict domain for radiologists, but soon emergency room physicians across the country were performing the procedure, and a dispute over who could perform the procedure, and thus get reimbursed for it, commenced (Cohen & Moore, 2004).

In nursing, there are ongoing concerns over the issue of advanced practice nurses, especially NPs, practicing outside the boundaries of their specific specialty area or outside their scope of education and practice (Klein, 2005; Reel & Abraham, 2007). Examples include scenarios where the acute care NP is practicing primary care, the domain of the family NP, or where the pediatric NP is caring for neonates,

---

[9]The answer is no. Botox injection is permitted for dental-related procedures only.

the rightful domain of the neonatal NP. The National Council State Boards of Nursing (NCSBN) has addressed these concerns and also the proliferation of new NP specialties/subspecialties in their *Consensus Model for Advanced Practice Registered Nurse (APRN) Regulation: Licensure, Accreditation, Certification & Education* (NCSBN, 2008). While a detailed discussion of this document is perhaps better suited for a graduate role development course, we believe the NCSBN has clearly proposed a very detailed regulatory model that is designed to establish more of a national standard for the advanced practice registered nurse with less state-to-state variability in the various nurse practice acts. The goal is for there to be less ambiguity and more legal protection (and thus fewer malpractice claims) for advanced practice nurses and increased protection of the health of the public by enhanced regulation to promote safe nurse practice.

The Nature of Practice: An Emphasis on the Interpersonal

In 1986 Whan, a social work scholar, attempted to make a distinction between the notion of the practical and the technical. He argued that the *practice* of social work was one of practical, moral engagement, and not primarily a matter of technique. In some ways this sounds very similar to the long, but ongoing discussion as to whether nursing is more an art or a science (Bishop & Scudder, 1997; Mitchell & Cody, 2002; Peplau, 1988). However, social work and nursing are different disciplines. Furthermore, the nature of practice is much more complex, and we favor an argument that *practice* is more interpersonal than artistic or merely scientific (or technical). It is the interpersonal skills of the professional[10] (nurse, minister, physician, social worker, occupational therapist, etc.) that give rise to higher-level expectations from the visible and measurable direct outcomes of their practice.

Part of the theoretical support for the primacy of interpersonal skills, which manifests as effective communication between the health professional and the patient (client) or in the therapeutic nurse–patient relationship, can be pooled from multiple disciplines. From nursing, Peplau's Theory of Interpersonal Relations[11] (1952; 1997) and Travelbee's Human-to-Human Relationship Model[12] (1966) are both particularly useful in conceptualizing that the practice of the professional nurse really flourishes (lives) or stagnates (dies), depending on the relationship between the nurse and the patient. While Travelbee's work was really articulated before the advanced nursing practice movement, both theorists' works have application to advanced and doctoral advanced practice and implications for other health profession

---

[10]It is also the *status* of the professional (versus the nonprofessional) and their *trustworthiness* that allows the individual/person being *practiced on* to be open to the impact of the professional's interpersonal skills. Whether the interpersonal skills of the respective professional are effective is another question, but the expectations are that they should be.

[11]The focus of Peplau's (b. 1909, d. 1999) theory is on the nurse–patient relationship and its phases: orientation, identification, exploitation, and resolution (Peplau, 1952).

[12]According to Travelbee's (b. 1926, d. 1973) theory, in her *Human-to-Human Relationship Model*, the nurse–patient relationship is the essence of the purpose of nursing (1966).

disciplines too.[13] From medicine, the literature on the skills necessary for physicians to deliver bad news or "death notification" expertly and with compassion is an example of an interpersonal professional practice (Leash, 1994; Lord, 2008). Delivering bad news is a professional skill that requires enormous maturity as over time the medical student, then intern, perhaps resident, and then finally attending physician, learns what to say, what not to say, and how to best communicate sensitive and usually painful news to individuals and families (Ptacek & McIntosh, 2009; Rosenbaum, Ferguson, & Lobas, 2004). There is even a contemporary body of litera-ture in dietetics that describes the importance of the dietician–patient relationship (Cant, 2009; Cant & Arroni, 2008). This was not a surprising finding since both pro-fessional nurses and advanced practice nurses are often challenged to successfully motivate patients to lose weight or follow a specific diet (Dreher, 2008).

Ultimately, it is the nature of practice, what the professional says and does for others that differentiate the work in health professions disciplines like nursing from the work of the aviator, banker, or chemist. We attest that it is also the emphasis of the interpersonal relationship the professional has with individual patients/clients and their families, more so than technical competency, that best distinguishes the prac-tice of the professional. Dreher has spent most of his early career in cardiovascular nursing. It was observed during graduate school that the CNS in cardiac rehabilitation [working primarily with patients post-Myocardial infarction (MI) and post-coronary artery bypass graft (CABG)] had distinct advantages over the masters-prepared exer-cise physiologists who were performing the same work. What was the most obvious advantage? The clinical nurse specialists appeared to have more advanced interperso-nal skills and were more comfortable talking to patients, building relationships, and likely motivating them. Were they perhaps as knowledgeable as the exercise physiol-ogists about the technical content of the specialty? Without making assumptions, one objective difference would likely be that the exercise physiology curriculum has a greater emphasis on applied kinesiology, biomechanics, and motor learning for example. Therefore, it is not unlikely that the exercise physiologist may have a greater knowledge base of the discipline on average. However, as described in Malcolm Gladwell's bestselling book *Outliers* (2008), success is not necessarily about having the most intelligence [or having the most knowledge], but having *enough intel-ligence*. Gladwell outlines the advantage that *practical intelligence* can have over *analyti-cal intelligence* and how factors other than mere IQ are correlated with success. One can only imagine a minister with no (or weak) interpersonal skills, a psychiatric nurse with poor therapeutic communication techniques, or an advanced practice nurse who is merely average at encouraging successful behavioral changes in her patients.

How would you describe the nature of practice? How important do you think it is to properly conceptualize the context of *practice* to the discipline of nursing? Does society perceive or value the practice of the physician, the practice of the physical therapist, or the practice of the advanced practice or doctoral advanced practice nurse differently? We contend that more emphasis should be given to the training of

---

[13]Peplau's work also preceded the advanced practice nursing movement too, but her longevity allowed her work to have direct application to advanced practice psychiatric nursing.

interpersonal skills of the professional practitioner and its central relationship to enhancing "practice." Thus the importance of *practice knowledge* will be explored in Chapter 16.

WHAT IS A *DISCIPLINE*?

A discipline is foremost a field of study. It is the generated knowledge of a collective of scholars/practitioners (usually residing in a university where the generation of knowledge and teaching and disseminating this new knowledge is the mission) that leads to the formation of a discipline. Some of the first scholarly discussions surrounding the meaning of an academic discipline began in the 1960s when Phenix indicated, "The distinguishing mark of any discipline is that the knowledge which comprises it is instructive—that it is peculiarly suited for teaching and learning" (1962, p. 58). Discipline is defined by the *Oxford English Dictionary* as "a branch of learning or scholarly instruction" (p. 244). King and Brownell further state, "Each discipline, at any time in history ... is best described as a 'community of discourse,' a company of persons moving in modest disarray toward its own goal. There have been and are now many such companies, more all the time. We attempt to institutionalize them in schools, colleges and universities" (1966, p. 62). Even today the Carnegie Foundation for the Advancement of Teaching confirms this, forcefully emphasizing in *Envisioning the Future of Doctoral Education: Preparing Stewards for the Discipline* (Golde & Walker, 2006) that "Disciplines continue to change, as do universities, the job market, the character of professional work, and the student population" (p. 4).

The first degree-granting university in medieval Europe was the University of Bologna founded in 1088 and then in 1150 the University of Paris (which later became La Sorbonne). Oxford (1167) and Cambridge (1209) were founded shortly thereafter. At the University of Paris and these early universities, there were faculties in only four disciplines: Theology, Medicine, Canon Law (Ecclesiastical or Catholic Church Law), and the Arts (largely grammar, rhetoric, logic, arithmetic, music, and astronomy). Most modern academic disciplines have their roots in the mid- to late-19th century secularization of universities. One example is the origins of the discipline of psychology (mostly attributed to Wilhelm Hundt[14] and William James[15] who both probably founded the first psychology lab around 1875) which evolved from integrating knowledge from medicine, physiology, neurology, and philosophy. Indeed, reminding ourselves how young psychology as a discipline is comparatively should give some comfort to nursing's own struggles with being a young and still maturing discipline. As one nursing scholar has stated, "While the practice of nursing is as old as humanity, the discipline of nursing is quite young" (O'Shea, 2001).

We know what a discipline is, but maybe the more important questions are: What defines a discipline? Are there criteria for what a discipline is? For instance,

---

[14]Wilhelm Hundt (b. 1832, d. 1920).

[15]William James (b. 1842, d. 1930).

nursing began as practice[16] and evolved eventually into an academic discipline, but by what standards? King and Brownell's 1966 book *The Curriculum and the Disciplines of Knowledge* has provided a classical list of criteria for what constitutes an academic discipline:

1. A discipline is a community: scholars, teachers, and learners form a specialized dynamic group.
2. A discipline is an expression of human imagination: there is almost a spontaneous generation of ideas that evolve as "germinal concepts" and "intellectual challenges" (p. 71) by various individual members.
3. A discipline is a domain: "that natural phenomenon, process, material, social institution, or other aspect of man's concern on which members of the discipline focus their attention" (p. 74).
4. A discipline has a history and traditions: a record of discourse of its forebears and the evolutionary intellectual craftsmanship.
5. A discipline has a conceptual structure: the dynamic and developmental full set of ideas in a discipline at any one time.
6. A discipline has a syntactical structure (mode of inquiry): the interrelated ensembles of principles in a field of inquiry.
7. A discipline has a specialized language or other system of symbols: the vocabulary, common language, and representative accumulated connotative meanings of the field and its members.
8. A discipline has a heritage of literature and a communications network: "the working materials of the community of discourse are the heritage of writings, paintings, composition, musical scores, artifacts, recorded interviews, and other symbolic expressions of the membership" (p. 86).
9. A discipline is a valuative and affective stance: the capacity for a field of inquiry to move beyond its mere rational attributes and to reflect various characteristics of man, reflect emotional dynamism, and exhibit aesthetic qualities.
10. A discipline is an instructive community: whereby a path for progression of learning in a discipline is created and communicated theoretically through curricula.

These criteria will be reexamined in the next chapter as we analyze whether nursing as a maturing discipline, and particularly as a *practice discipline*, has met these criteria. Dorothea Orem (a noted nurse theorist),[17] however, has documented that historically neither King and Brownell, nor Phenix had yet conceptualized the term *a practice discipline* in the 1960s, and it was not until October 7, 1967 that Dickoff and James introduced the term relative to nursing at a "Theory Development in Nursing" symposium at Case Western Reserve University (Orem, 1988).

---

[16]It could also be said that historically, humans engaged in nursing behaviors or *lay nursing* before it even became a rudimentary formalized practice at the time of Nightingale. So the time trajectory from a human behavior to a formal discipline was indeed long, even given the time from the origins of the first university academic disciplines.

[17]Dorothea Orem (b. 1914, d. 2007) was the founder of the *Self-Care* Model of Nursing. Her chief contribution, The Self-care Deficit Theory of Nursing, essentially states that nurses have to supply care when patients cannot provide it themselves (1995).

Disciplinary Boundaries

Disciplinary boundaries are similar to the description of practice boundaries in our previous discussion. However, in many ways, the disciplinary boundaries of a practice discipline are more fluid than nonpractice disciplines. In this discussion, we will examine disciplinary boundaries in two different, but important contexts: (1) Who is a legitimate member of the discipline? (2) Who can legitimately produce knowledge for the discipline?

Who is a Legitimate Member of a Discipline?

At first glance, this is an easy question, but in reality it is not. Members of a discipline have the responsibility to determine the qualifications for students to enter their program, the course of study to obtain a degree in the discipline, and the level of knowledge, psychomotor skill acquisition (where applicable), and socialization to graduate from the program. Individual university faculties are ordinarily replete with members with degrees *in the respective discipline*. However, there are often faculty with terminal degrees in other disciplines who are duly members of a respective department. In any given divinity school, for example, there are usually faculty in moral theology who have doctorates in philosophy or biomedical ethics, but who are not necessarily ordained and do not belong to a ministerial profession. In nursing, the faculty might include nurses who may have a graduate degree in nursing, but who have doctorates in non-nursing fields. Further, in nursing, some faculty may indeed actually be trained pharmacologists or physiologists who teach the pharmacology and anatomy and physiology courses or they could also be based in their home disciplinary department. These persons, however, do not have the educational background or socialization as part of the discipline of nursing. Del Favero (2010) has suggested, perhaps more radically, that a legitimate member of a discipline is simply one who professes primary allegiance to a discipline. Nevertheless, we would contend that graduates with at least a baccalaureate degree in a specific discipline should be considered *de facto* members of a discipline. But whether individuals with a graduate degree in one discipline and a terminal doctorate in another are best positioned to advance knowledge in their nondoctoral discipline is another question.

Who Can Legitimately Produce Knowledge for the Discipline?

After discussion of membership, the next important argument is who can legitimately produce knowledge for the discipline or who is best positioned to do so? Golde and Walker take a very traditionalist approach and state, "we believe that PhD recipients bear responsibility for the integrity of their discipline" (2006, p. 10). However, it is with certainty, in light of the relatively new DNP movement, that *doctoral graduates* bear the responsibility for the integrity of the discipline. In many ways, those who are a member and those who generate the knowledge for a discipline are both very much aligned. In other cases, it is not. For instance, it would be highly uncommon (if not outright unacceptable in many cases) if a student in a typical university sociology class was taught by someone without a doctorate in sociology (but another field). The point here is not to disparage individuals who have an identity as a member of a discipline, but a doctorate in another. It is to emphasize that the formal members in any given discipline are the ones most credible to advance disciplinary knowledge and establish the disciplinary boundaries. In this example, the assumption is that the guardians of knowledge for the discipline of sociology are logically faculty *with a doctorate in that discipline,* and not another.[18] First, distinctions have to be made between new disciplines, maturing disciplines, or traditional, established disciplines. For instance, the discipline of Knowledge Management is only 15 years old (Stankovsky, 2005). Male Studies (as opposed to Men's Studies which has been around since the 1970s) is even newer and was just proposed in 2009 at Wagner College in New York (Epstein, 2010). It will formalize itself with the first International Conference on Male Studies scheduled for October 2010 and the launch of a *Male Studies Journal* (Elam, 2010). Some controversy has surrounded this new discipline, and Goudreau reports from one of the new discipline's founders:

> 'This came out of the contentious business of gender studies,' says Lionel Tiger, professor of anthropology at Rutgers University. 'It's not men's studies as contrasted with women's studies. It's a study of males without all the ideology and self-righteousness of feminists about turning over patriarchy'
>
> —*Goudreau, 2010, p. 1.*

For these disciplines, the founders are obviously scholars in other fields who have begun to create a body of scholarly work that is indeed distinctive and different. These new disciplines either have broken away from a parent discipline and have become independent, or have likely emerged by drawing on scholars from multiple disciplines to create something entirely new.[19]

If one traces the history of modern nursing from Nightingale (the first nursing school, the Nightingale Training School at St. Thomas' Hospital, was founded in 1860), then nursing is around 150 years old, but its precise arrival as a formal discipline remains murky and unclear. Thus, for maturing disciplines like nursing (the first nursing doctorate was an EdD at Teacher's College, Columbia University in 1924), the founding scholars obviously had doctoral preparation outside the discipline (Robb, 2005).[20] Over time the overwhelming majority of scholars are then prepared inside the discipline in the respective doctoral programs. In 1961 the Nurse-Scientist Training Program was formed to prepare nurses in PhD programs *outside of nursing*

---

[18]This author has often fielded such questions as "Should I get my doctorate in nursing, or maybe education, or perhaps public health, or informatics, etc.," over the years from masters-prepared nursing faculty pondering seeking a doctorate. My default response has almost always been to advocate that the best way to generate evidence for the profession of nursing is to ground oneself in the science of the discipline.

[19]Biomedical engineering is likely an example of the first type. While its roots as a discipline began during WWII with a merging of biology, medicine and engineering, it mostly became a branch of engineering until its stature surged. Knowledge management arose more recently from artificial intelligence, decision-support systems, informatics, and other related fields (Whitaker Foundation, 2002).

[20]The first *chartered nursing school* in America, the Training School of the Woman's Hospital in Philadelphia, was founded in 1863 by a physician, Emmeline Horton Cleveland, MD, a 1855 graduate of the Woman's Medical College of Pennsylvania, the first medical college in the world for women (Robinson, 1946).

(Gortner, 1991). While this may sound odd, in fact the program began since there was a dearth of PhD in Nursing programs at the time, and a critical mass of doctoral-prepared nurses was needed in order to jump-start the research underpinnings of the discipline. Many of these graduates indeed went on to form new doctoral research programs in nursing, including the PhD, DNSc (Doctor of Nursing Science), DSN (Doctor of Science in Nursing), and DNS (Doctor of Nursing Science) degrees, and subsequently there were a spur of new doctoral nursing programs in the late 1960s and 1970s. Other examples of maturing disciplines include Occupational Therapy (founded in 1917) and Physical Therapy (founded in 1921). Although there were earlier historical developments in both disciplines, these dates appear to be land-marks in the formalizing of each of these new health professions (Punwar & Peloquin, 2000).

The practice discipline of occupational therapy has a very interesting history. What is not widely known is that occupational therapy had its earlier roots in nursing, not physical therapy as widely believed (Gibson & Serrett, 1985). In some ways it emerged in the 20th century as *health* and *work* (occupation) became so inter-related (Sensory-processing-disorder.com, 2009). If one was not healthy, then one could not work and make a living. As a result, those rehabilitative efforts that could best assist a person to return to function (and work) were termed *occupational therapy*. In the early 1900s, a nurse named Susan Tracy coined the term *occupational nurse* as she became involved in initiating training for people with mental illness to perform work tasks and be more productive to society (Bing, 2005; Sensory-processing-disorder.com). She even began to train other student nurses in this new endeavor and in 1910 wrote the first known book on occupational therapy, a man-ual introducing nurses to invalid occupations (Reed, 1993). In 1914, George E. Barton, an architect, and Dr. William R. Dunton, Jr., who were interested in the response of the human body to the therapeutics of occupation, began to explore the formation of an organization for individuals interested in *Occupation Work* (as Occupational Therapy was originally known until this time) (Reed, 2005). On March 15, 1917, the National Society for the Promotion of Occupational Therapy (NSPOT) was founded and the charter members included a partially trained social worker, two architects (including Barton), a secretary (who later became Barton's wife), a psychiatrist, a teacher/philanthropist, and nurse Susan Tracy (Sensory-processing-disorder.com).

Finally, there are the traditional, mature disciplines like psychology and social work (both founded in the late 19th century), and medicine which is much older. Modern medicine in the United States can be traced to the establishment of the American Medical Association in 1847. However, medicine only established reformed educational standards for their profession in 1910 with the publication of the highly influential Flexner Report, which led to the closure of inferior medical schools (largely homeopathic medical colleges) and to more standardization in the medical curricula (Flexner, 1910).[21] Nevertheless, each of these disciplines has a long history

---

[21]Flexner also exposed the seedy practice of medical schools operating as proprietary schools "which were usually owned by the faculty [often just local doctors and not even professors] and operated for profit" (Hiatt, 1999, p. 21).

of well-advanced knowledge development. In these established disciplines (all over 100 years), it is a foregone conclusion that in the circles of academia, the contemporary producers of knowledge for each respective discipline are educated in very traditional, and usually long-established doctoral programs. One example of medicine's maturity and influence as a discipline is exhibited in the leadership medicine has taken in the evidence-based medicine and evidence-based practice movements, which have had great impact on other health-related disciplines, including nursing (Melnyk & Fineout-Overholt, 2005; Sackett & Rosenberg, 1995; Strauss, Richardson, Glasziou, & Haynes, 2005).

We further raise this issue of who is the legitimate steward of the discipline from the relatively new (albeit not widespread) practice of allowing non-nurses (students who are not even registered nurses [RNs]) to enroll in PhD degree programs in nursing (Robb, 2005).[22] Regardless of your own initial response to this—whether you agree or disagree—could it be imagined that some program would conceivably permit non-nurses to enroll in a DNP degree? In this author's own DrNP program, one of our first doctoral comprehensive exam questions was for the doctoral student to describe how the doctorally prepared advanced practice nurse should differ from the masters-prepared advanced practice nurse. Of course the examining faculty expected a plethora of very scholarly written (and oral) responses, but one response in particular led to a great discussion among the faculty: the masters-prepared APRN generally has a responsibility to their patients or clients, but the doctoral-prepared APRN has an additional and particular responsibility *to the discipline of nursing.* Aside from the controversy over whether the DNP ought to generate empirical knowledge for the discipline or not (Dreher, Donnelly, & Naremore, 2005; Florczak, 2010), other scholars do support this mandate of more disciplinary responsibility for the DNP graduate (Chism, 2009; Clinton & Sperhac, 2009).

Is nursing there yet? Are we a mature discipline like psychology, social work, or medicine? Certainly nursing does not have to struggle anymore to establish consensual credibility as a profession like chiropractic does (Cooper & McKee, 2003). While we explore this in more detail in the next chapter, the answer may be "perhaps, but not quite yet." Our concern is how we take our next steps to properly socialize new members of the discipline appropriately and educate them to be legitimate stewards of the discipline. In some ways, the linkage of a practice discipline to its inherent ability to transform health care practice and thus make a visible impact on society is whether it is likely to be considered a true discipline or not.

---

[22]As of this writing, the University of Washington (Seattle) and the University of Rochester (and perhaps others) permit non-nurses to enroll in their PhD in Nursing programs. Actually, despite the course titles having the *NURS* prefix, the official title of the degree at the University of Rochester is a "PhD Program in *Health Practice Research*"! The question is: Whether this degree will advance nursing practice/nursing science? Startling as this may be to some, a current AACN Task Force on *The Future of the Research-Focused Doctorate in Nursing* is considering formalizing entry of non-nurses in PhD in Nursing programs as one possible pathway to the PhD (Dunbar-Jacob, 2010).

A PRACTICE DISCIPLINE AS A PROFESSION: AN EMPHASIS ON THE ETHICAL

A profession has the following characteristics: (1) it has exclusive powers to recruit, educate, and train new members as it sees fit; (2) it has exclusive powers to judge who is qualified; (3) it is responsible for regulating the quality of professional work; (4) it has high social prestige; and (5) it is grounded in an esoteric and complex body of knowledge (Light, Jr., 1974). New professions do not easily meet these criteria, and it is often a historic path from a discipline's first foray into the workforce and public consciousness to its proven path of establishing full legitimate credibility as a profession. Wright's (1951) very classical legal definition of a profession is:

> A profession is a self-selected, self-disciplined group of individuals who hold themselves out to the public as possessing a special skill derived from education and training and who are prepared to exercise that skill primarily in the interests of others.
>
> —*Wright, 1951, p. 748.*

The early practice disciplines of divinity, law, and medicine were clearly practice professions, but they were not identified as such (Klass, 1961). However, it is clear from our earlier explorations of the origins of practice that indeed these professions have a practice orientation. This would confirm that there need to be guidelines and boundaries for practicing professionals, and that there need to be codes of ethics that guide the respective practitioner. For this reason, there has developed a very large body of literature that has critically examined "ethics in the professions" or in the *helping professions* (Corey, Corey, & Callanan, 2006; Rowan & Zinaich, Jr., 2002). As a practice discipline, nursing has always had an emphasis on ethics in both undergraduate and graduate curricula, especially surrounding the American Nurses Association (ANA) Code of Ethics (Crawford, 1926; Fry, 2004; Silva & Guillet, 1996). However, the movement to more formal instruction in ethics for nurses began largely in the 1980s (Aroskar, 1977, 1980). There is an ongoing debate as to who should be teaching (who is properly qualified/credentialed) ethics to nurses or even whether philosophers can teach professional ethics (Kalb & O'Conner-Vonn, 2007; Krawczyk, 1997; Shotton, 1997; Weil, 1989). This issue was a very prominent sidebar debate at a recent International Center for Nursing Ethics Conference held at Yale University School of Nursing in 2008. Should nurses with no formal training in ethics be teaching it?[23] Ethics is foremost a branch of philosophy. There is also the field of clinical ethics[24]

---

[23]The first author of this text attended this conference and there were several diverse camps with different perspectives on this issue: (1) nurses with classical doctorates in philosophy/ethics (a minority); (2) nurses with masters degrees in ethics, but doctorates in nursing or other fields; (3) non-nursing scholars with doctorates in philosophy/ethics who taught nurses; and (4) nurses who taught ethics with either modest nondegree training in ethics (a certificate in postgraduate study) or those simply without any formal training (likely the plurality).

[24]There is also ongoing tension between those classically trained in ethics/philosophy and those who believe the field of clinical ethics is *distorted* (Murray, Koenig, & Ross, 1996). There are also those who believe the field of *applied ethics* is similarly simplified for students, especially when students take applied ethics courses (i.e., a course in *nursing ethics*) before even a basic philosophy or basic ethics class. For instance, one author criticizes the teaching of moral theory in applied ethics courses whereas another is not so sure (Benatar, 2007; Lawlor, 2007).

where many formal recognized members and practitioners in this field are not entirely classically trained in philosophy or ethics. This issue returns us to the central issues in this chapter: Who is a formal member of a discipline? Who has the credibility or right to conduct disciplinary knowledge development? The teaching of ethics in a practice discipline is important. Which discipline should teach it or who is the ideal academic to teach this? What should their ideal preparation be?

In 2001, the world-renowned ethicist Peter Singer, along with colleagues Pellegrino and Siegler, called for an increased research focus on the ethical problems facing clinical medical ethics. They suggested a different focus to these problems, which included approaches that were:

- *Multidisciplinary*: where researchers work in parallel or sequentially from a disciplinary-specific base to address a common problem.
- *Interdisciplinary*: where researchers work jointly, but still from a disciplinary-specific base, to address a common problem.
- *Transdisciplinary*: where researchers work jointly using a shared conceptual framework drawing together disciplinary-specific theories, concepts, and approaches to address a common problem.

We contend that there ought to be a heavy emphasis on ethics education in any practice discipline. Practice disciplines, particularly those that have earned professional status, have a responsibility to educate their practitioners to practice with the highest ethics. In the last decade, there have been many episodes of gross unethical practice in society. It began with the Enron debacle in the early 2000s and culminated at the end of the decade with the fall of Wall Street and the resulting near-economic depression that befell the United States and the globe (Kidder, 2009; Kienzler & David, 2003). Ethical issues in society this decade related to the health professions include the enormous impact of the Terry Schiavo case and continuing debate over the right to die (Gastmans & De Lepeleire, 2010; Quill, 2005). To manage these contemporary and complex ethical issues effectively, practice disciplines must enhance the emphasis on ethics and clinical ethics in their various curricula. DNP programs in particular should continue the ethics education that nurses first complete in their undergraduate education and sometimes formally continue during their masters study. This is one area where AACN's *The Essentials of Doctoral Education for Advanced Nursing Practice* may already be out of date (2006).[25] This document focuses on eight essentials of [doctoral] advanced nursing practice, but only three of the eight essentials have curricular objectives that address ethical issues in DNP curricula. We could easily support a modernization of the document with an inclusion of a separate essential that recognizes the critical need for the doctoral advanced practice nurse to have expert skills to better collaborate across disciplinary lines to solve ethical issues in practice. At this [doctoral]

---

[25]This is the leading document that guides the curricula of most DNP programs. Our concern is that since it was authored in 2006, well before the surge of most DNP programs and before the actual practice of DNP/DrNP graduates could be evaluated, it may already be out of date. We urge its use as a blueprint, but not as a set of rigid curricular prescriptions.

level, ethical issues and their resolution in health care are rarely ever the decision of a single individual or single practice discipline. Thus, more skill at multidisciplinary collaboration is essential.

MOVING TOWARD A DEFINITION OF A CONTEMPORARY *PROFESSIONAL PRACTICE DISCIPLINE*

If we take a look at the average hospital or large medical center, we see a lot of practice disciplines working together on a daily basis: nursing, medicine, pharmacy, physical therapy, occupational therapy, social work, psychology, respiratory therapy, divinity, and others. The health sciences literature is in agreement on one central point: multidisciplinary care and practice are far superior to narrow practice from disciplinary silos (Bell, Corfield, Davies, & Richardson, 2010; Yeager, 2005). The Cochrane database is full of such health outcome evidence (Handoll, Cameron, Mak, & Finnegan, 2009; Ng, Khan, & Mathers, 2009). Therefore, nursing (particularly doctoral advanced practice nurses) should maximize *interprofessional care*[26] with more skillful communication and consultation to enhance the health outcomes of the patients and families under their care. A recent scholar (Copnell, 2010) has called for a modernizing of the contemporary allied health professions with more enhanced development of the professional's knowledge and skills. In many ways, the current movement toward health reform in the United States actually implores the practice-based professional to do more to increase positive health outcomes. An argument can be made that this was one of the chief reasons for the creation of the DNP degree — to provide the public with a more highly educated and skilled advanced nursing practitioner.

In conclusion, a new definition for a practice discipline is proposed which can be placed into a contemporary health context and embraces the global health challenges that practice disciplines and their practitioners face. In our view, a professional practice discipline has the following characteristics:

1. A recognized role and work product highly valued by society.
2. A legitimate claim to certain boundaries in the field.
3. A distinct body of knowledge that is both practical and theoretical.
4. A critical mass of knowledge generators *within the domain of the formal field*.
5. Regulations and standards for membership that includes rigorous educational preparation.
6. A formal organization of the community of practitioners and scholars.
7. An emphasis on the interpersonal aspects of the role and work.
8. A highly developed code of ethics and behavior.

---

[26]The word *interprofessional care* can be defined as: (1) the provision of comprehensive health services to patients by multiple health caregivers who work collaboratively to deliver quality of care within and across settings (Ministry of Health & Long-terms Care, Province of Ontario, 2007) and (2) occasions when two or more professions learn with, from, and about each other to improve collaboration and the quality of care (Centre for the Advancement of Interprofessional Education, 1997).

New disciplines, such as Male Studies, will continue to develop. But the emergence of a new practice discipline means that certain standards and expectations (including its safe practice by competent practitioners) must be met incrementally if a practice discipline is indeed destined to be *professional* and so recognized in society. It also takes a historical trajectory for many of the aforementioned criteria to fully evolve. As Joel has written, "professions progress through an expected evolutionary process" (2002, p. 1). This indeed takes time.

SUMMARY

This chapter has attempted to examine the real frameworks of what constitutes *practice* and what defines a *discipline*. In nursing's quest to be fully recognized as a professional discipline, it may be that nursing and its practitioners and scholars need to revisit the meaning of practice to more formally understand the uniqueness of what is a practice discipline. The discipline of nursing should not model itself after nonpractice disciplines in order to be more like other traditional members of the academy like the neuroscientist or biochemist. Our position and uniqueness as a community of practitioners and scholars depends on agreement on what kinds of knowledge development is needed to advance our discipline. This will be more fully discussed in Chapter 16. However, none of this can take place without some adherence to the principles of philosophy of science as an underpinning for all knowledge construction—whether practice-oriented or theoretical. As a practice discipline, it is essential that it is established by what criteria an individual becomes a member and by what standard does one legitimately claim to be a generator of knowledge *within the domain of the discipline.* There also needs to be a thorough delineation of practice boundaries which helps establish legal contexts of practice. We also propose that a more constructed focus on the interpersonal aspects of practice and ethics is what distinguishes the active practice of health professions disciplines. In the next chapter, the focus will be on a more intricate exploration of the practice of nursing, but it will become obvious to the reader that nursing and other practice disciplines have much in common, despite the disciplinary differences.

CRITICAL THINKING QUESTIONS

1. Reflect and describe how your *practice* has changed and evolved over your nursing career.
2. How is *nursing practice* valued by society?
3. Provide other examples of where NPs or other advanced practice nurses may be practicing outside the proscribed domain of their practice for which they were educationally prepared.
4. Which disciplines (and in what proportion) do you think have contributed to the evolution of nursing practice and nursing science?
5. Debate the following: Resolved, "Is nursing a profession?" Make a case for nursing as a formal profession and make a case that it is not.
6. How are practice professions different from some other nonpractice professions?

7. Discuss the argument made that there should be more emphasis on the interpersonal aspects of practice in *practice disciplines.*
8. Discuss whether the current ethics education you received over your previous nursing education was adequate to support your practice.
9. How important will interpersonal care and multidisciplinary collaboration be to you as you commence your doctoral advanced nursing practice?
10. Do some research and examine the state of academic dentistry practice and science (or look at another practice discipline). Do you find any parallel disciplinary issues?

REFERENCES

American Association of Colleges of Nursing. (2006). The essentials of doctoral education for advanced nursing practice. Retrieved from http://www.aacn.nche.edu/DNP/pdf/Essentials.pdf.

Apold, S. (2008). The doctor of nursing practice: Looking back, moving forward. *The Journal for Nurse Practitioners, 4*(2), 101–107.

Aroskar, M. A. (1977). Ethics in the nursing curriculum. *Nursing Outlook, 25*(4), 260–264.

Aroskar, M. A. (1980). *Arguments for ethics in the nursing curriculum. ANA Publication, 145,* 31–38.

Bayhham, M. (2002). Academic writing in new and emergent discipline areas. In R. Harrison, F. Reeves, A. Hanson, & J. Clarke (Eds.), *Supporting lifelong learning, Vol. 1. Perspectives on learning* (pp. 189–202). London: Routledge Falmer.

Bell, A., Corfield, M., Davies, J., & Richardson, N. (2010). Collaborative transdisciplinary intervention in early years—Putting theory into practice. *Child: Care, Health & Development, 36*(1), 142–148.

Benatar, D. (2007). Moral theories may have some role in teaching applied ethics. *Journal of Medical Ethics, 33,* 671–672.

Bing, R. K. (2005). Looking back, living forward: Occupational therapy history. In S. E. Ryan, & K. Sladyk (Eds.), *Ryan's occupational therapy assistant: Principles, practice issues, and techniques* (4th ed.) (pp. 2–13). Thorofare, NJ: Slack Incorporated.

Bishop, A., & Scudder, J. (1997). Nursing as a practice rather than an art or a science. *Nursing Outlook, 45*(2), 82–85.

Bouck, L. (2008). Injection question: Should general dentists administer Botox? *AGD Impact, 26*(12), 1.

Buppert, C. (2006). The legal powers of the boards of nursing. *Journal for Nurse Practitioners, 2*(10), 660–661.

Cant, R. (2009). Constructions of competence within dietetics: Trust, professionalism and communications with individual clients. *Nutrition & Dietetics, 66*(2), 113–118.

Cant, R., & Arroni, R. A. (2008). Exploring dietitians' verbal and nonverbal communication for effective dietitian–patient communication. *Journal of Human Nutrition & Dietetics, 21*(5), 502–511.

Chism, L. (2009). Toward clarification of the doctor of nursing practice degree. *Advanced Emergency Nursing Journal, 31*(4), 287–297.

Clinton, P., & Sperhac, A. (2009). The DNP and unintended consequences: An Opportunity for dialogue. *Journal of Pediatric Health Care, 23*(5): 348–351.

Cohen, H. L., & Moore, W. H. (2004). History of emergency ultrasound. *Journal of Ultrasound Medicine, 23,* 451–458.

Conway, J. (1994). Reflection, the art and science of nursing and the theory-practice gap. *British Journal of Nursing, 3*(3), 114–118.

Cooper, R. A., & McKee, H. J. (2003). Chiropractic in the United States: Trends and issues. *The Milbank Quarterly, 81*(1), 107–138.

Copnell, G. (2010). Modernising allied health professions careers: Attacking the foundations of the professions? *Journal of Interprofessional Care, 24*(1), 63–69.

Corey, G., Corey, M. S., & Callanan, P. (2006). *Issues and ethics in the helping professions.* Florence, Kentucky: Brooks, Cole Publishers.

Crawford, B. (1926). How and what to teach in nursing ethics. *The American Journal of Nursing, 26*(3), 211–215.

Cronin, P., & Rawlings-Anderson, K. (2004). *Knowledge for contemporary nursing practice.* London: Elsevier Limited.

Del Favero, M. (2010). Academic disciplines: Disciplines and the structure of higher education, discipline classification systems, discipline differences. *StateUniversity.com.* Retrieved on 2/3/2010, from http://education.stateuniversity.com/pages/1723/Academic-Disciplines.html

Dreher, H. M. (2008). Is poor weight management a failure of primary care? *Holistic Nursing Practice, 22*(6), 312–316.

Dreher, H. M., Donnelly, G., & Naremore, R. (2005). Reflections on the DNP and an alternate practice doctorate model: The Drexel DrNP. *Online Journal of Issues in Nursing, 11*(1), www.nursingworld.org/ojin/topic28/tpc28_7.htm

Dreher, H. M., & Montgomery, K. E. (2009). Let's call it "doctoral" advanced practice nursing. *The Journal of Continuing Nursing Education, 40*(12), 530–531.

Dunbar-Jacob, J. (2010). *AACN Webinar on 'The Future of the Research-Focused Doctorate in Nursing.'* May 12, 2010. The American Association of Colleges of Nursing: Washington, DC.

Elam, P. (2010). Male studies, media and misunderstandings. *MND: mensnewsdail.com.* Retrieved on 9/2/2010, from http://mensnewsdaily.com/2010/03/31/male-studies-media-and-mis-understandings/

Epstein, J. (2010). Male studies vs. men's studies. *Insidehighered.com.* Retrieved on 9/2/2010, from http://www.insidehighered.com/news/2010/04/08/males

Flexner, A. (1910). *Medical education in the United States and Canada: A report to the Carnegie Foundation for the Advancement of Teaching; Bulletin No. 4.* New York, NY: Carnegie Foundation for the Advancement of Teaching.

Florczak, K. (2010). Research and the doctor of nursing practice: A cause for consternation. *Nursing Science Quarterly, 23*(1): 13–17.

Frank, et al. v. South, et al. (1917). Court of Appeals of Kentucky 175 Ky. 416; 194S.W.375; 1917Ky. LEXIS 336.

Fry, S. T. (2004). Nursing ethics. In G. Khushf (Ed.), *Handbook of bioethics* (pp. 489–505). The Netherlands: Kluwer Academic Publishers.

Gastmans, C., & De Lepeleire, J. (2010). Living to the bitter end? A personalist approach to euthanasia in persons with severe dementia. *Bioethics, 24*(2), 78–86.

Gibson, D., & Serrett, K. D. (1985). *Philosophical and historical roots of occupational therapy.* New York, NY: Routledge Publishers.

Gladwell, M. (2008). *Outliers: The story of success.* New York, NY: Little, Brown and Company.

Golde, C. M., & Walker, G. E. (2006). *Envisioning the future of doctoral education: Preparing stewards for the discipline.* San Francisco, CA: Jossey-Bass.

Gortner, S. (1991). Historical development of doctoral programs: Shaping our expectations. *Journal of Professional Nursing, 7*(1), 45–53.

Goudreau, J. (2010). Is feminism getting in the way of "Male Studies?" *Forbes.com.* Retrieved on 9/2/2010, from http://blogs.forbes.com/work-in-progress/2010/04/09/is-feminism-getting-in-the-way-of-male-studies/

Hamrin, E. (1997, June 17). *Models of doctoral education in Europe.* Paper presented at the Conference on International Network for Doctoral Education in Nursing: Vision and Strategy for the International Doctoral Education, University of British Colombia, Vancouver, Canada. Co-sponsored by the University of Michigan and University of British Columbia.

Handoll, H. H., Cameron, I. D., Mak, J. C., & Finnegan, T. P. (2009). Multidisciplinary rehabilitation for older people with hip fractures. *Cochrane Database of Systematic Reviews,* (4), Art. No. CD007125.

Hiatt, M. D. (1999). Around the continent in 180 days: The controversial journey of Abraham Flexner. *The Pharos,* Winter, *62*(1), 18–24.

Joel, L. (2002). Education for entry into nursing practice: Revisited for the 21st century. *Online Journal of Issues in Nursing, 7*(2), Manuscript 4. Retrieved on 5/5/2010, from www.nursingworld.org/MainMenuCategories/ANAMarketplace/ANAPeriodicals/OJIN/TableofContents/Volume72002/No2May2002/EntryintoNursingPractice.aspx

Journal of Applied Physics. (2010). *About the Journal.* Retrieved on 9/2/2010, from http://jap.aip.org/about/about_the_journal

Kalb, K. A., & O'Conner-Vonn, S. (2007). Ethics education in advanced practice nursing: Respect for human dignity. *Nursing Education Perspectives, 28*(4), 196–202.

Kendall, J. L., Blaivas, M., Hoffenberg, S., & Fox, J. C. (2004). History of emergency ultrasound. *Journal of Ultrasound Medicine, 23,* 1130–1135.

Kentucky, 1917. *Frank v. South,* 175 Ky. 416.

Kidder, R. M. (2009). *The ethics recession: Reflections on the moral underpinnings of the economic crisis.* Rockland, ME: Institute of Global Ethics.

Kienzler, D., & David, C. (2003). After Enron. *Journal of Business and Technical Communication, 17*(4), 474–489.

King, A. R., & Brownell, J. A. (1966). *The curriculum and the disciplines of knowledge: A theory of curriculum practice.* Hoboken, NJ: Wiley.

Klass, A. A. (1961). What is a profession? *Canadian Medical Association Journal, 85,* 698–701.

Klein, T. A. (2005). Scope of practice of the nurse practitioner: Regulation, competency, expansion, and evolution. *Topics in advanced practice e-journal, 5*(2). Retrieved from http://www.oregon.gov/OSBN/pdfs/KleinMedscapeArticle.pdf

Krawczyk, R. M. (1997). Teaching ethics: Effect on moral development. *Nursing Ethics, 4*(1), 57–65.

Lawlor, R. (2007). Moral theories in teaching applied ethics. *Journal of Medical Ethics, 33*(6), 370–372.

Leash, R. (1994). *Death notification: A practical guide to the process.* Hinesburg, VT: Upper Access.

Light, D. (1974). The structure of the academic professions. *Sociology of Education, 47*(1), 2–28.

Lobo, M. L. (2005). Research in PhD in nursing programs. *Nursing Science Quarterly, 18*(1), 16–17.

Long, N. (1992). Introduction. In N. Long, & A. Long (Eds.), *Battlefields of knowledge: The interlocking of theory and practice in social research and development* (pp. 3–15). Abingdon, Oxon, UK: Routledge.

Lord, J. H. (2008). *I'll never forget those words: A practical guide to death notification.* Burnsville, NC: Compassion Press.

Melnyk, B. M., & Fineout-Overholt, E. (2005). *Evidence-based practice in nursing and healthcare: A guide to best practice.* Philadelphia, PA: Lippincott Williams & Wilkins.

Merriam–Webster Online Dictionary. (2010). Definition of 'practice.' Retrieved from http://www.merriam-webster.com/dictionary/practice

Mitchell, G., & Cody, W. (2002). Ambiguous opportunity: Toiling for truth of nursing art and science. *Nursing Science Quarterly, 15*(1), 71–79.

Murray, T. H., Koenig, B. A., & Ross, J. W. (1996). Does clinical ethics distort the discipline? *The Hastings Center Report, 26*(6), 28–29.

National Council of State Boards of Nursing (NCSBN). (2008). *Consensus Model for APRN Regulation: Licensure, Accreditation, Certification & Education.* Retrieved from https://www.ncsbn.org/7_23_08_Consensue_APRN_Final.pdf

Ng, L., Khan, F., & Mathers, S. (2009). Multidisciplinary care for adults with amyotrophic lateral sclerosis or motor neuron disease. *Cochrane Database of Systematic Reviews, 4.* Art. No.: CD007425.

Olsen, D. (2009). Planned parenthood to offer abortion pills. *SJ-R.com.* Retrieved on 9/2/2010, from http://www.sj-r.com/health/x576519774/Local-Planned-Parenthood-to-offer-abortion-drugs

Orem, D. (1988). The form of nursing science. *Nursing Science Quarterly, 1*(2), 75–79.

Orem, D. (1995). *Nursing: Concepts of practice* (5th ed.). St. Louis, MO: Mosby.

O'Shea, H. (2001). The state of the discipline in nursing: Science, technology, and culture have stirred rapid change. *The Academic Exchange,* October/November. Retrieved on 2/2/2010, from http://www.emory.edu/ACAD_EXCHANGE/2001/octnov/oshea.html.

Ousey, K., & Gallagher, P. (2007). The theory–practice relationship in nursing: A debate. *Nurse Education in Practice, 7*(4), 199–205.

Oxford American Dictionary. (1980). E. Ehrlich, S. B. Flexner, G. Carruth, J. M. Hawkins (Eds). New York, NY: Avon.

Parse, R. (2005). Symbols and meanings in academia. *Nursing Science Quarterly, 18*(3), 197.

Peplau, H. (1952). *Interpersonal relations in nursing.* New York, NY: G.P. Putnam's Sons.

Peplau, H. (1988). The art and science of nursing: Similarities, differences, and relations. *Nursing Science Quarterly, 1*(1), 8–15.

Peplau, H. (1997). Peplau's theory of interpersonal relations. *Nursing Science Quarterly, 10*(4), 162–167.

Phenix, P. (1962). The use of the disciplines as curriculum content. *The Educational Forum, 26*(3), 273–280.

Ptacek, J. T., & McIntosh, E. G. (2009). Physician challenges in communicating bad news. *Journal of Behavioral Medicine, 32*(4), 380–387.

Punwar, A. J., & Peloquin, S. M. (2000). *Occupational therapy: Principles and practice.* Philadelphia, PA: Lippincott Williams & Wilkins.

Quill, T. E. (2005). Terri Schiavo—A tragedy compounded. *New England Journal of Medicine, 352,* 1630–1633.

Reed, K. L. (1993). The beginning of occupational therapy. In H. L. Hopkins & H. D. Smith (Eds.), *Willard and Spackman's occupational therapy* (8th ed.) (pp. 26–43). Philadelphia, PA: Lippincott.

Reed, K. L. (2005). Dr. Hall and the work cure. *Occupational Therapy in Health Care, 19*(3): 33–50.

Reed, P. (2006). The dialogue within nursing theory-guided practice: A frontier of knowledge development. *Nursing Science Quarterly, 19*(4), 328–329.

Reel, S., & Abraham, I. (2007). *Business and legal essentials for nurse practitioners: From negotiating your first job through owning a practice.* Philadelphia, PA: Elsevier Health Sciences.

Robb, W. J. W. (2005). PhD, DNSc, ND: The ABCs of nursing doctoral degrees. *Dimensions of Critical Care Nursing, 24*(2), 89–96.

Robinson, V. (1946). *White caps: The story of nursing.* Philadelphia, PA: J.B. Lippincott.

Rosenbaum, M., Ferguson, K., & Lobas, J. G. (2004). Teaching medical students and residents skills for delivering bad news: A review of strategies. *Academic Medicine, 79*(2), 107–117.

Rowan, J. R., & Zinaich, S. Jr., (2002). *Ethics for the professions.* Florence, KY: Wadsworth.

Sackett, D. L., & Rosenberg, W. M. C. (1995). On the need for evidence-based medicine. *Journal of Public Health, 17*(3), 330–334.

Sensory-processing-disorder.com. *The history of occupational therapy: Where did we come from? How did we get here?* Retrieved on 12/4/2009, from http://www.sensory-processing-disorder.com/history-of-occupational-therapy.html

Shotton, L. (1997). The ethics of teaching nursing ethics. *Healthcare Analysis, 5*(3), 259–263.

Silva, M. C., & Guillett, S. E. (1996). Teaching ethics in nursing education: National curriculum trends. *Nursing Connections, 9*(3), 26–28.

Singer, P., Pellegrino, E. D., & Siegler, M. (2001). Clinical ethics revisited. *BioMed Central Medical Ethics, 2*(1). Retrieved on 2/8/2010, from http://www.ncbi.nlm.nih.gov/pmc/articles/PMC32193/

Smith, L. (2007). Said another way: Is nursing an academic discipline? *Nursing Forum, 35*(1), 25–29.

Stankovsky, M. (2005). *Creating the discipline of knowledge management: The latest in university research.* Burlington, MA: Butterworth-Heinemann.

Strauss, S. E., Richardson, W. S., Glasziou, P., & Haynes, R. B. (2005). *Evidence-based medicine: How to practice and teach EBM* (3rd ed.). London: Churchill Livingstone.

Travelbee, J. (1966). *Interpersonal aspects of nursing.* Philadelphia, PA: F.A. Davis.

Weil, V. (1989). How can philosophers teach professional ethics? *Journal of Social Philosophy, 20*(1–2), 131–136.

Whan, M. (1986). On the nature of practice. *British Journal of Social Work, 16*(2), 243–250.

Whitaker Foundation. (2002). A history of biomedical engineering. Retrieved on 9/2/2010, from http://bmes.seas.wustl.edu/WhitakerArchives/glance/history.html

Wright, P. (1951). Definition of a profession. *Canadian Bar Review, 29,* 748.

Yeager, S. (2005). Interdisciplinary collaboration: The heart and soul of health care. *Critical Care Nursing Clinics of North America, 17*(2), 143–148.

2

Nursing as a Practice Discipline

The untrained nurse is as old as the human race; the trained nurse is a recent discovery.

INTRODUCTION

The words that first describe nursing as a *practice discipline* are largely attributed to the seminal work of Dickoff, James, and Wiedenbach in their 1968a,b two-part article *Theory in a Practice Discipline*.[1] While this paper will relate more to the content in Chapter 16, the authors[2] emphasized (remember this is 1968, well before the founding of almost all of our current nursing doctoral programs) that *nursing theory, nursing practice*, and *nursing research* are mutually interrelated and interdependent. Today, some 40 years or more later, is this still true? It is very likely that most nurses, even professional nurses, would agree that nursing practice and nursing research are very interrelated. The evidence-based nursing practice movement is obviously confirmation of this (Kramer, 2010; Mantzoukas, 2007; Melnyk & Fineout-Overholt, 2005). However, as mentioned in Chapter 1, the recognized relevance of nursing theory to nursing practice today (at least the historical nursing theories) remains controversial (Apold, 2008; Mawdsley, 2005). Timpson has written, "nursing theory has a reputation for abstraction, even irrelevance in the minds of many practitioners" (1996, p. 1030). More recently, Stew (in press) has stated, "Nursing theory created by academics away from the clinical setting (on the *high, hard ground* of technical rationality) cannot be easily incorporated into practice (in the *swampy lowlands*) in the same way that oil

---

[1]This article is one of the classical, influential publications in the nursing discipline. It has been a stalwart required reading in PhD in Nursing programs for decades. It may now have new relevance for DNP programs, especially those that consider the theoretical exploration of nursing practice important to carve out the proper practice domain and boundaries for inquiry for graduates with practice nursing doctorates.

[2]Dr. Dickoff and Dr. James were both philosophers and Professor Ernestine Wiedenbach (b. 1900, d. 1998) was an Emeritus Associate Professor of Maternal and Newborn Nursing at Yale University School of Nursing at the time of the article's publication.

and water cannot mix" (p. 10). In this characterization, the philosopher Jürgen Habermas's (1971) use of *technical rationality* represents the triumph of theory over practice (largely by academics and scholars). This predominance of technical rationality among nursing academics has largely contributed to the *theory–practice gap* that has plagued educators and practitioners in nursing since the 1960s (McCaugherty, 2006).

We are not suggesting that nursing theories have no absolute relevance to nursing practice today. Indeed a review of the articles in any recent issue of the *Journal of Advanced Nursing, Advances in Nursing Science*, or *Nursing Science Quarterly* would indicate a very healthy use of theory, at least in the published nursing literature and by academicians and scholars. Dekeyser and Medoff-Cooper also take a nontheorist perspective on nursing theory and indicate, "As the discipline has matured, the focus of theory development has changed to more realistically reflect the practice and research environment" (2001, p. 341). However, this is a text about philosophy of science in nursing practice, and these introductory chapters are focused on the context of nursing as a practice-focused discipline. A careful examination of any contemporary baccalaureate or masters nursing curricula is very "truth-telling" about the degree to which nursing theory is emphasized in the curricula and the importance it is accorded. Donaldson and Crowley's (1978) seminal article on the discipline of nursing explored some of the earliest discussions on the differences between *nursing* as a discipline, as a science, and nursing as practice. Today, however, the tensions between the theoretical and the practical are still evident in a noted nursing scholar's linguistic preference to describe nursing as a *scientific discipline* rather than a *practice discipline* (Chinn, 2008, p. 1). Similarly, don't we more often hear the phrase *the practice of medicine* rather than the *science of medicine/medical science* or the *scientific discipline of medicine*? Chinn writes that a *discipline* is "distinguished by the social and cultural constraints that are imposed both externally and internally. The definition of the science, the phenomena of concern, the group's collectively accepted knowledge, the accepted methods and practices—all form a structure, without which the discipline would be indistinguishable" (p. 1). It is very likely Chinn recognizes nursing as both a scientific *and* practice discipline. We are just making observations about how there is a proclivity for nursing scholars and nursing educators to emphasize nursing as *science* (nursing science), whereas practitioners (RNs, APRNs) seem more inclined to emphasize nursing as *practice* (nursing practice). Our guess is that graduate nursing students (at least at first) may be somewhere in between. Thus, this chapter will further examine nursing as a practice discipline, recognizing that nursing practice *cannot* evolve without nursing science.[3] Conversely, as a practice discipline, any nursing science far removed from the context of practice is likely to be minimized, dismissed, or ignored by the masses of practitioners. Whether this is good for the discipline is certainly fodder for discussion, especially among DNP students and faculty. Whether

---

[3]We would even be so bold as to say unless there is more emphasis on creating nursing science (knowledge) or more respect for those who seek to create the *evidence* of evidence-based and practice-based nursing practice, that ultimately the discipline will stagnate and not prosper. Contemporary and future DNP programs are going to have to retackle the issue as to whether DNP graduates ought to be generating evidence (or practice evidence) for the profession (Florczak, 2010; Smith Glasgow & Dreher, 2010).

there is a rightful or practical place for entirely theoretical nursing today or whether we need new contemporary nurse theorists is beyond the scope of this text but interesting to consider nonetheless.[4]

THE EVOLUTIONARY IDENTITY OF NURSING AS A PRACTICE DISCIPLINE

1910: First a "Field"

The image of nurses and nursing is a complicated one. The identity of nursing is grounded in a historical caricature of both the public's perception of nursing and nurses and the professions' own internalized perceptions and beliefs about itself. In other words, the status and stature of nursing in 1910 was very different from the status and stature of nursing in 2010. For an examination of 1910, Sussman published an interview which was based on a 101-year-old nurse's recollections of her early days in nursing school. Much of what is described below was based on her interview and the commentary of Joan Lynaugh, a noted nurse historian:

> "You have these young women who left home and are living with other women and working with doctors," Lynaugh said. "Like it or not, there was a lot of fun going on. At the same time, she's learning helpful things and learning to do the right thing." She learned to do the right thing as a nurse only after months of menial labor: scrubbing floors, making beds, carrying bedpans, preparing meals, and arranging trays. Only then did students progress to giving medication, recording vital signs, and other "scientific things," as the woman called them. Those "scientific things" meant anatomy, physiology, bacteriology, urinalysis, materia medica, gynecology, and medicinal "solutions," as well as ethics, massage, cookery, and hygiene. "We tend to think they didn't know that much, but it's not true," Lynaugh said. "What nurses knew in 1910 was quite a lot, really. They knew anatomy and about drugs—quinine, morphine, stimulants, emetics, cathartics, sedatives." Besides the heavy course work, usually taught in a stern authoritarian manner, students worked 12-hours shifts with time off for meals and rest. For their labor—and students made up the bulk of the nursing work force in hospitals—they received about $50 a year, room, board, and uniforms. Once out of school, large numbers of nurses became private duty nurses. For days, weeks, or even months at a stretch—until the pneumonia or TB they had been hired to treat resolved—the nurses would single-handedly keep the patient hydrated, supervise meals, dress wounds, and clean the room and equipment. "They never left," Lynaugh said.
>
> —*Sussman, 1999, p. 1.*[5]

Nursing practice in 1910 was certainly extremely different from what it is today. Ask yourself, was nursing a discipline yet? Or was it more of a *field*, a good description

---

[4]Additionally ask yourself, aren't medicine and pharmacology both practice disciplines? Are they theory driven? Do physicians or pharmacologists practice with a theoretical lens? We agree that psychologists, likely social workers, practice more theoretically than most. Whether nurses really do is still up for debate.

[5]Reprinted with permission. Copyright 1999 Gannett Healthcare Group.

of what a discipline is in its formative, less established, early stages (Hongcai, 2007)? A quick historical overview of what was happening in nursing around 1910 is as follows:

- 1908: The National Association of Colored Graduate Nurses (NACGN) was established, largely by Martha Minerva Franklin.
- 1909: The School of Nursing of the University of Minnesota (largely under the direction of Dr. Richard Olding Beard) becomes the first nursing school organized as an integral part of a university, but would not offer a degree granting basic nursing program until 1919.
- 1910: M. Adelaide Nutting becomes the first professor of nursing in the world at Teacher's College, Columbia University in New York.
- 1910: Isabel Adams Hampton Robb (b. 1859), the first president of the Nurses Associated Alumnae, who is described as the architect of American nursing organizations, dies in a traffic accident.
- 1911: The ANA becomes the successor to the Nurses Associated Alumnae.
- 1911: Linda Richards, America's first trained nurse dies.
- 1912: National League of Nursing Education (NLNE) is founded.
- 1912: National Organization for Public Health Nursing (NOPHN) was founded with Lillian D. Wald as the first president—in 1895 she founded the renowned Henry Street Settlement House in New York City.
- 1912: The first comprehensive survey of schools of nursing in the United States. *The Educational Status of Nursing* was published by the Federal Bureau of Education and M. Adelaide Nutting.

Nurse historian Donahue (1996) actually describes this era as the "rise of organized nursing" (p. 318). Our own particular interest in these events are those that signal the rise of a discipline as it shifts and evolves from a field to a recognized discipline of study. We usually see this with the progression of a heritage of literature typical of a discipline described in Chapter 1. Examples include the publication of the first nursing journal *Nightingale* (1886), followed by *The Trained Nurse and Hospital World* (1888) and in 1900 *The American Journal of Nursing*, which is still in existence today (American Association for the History of Nursing, 2008; Flaumenhaft & Flaumenhaft, 1989). The emergence of new schools of nursing also meant there was great demand for nursing textbooks. The first nursing textbook was Clara S. Weeks-Shaw's *A Textbook of Nursing for the Use of Training Schools, Families, and Private Students* in 1885 and shortly thereafter Isabel Adams Hampton Robb's *Nursing: Its Principles and Practice for Hospital and Private Use* (1893).

A closer examination of these historical landmarks during the rise of organized nursing in the late 20th and early 21st centuries indicates to us that nursing was in its formative stage as a field, and had yet to fully emerge as a complete discipline. The practice orientation of the work of early American nursing students was also codified by very strict behavioral and moral guidelines for an overwhelmingly middle-class, female student population (Tomes, 1978).[6] These principles, by which student

---

[6]From 1900 to 1930 men were actually excluded from all nursing schools. A survey of nursing schools published in 1934 indicated only four allowed males to enroll (Witte, 1934).

nurses were socialized, meant that the mission of the first nursing schools in the late 1800s and early 1900s (and for many subsequent decades of nursing education) was to ensure that each nursing school's mission was "to establish and maintain a code of ethic"[7] (Walker, 1900, p. 203). Most academic disciplines in their evolution are not burdened in the very public way practice disciplines are. Did the very visible, often unglamorous practice of nursing that was seen (and perceived) in the hospital ward, the settlement house, or the home (the domain of the private duty nurse) make it more difficult for the field to establish respect for its scientific base and to emerge as a discipline? Did the burden of nursing, being an occupation of women, also hamper its slow acceptance as a "proper academic discipline" as many have suggested? (Thompson, 2009; Wuest, 1994) Or was nursing's early legitimacy as a discipline hampered more by its lack of advanced educational opportunities which left it dangling at the door of the academy (Emerson & Records, 2005)?

1960s: A Practice Discipline Begins to Emerge

If we shift 50 years later to 1960, we can take a brief glimpse into the state of the discipline as it emerges from the shadows of a field, and the first tangible signs of an emerging discipline appear. Largely because of the important public and very visible role nurses had in WWII, nursing's image was certainly elevated, and the forces to improve the status of nursing in society began to take place (Breakiron, 1995; Stevens, 1990). Famed nurse historian Beatrice Kalisch has stated of the role of nurses during WWII that, "There was a flow of wartime films showing heroic nurses; there were autobiographical films and books about nurses" (Schmidt, 2001, p. 1). The heroism of nurses during WWI and WWII was also replicated with the war effort of nurses in the Vietnam War where nurses first served as commissioned officers. Many women, including eight nurses, died in the Vietnam War, and their heroism and service formed the basis for the Vietnam Women's War Memorial commemorative statue erected in Washington, DC in 1993 (Sheehy, 2007).

The 1960s began as a decade where nursing's scholarship began to flourish. It was also the decade when the first real discussion about what kind of minimal educational preparation RNs should possess. In 1965, only 22% of RNs had been prepared in an academic program (this included RNs with an associate, baccalaureate or higher degree), with 85% of all nurses still prepared in diploma programs (Nelson, 2002). In response to this need to elevate the educational level of the profession, the ANA proposed in 1965 to require the bachelor's degrees in nursing (BSN) degree for entry into professional nursing. With regard to higher education in nursing, this was still the era before the beginning of the advanced practice nursing movement. Advanced practice nursing would begin to evolve with the first certificate pediatric NP program at the University of Colorado (Denver) in 1965 (Silver, Ford, & Steanly, 1967). At the beginning of the decade there were only three nursing doctoral programs in existence — at Teacher's College, Columbia University (1924), New York University (1934), and the University of

---

[7]*Ethic* is spelled correctly in this reference.

Pittsburgh (1954) (Dreher, 2009a; Robb, 2005). As mentioned in Chapter 1, a larger critical mass of nurse scientists was created through the Nurse-Scientist Training Program at the National Institutes of Health (Gortner, 1991). Formed early in the decade (1961), it helped prepare competent nursing scientists who pursued doctorates in the basic sciences, physical sciences, and social sciences, with the goal of using this interdisciplinary knowledge to create nursing knowledge while maintaining a nursing identity (Gortner, 1986). In 1962, an experimental Division of Nursing Field Research Center was founded in San Francisco (Nursing Research, 1962). According to Gortner "The late 1960's began an important reorientation of the Federal interest in nursing research with particular attention being given to studies that would be relevant to patient care issues and problems" (1986, p. 124). She further indicated that "Following establishment of the National Center for Health Services Research in 1967, some nursing research grant project investigators moved their research efforts into the field of health services research[8] in general" (1986, p. 124).

Interestingly, the value of health services research has steadily increased over time and the standards and protocols of care and practice that are reported by the Agency for Healthcare Research and Quality (AHRQ) have become so important that funding decisions for health care at the federal level are often based on these expertly produced mostly multidisciplinary research studies. Unfortunately, aside from the brilliant nursing health services research work of Dr. Linda Aiken[9] (also a sociologist), we see a decline in nursing health sensitive health services research and fewer nurse scientists properly trained in these methods. This decline, which includes research that explores the *cost effectiveness* of nursing interventions (Shever et al., 2008; Spetz, 2005), will impact the practice of DNP graduates who, many indicate, should be the leaders of evaluating and implementing best-practice protocols of care (AACN, 2006; Fitzpatrick, 2008).[10] This movement toward the study of the efficacy of nursing and nursing interventions, nevertheless, was indeed in its infancy in the late 1960s.

By the end of the decade there would be three additional nursing doctoral programs founded nationally and many more in the early 1970s (see Table 2.1). These institutions would cement their reputations over time by producing the chief nursing science graduates that would help nursing crystallize itself as a practice discipline. It should be noted that Table 2.1 reflects three different doctoral nursing degrees—DNSc (Doctor of Nursing Science), PhD (Doctor of Philosophy in Nursing

---

[8]*Health services research* can be defined as "the multidisciplinary field of scientific investigation that studies how social factors, financing systems, organizational structures and processes, health technologies, and personal behaviors affect access to health care, the quality and cost of health care, and ultimately our health and well-being" (Lohr & Steinwachs, 2002, p. 16). Its domains include research on individuals, families, organizations, institutions, communities, and populations.

[9]Dr. Linda Aiken is widely known for her high impact 2003 study published in the *Journal of the American Medical Association (JAMA)* which reported that hospitals that employed a higher proportion of nurses with at least a bachelor's degree had lower rates of death for surgical patients compared to nursing care from RNs with either a diploma or associate degree. She has also published on advanced practice nursing workforce policy (2003).

[10]Again, we do not want to exclude those who also believe DNP graduates should also generate nursing knowledge too, not just translate and disseminate it. This debate is likely to continue.

TABLE 2.1
Doctoral Nursing Programs Founded in 1960–1975

University	Type of Doctoral Degree	Year
Boston University	DNSc	1960
University of California at San Francisco	DNSc	1964
Catholic University	DNSc	1967
Texas Women's University	PhD	1971
Case Western Reserve University	PhD	1972
University of Pennsylvania	DNSc	1974
University of Texas at Austin	PhD	1974
University of Alabama at Birmingham	DSN	1975
Wayne State University	PhD	1975
University of Illinois at Chicago	PhD	1975
University of Michigan	PhD	1975
University of Arizona	PhD	1975

Dreher (2009a) and Leininger (1976).

or Nursing Science), and DSN (Doctor of Science in Nursing). Much has been written about the origins of the DNSc, DSN (first approved at the University of Alabama-Birmingham in 1975), and DNS (first approved at the University of Indiana in 1976) degrees. Unfortunately much of the literature that describes these degrees, their purpose and historical trajectory, is very muddled and confusing. Joyce Fitzpatrick (2003), the former Dean of the Frances Payne Bolton School of Nursing at Case Western Reserve University, makes this case quite nicely in her plea for nursing to embrace a clinical doctorate as a credible alternative to the PhD and the other multiple nursing research degrees. Essentially, the DNSc, DSN, and DNS were all designed as clinical doctorate degrees for the nursing discipline. The first, the DNSc at Boston University founded in 1960 with the first graduate in 1963, was designed to focus on clinical practice and scholarship in psychiatric nursing. But over time all three of these degrees lost their original *clinical doctorate mission* and practically everyone is in consensus that they indeed all became *de facto* research degrees, just like the PhD in Nursing (AACN, 2006).

One question largely absent from the nursing literature is why the early PhD programs at NYU and University of Pittsburgh did not lead the way for more subsequent PhD programs instead of the DNSc? Some have declared there was too little political support in many universities or among the standing faculty to support the awarding of a PhD in Nursing (Veeser, Stegbauer, & Russell, 1999). Others reasoned that even many nursing scholars at the time did not consider nursing science mature enough to award the PhD (Carter, 2006). Aside from some of the leading nursing schools in the nation that first established DNSc degree programs instead of the PhD (see Table 2.1), there were other nursing schools that began as DNSc programs before converting to a PhD: Columbia University (DNSc 1993 to PhD 2008), Yale University (DNSc 1994 to PhD 2006), Rush University (DNSc 1977 to PhD 2008), UCLA (DNSc 1986 to PhD

1995), and Widener University (DNSc 1984 to PhD 2008) (AACN, 2009). Why did these first doctoral programs and those above founded years later start DNSc degrees instead of the PhD? We believe there has been a historical prejudice against the recognition of nursing as a legitimate discipline. We further surmise that many faculty in other disciplines historically just could not accept that nursing was credible enough to award a PhD degree.[11] In rare cases, the university may not have initially had a state charter to award a PhD degree (Widener University's first doctoral degree was the DNSc and was not permitted to award any PhD until the charter was amended), but this reason was indeed an anomaly. The question we are faced with today is whether nursing has sufficiently established itself as a discipline today and whether its scholars fully embrace its identity as a "practice discipline" or not? Further, are our doctoral nursing graduates good stewards of the discipline and creating enough evidence to keep current with a rapidly changing, highly technological health care system? What do you think?

2010: New Energy, New Tension: A DNP Degree Surges

Now we arrive at 2010. A new nursing doctorate, a practice doctorate, has been around formatively since 2005, although the first DNP degree was founded at the University of Kentucky in 2001. Startlingly, it was recently projected that by the end of 2009 there would be more DNP than PhD programs, and while this did not quite happen, it is very likely to occur by the end of 2010 (Dreher, 2009a). Indeed, there is new energy in doctoral nursing education, but also new tension. Can it be that the sudden, if not surprising growth curve of new DNP programs will force nursing to revisit its origins as a practice field? Will scholars teaching in both DNP programs and PhD programs be challenged to reflexively and honestly examine how nursing, now *as a more mature discipline*, is going to generate the necessary practice knowledge it needs for the future? According to noted nursing Deans Afaf Meleis (University of Pennsylvania School of Nursing) and Kathleen Dracup (University of California, San Francisco), "Practice drives knowledge development in nursing" (2005, p. 1). With a decade of stagnant enrollments in PhD programs from 1996 to 2006 (with future declines in overall PhD enrollments and graduations quite possibly on the horizon)[12] and with surging enrollments in DNP programs, nurses with practice doctorates cannot be excluded from the knowledge-generating enterprise for a practice discipline (AACN, 2009b; DeMarco, Pulcini, Haggerty, & Tang, 2009). Or can they?

---

[11]Except in rare cases, all new university or college-based doctoral degrees must be approved by a vote of a respective faculty senate—often primarily senior faculty with tenure who may have very traditional viewpoints.

[12]Since 1996 there appears to be a slight increase in both PhD enrollments and graduations. New 2009–2010 AACN data indicate overall PhD in Nursing enrollment was up 5.1% and graduations was up 2.2%, but full-time post-doc enrollment was down 6.1% (Fang, Tracy, & Bednash, 2010). This latter number is particularly concerning as it is this population that is most likely to replace retiring nurse scientists. Further, we contend these slight improvements in enrollment are not enough to overcome the much larger number of retirements from the nursing professoriate now and which are predicted to surge in the coming years (McNeil, 2010).

Moreover, if practice doctorate nurses are going to generate knowledge (or science) for the discipline, grounding in philosophy of science will be essential if the methods of inquiry are going to be reputable. Again, the issue for the future, we boldly predict, is not *if* the practice doctorate graduate will produce knowledge for the nursing discipline, but how will this *practice knowledge* be different from what is traditionally produced by the PhD graduate (Coghlan, 2007; Sheriff & Chaney, 2007; Smith Glasgow & Dreher, 2010). This important issue will be addressed more fully in Chapter 16.

In many ways, the relatively new doctor of nursing practice degrees in nursing (both DNP and DrNP) are perhaps best described as third-generation practice doctorates for the nursing discipline. It has been noted earlier that the first generation of clinical doctorates[13] (DNSc, DSN, and DNS) originally conceived in the 1960s and 1970s really never fully became clinical doctorates and ended up being very reputable *de facto* research doctorates like the PhD (AACN, 2006; Bellack, 2002; Dreher, Donnelly, & Naremore, 2005). The second-generation clinical or practice doctorate for the nursing profession was the Doctor of Nursing (ND) degree, founded at Case Western Reserve University in 1979 (Bellack, 2002; Dreher, 2009a; Sakalys & Watson, 1986). The ND was created as a professional doctorate, much like the MD degree, where any typical college graduate[14] would complete three years of full-time study and exit as an RN with a clinical/professional doctorate. Unfortunately, whether this was indeed a visionary degree for the nursing profession or not, is still up for debate—especially since the nursing profession had never even fully implemented the requirement for the BSN to be required for entry level (Donley & Flaherty, 2008). For some, even the suggestion that the nursing profession should move to doctoral level entry in 1979 was preposterous. Nevertheless, the ND degree was a failure of innovation, with only four degree programs ever established (1979: Case Western Reserve University; 1987: Rush University; 1990: University of Colorado at Denver; and 1999: the University of South Carolina) (Dreher, 2005; Mundinger, 2005). All four ND programs subsequently closed between 2004 and 2005 and converted to DNP programs (AACN, 2009). The real question for history is why did this second-generation "practice nursing doctorate" fail, although Lenz (2005) has indicated that they actually paved the way for the current and third-generation nursing practice doctorate—the DNP.

The emergence of the current practice doctorate for the discipline of nursing began with the work of Dean Mary Mundinger at the Columbia University School of Nursing in the late 1990s. In 2000, Mundinger and colleagues published a very

---

[13]There is a solid case that the words *clinical doctorate, practice doctorate* and *professional doctorate* are now relatively interchangeable. One distinction perhaps is that all practice doctorates include an actual requirement for *practice* (additional clinical hours, practica, internships, or residency hours). We have found many cases where additional practice hours (beyond the classroom) are, however, *not* universally required in clinical or professional doctorates. Finally, it should be noted that at the time of the first ND degree, the term *practice doctorate* was not in use, and the ND was more like a professional doctorate (again akin to a medical or dental school degree model) than a clinical doctorate like the first DNSc.

[14]Originally, BSNs did not enter the ND programs but eventually they did—including nurses with MSN degrees—and thus the muddying of the original intent of the degree model (to replicate the MD) helped lead to its demise.

provocative study in the prestigious *Journal of American Medical Association (JAMA)* where her team conducted a randomized trial and reported:

> In an ambulatory care situation in which patients were randomly assigned to either nurse practitioners or physicians, and where nurse practitioners had the same authority, responsibilities, productivity and administrative requirements, and patient population as primary care physicians, *patients' outcomes were comparable.*[15]
>
> —*Mundinger, 2000, p. 59*

This was the first study in the United States of its caliber to indicate that under certain conditions physician medical care and NP care (with MSNs!) were equivalent.[16] These findings led Dean Mundinger to introduce the first DrNP degree program at Columbia University in 2005 after first piloting the degree with a cohort of internal faculty in an intensive format in 2004 (Honig & Smolowitz, 2009). Described initially as a *clinical doctorate*, the Columbia DrNP program was created as a very clinically based 30-credit doctoral program that required a one-year, full-time residency as well as a portfolio of case studies (but no clinical research project or clinical dissertation) (Mundinger, 2005). Despite its converting to a DNP program in 2008,[17] the historical impact of Columbia University's practice doctorate model has largely surpassed the impact of the first DNP program at the University of Kentucky in 2001. While they were both DrNP programs with different initials, the Kentucky DNP did not prepare clinicians or practitioners, but only clinical executives. Further, its creators never published their rationale as to why their DNP model was superior to the established ND which had by this time largely become both an entry-level doctorate and post-masters degree model.

The rapid surge in new doctor of nursing practice programs in 2005 (Table 2.2 lists the first DNP/DrNP programs established as of August 2005) has led us to today where according to the AACN there are reported 118 DNP (including 1 DrNP program) and 118 research doctoral programs in nursing (114 PhD, 3 DNS, and 1 EdD) (Fang, Tracy, & Bednash, 2010).[18]

The implication for so many DNP programs appearing so suddenly is enormous, and its ultimate impact on the discipline is unknown.[19] Unlike 2005 (when there were

---

[15]Italics mine.

[16]A subsequent Cochrane systemic review published in the *British Medical Journal* also found no differences in prescriptions, return consultations, or referrals between nurse practitioners' care and physicians in primary care settings. Perhaps more astounding, this review found quality of care, in some ways, was better for nurse practitioner consultations (Horrocks, Anderson, & Salisbury, 2002)

[17]Largely out of fear of the historical conundrum of multiple doctoral nursing degrees, the AACNs Collegiate Commission on Nurse Accreditation (CCNE) voted in 2006 to only accredit programs that use the initials "DNP" not "DrNP." However, nursing's other accrediting organization, the National League for Nursing Accrediting Commission (NLNAC), is not adhering to this restriction. The second author of this text was informed Columbia made the change from DrNP to DNP to seek CCNE accreditation.

[18]This 2010 report also indicates one ND program, while closed to new students, has students still matriculating.

[19]According to the AACN, as of October 2009 there are 100 additional schools planning DNP programs and a few schools (far fewer) planning PhD programs.

TABLE 2.2
Inaugural DNP/DrNP Programs in the United States (as of August 1, 2005)

University	Year Founded	Type of Program	Notes
Case Western Reserve University	2005	DNP	Founded as ND and converted to DNP
Columbia University	2005	DrNP	Founded as DrNP and converted to DNP in 2008
Drexel University	2005	DrNP	Founded as a hybrid professional doctorate combining the practice doctorate and the research doctorate
Rush University	2005	DNP	Founded as ND and converted to DNP
Tri-College University Nursing Consortium[a]	2005	DNP	Founded as joint-DNP program; NDSU left Consortium in 2007; Consortium disbanded in 2008
University of Colorado, Denver	2005	DNP	Founded as ND and converted to DNP
University of Kentucky	2001	DNP	First DNP—Clinical Leadership (only)
University of South Carolina	2005	DNP	Founded as ND and converted to DNP
University of Tennessee, Memphis	2005	DNP	Founded as DNSc and converted to DNP

[a]Concordia College; Minnesota State University, Moorhead; North Dakota State University.

lots of articles both pro and con written about the degree), this recent surge in programs the last two years has created a vacuum in which very few nursing scholars have publically written or hypothesized about this degree's impact on nursing science knowledge development.

A couple of developments with the doctor of nursing practice degree should be noted. Shortly after Columbia University in 2005, Drexel University also implemented a DrNP degree, but their degree model was a hybrid model (different from Columbia's DrNP) that combined a focus on advanced practice *with* clinical research and included a requirement to complete a clinical dissertation (Dreher, Donnelly, & Naremore, 2005).[20] The Drexel DrNP degree model was created to fall in between the PhD and DNP degrees with its graduates prepared to not just evaluate and disseminate, but to also conduct practical, practice-grounded, clinically oriented research. Figure 2.1 indicates the conceptual placement of this degree among the current nursing doctorates. Our description here of the DNP as a *Practice/Non-Research* doctorate is a

---

[20]This hybrid degree model was more similar to professional doctorates that traditionally include a research project in the form of a clinical dissertation or dissertation (e.g., PsyD, DrPH, DSW, and DScPT degrees). The DNP as conceived by the AACN is a nonresearch-oriented, practice/professional doctorate and is more like the MD, DPT, and PharmD degree models. There is usually a final doctoral project instead of a traditional empirical research study.

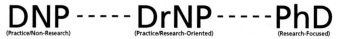

FIGURE 2.1
Practice/Nonresearch, practice/research-oriented, and research-focused
nursing doctorates

technical description as the AACN *Essentials of Doctoral of Education for Advanced Nursing Practice* still states "Doctoral program in nursing fall into two principle types: research-focused and practice-focused" (2006, p. 3).

While Drexel has been the only school to endorse the hybrid model at this time, there are several schools that have included a research requirement for the DNP degree, albeit with some controversy. Finally, having two models of the DNP and DrNP is also not without controversy as some (including the AACN) have indicated that it is confusing and again fear the previously mentioned doctoral nursing degree alphabet conundrum (AACN, 2006; Fulton & Lyon, 2005, 2006). Nevertheless, nurse anesthesia has not embraced the idea of a single practice doctorate for CRNAs and CRNAs may now pursue the DNP, DrNP, Doctor of Nurse Anesthesia Practice (DNAP) or Doctor of Management Practice of Nurse Anesthesia (DMPNA) (Hawkins & Nezat, 2009).

A second issue largely impacting the DNP degree is whether by 2015 all new advanced practice nurses should possess the DNP degree instead of the masters degree as voted by the AACN in 2004 (AACN, 2004a). While the AACN passed this resolution in 2004 by a vote of: 162 (yes), 101 (no), 13 (abstain), the question is whether this ruling has *any teeth* (Dreher, Donnelly, & Naremore, 2005)?[21] The correct answer is no, but the pragmatic response is: *it remains a goal.* In reality, in order for this to truly take place by 2015, several things must happen:

1. All 50 state Nurse Practice Acts would need to be changed to permit the entry of advanced practice nurses at the doctoral level—and many have not yet done so. Some still have codified regulation that *requires* an MSN for advanced practice nursing.
2. All major APRN organizations would have to go on record as supporting this—and so far none have agreed to the 2015 deadline.
3. The AACN/CCNE would need to cease accrediting MSN advanced practice programs as of 2015 and there is no indication that this will occur.
4. The NLN/NLNAC would need to cease accrediting MSN advanced practice programs as of 2015 and this appears certain not to occur.
5. All MSN advanced practice programs in the United States would need to close and convert to DNP programs by 2015—and this is highly unlikely.

---

[21]Further, only 53% of eligible schools voted, despite a membership of more than 500 schools, and no proxy voting was allowed. Our point is only to describe how controversial this 2004 vote was (Fulton & Lyon, 2005; National Association of Clinical Nurse Specialists [NACNS], 2005). Today, 6 years later, the controversy is more the direction of the degree than the degree itself.

First, Fulton and Lyon (2005) have affirmed that various Nurse Practice Acts will need to be modified if the MSN is no longer going to be required to sit for certification as an advanced practice nurse in any respective state. For instance, in 2006, the Pennsylvania State Nurses Association published a position paper against the requirement that all APRNs obtain a DNP instead of MSN by 2015, although the Nurse Practice Act in that state was modified to actually permit new advanced practice nurses to have either a masters or doctoral degree (instead of an MSN only) (Vogel & Gobel, 2006). One good question to ask yourself is what is the current language regarding the educational preparation of advanced practice nurses in your state? Second, the major advanced practice nursing organizations (American College of Midwives, NACNS, American Association of Nurse Anesthetists [AANA], and a cadre of NP organizations) all have taken different perspectives on the 2015 deadline. Most NP organizations have taken a progressive stance that approves of DNP education without diminishing or marginalizing current masters level NP education, but not explicitly endorsing the 2015 implementation date. A recent consensus statement of multiple NP organizations[22] stated the following:

> Current masters and higher degree nurse practitioner programs prepare fully accountable clinicians to provide care to well individuals, patients with undifferentiated symptoms, and those with acute, complex chronic and/or critical illnesses. The DNP degree more accurately reflects current clinical competencies and includes preparation for the changing health care system. It is congruent with the intense rigorous education for nurse practitioners. This evolution is comparable to the clinical doctoral preparation for other health care professions.
>
> —*Nurse Practitioner Roundtable, 2008, p. 1*

Similarly, the American College of Nurse Midwives (ACNM) attested in 2007 and reaffirmed in 2009 that the DNP may be an option for some midwifery programs, but should not be a requirement for entry into midwifery practice (ACNM, 2007, 2009).[23] In June 2007 the AANA Board of Directors unanimously adopted the position of supporting *doctoral education*[24] for entry into nurse anesthesia practice by 2025. In May 2009 the NACNS published the following as part of their *Position Statement on the Nursing Practice Doctorate*:

> Consistent with the conclusions of the NACNS *White Paper on the Nursing Practice Doctorate* (2005), the 2009–2010 NACNS Board of Directors affirms a position of neutrality with respect to the DNP. *Neutrality* means the board neither endorses nor opposes the DNP degree as an option for clinical nurse specialist (CNS) education. NACNS recognizes

---

[22]Endorsed by the following NP organizations: American Academy of Nurse Practitioners, American College of Nurse Practitioners, Association of Faculties of Pediatric Nurse Practitioners, National Association of Nurse Practitioners in Women's Health, National Association of Pediatric Nurse Practitioners, National Conference of Gerontological Nurse Practitioners, and National Organization of Nurse Practitioner Faculties (NONPF).

[23]The July 2009 American College of Nurse-Midwives *Position Statement on Midwifery Education and the Doctor of Nursing Practice* can be found at http://www.acnm.org/siteFiles/position/Midwifery_Ed_and_DNP_7_09.pdf

[24]Any doctorate (not restricted to a nursing doctorate either), and not just the DNP.

"the importance of advanced education and remains interested in participating in the national dialogue with other stakeholders and organizations representing CNS members" (p. 5). NACNS defines CNSs as "licensed registered professional nurses with graduate preparation (masters or doctorate) from a program that prepares CNSs" (NACNS Statement on Practice and Education, 2004, p. 12).

—NACNS, 2009, p. 1

Finally, since the AACN DNP model of *practice* also includes the executive role, it is worth noting that the most recent statement by the American Organization of Nurse Executives (AONE) attests "AONE supports the DNP as the terminal degree option for practice-focused nursing. However, AONE, at this time, believes nursing masters degree programs in both specialty and generalist courses of study should be retained" (2007, p. 3). One of the prime reasons for the AONE position was their belief that there was a lack of analysis and support that a doctoral educated manager/executive was needed across all aspects of the care continuum.

Overall, despite the cautious endorsements of the DNP degree by the major APRN organizations, it remains evident that with over 100 (and likely to push 200) current, planned, and future largely DNP programs, the degree is going to continue to evolve and proliferate. Its ultimate success, however, will be in the measurable outcomes of the graduates, their direct impact on the health care delivery system, and the overall reception of the new degree by the health care marketplace and important stakeholders—including academia. We must remember that the permanence of advanced practice nursing from the earliest certificate movement to the requirement of the masters degree took some 40 years to come to fruition (Dreher, 2008).[25] Further, and perhaps even more astonishingly, we have never resolved even the minimal educational entry-level question for basic nursing practice (Donley & Flaherty, 2008). So current DNP students should not despair as the profession and public (and health care system) try to figure this new degree out. As a DNP student (and forthcoming graduate) you are at the forefront of this movement. The critical mass of graduates will ultimately blaze the trail for this degree's future.

THE NATURE OF DISCIPLINARY NURSING PRACTICE

While this text is written largely for graduate nursing students (and chiefly for DNP students), some comments about the diverse nature (and complexity) of disciplinary nursing practice should be made.

Basic and Professional Nursing Practice

As has been noted by Nelson (2002), with the arrival of Associate Degree Nursing (ADN) programs (first conceived by Dr. Mildred Montag[26] of Adelphi University) in 1958, the resulting designation of two separate educational levels of nursing

---

[25]Dr. Ann O'Sullivan, past president of NONPF, has widely publicized this point in response to those who expect the DNP to be accepted and integrated immediately.

[26]Dr. Mildred Montag (b. 1908, d. 2004).

education did not ultimately differentiate practice between *technical* (ADN) and *professional* (BSN) nursing (Haase, 1990). Dr. Montag, however, never conceived that the ADN-prepared *technical nurse* would have absolute parity with the BSN-prepared *professional nurse*, but due to the shortage of nurses after WWII with a bustling postwar economy, that is exactly what happened. According to Nelson:

> The ANA position in 1965 was later supported by a resolution in 1978 by the ANA House of Delegates in which the requirement was set forth that by 1985 the minimum preparation for entry into professional practice would be the baccalaureate degree (2002, p. 1).

What this designation did was to essentially affirm and attempt to codify two levels of nursing practice, professional and technical. Nevertheless, over time the technical nurse label has never really been affixed to the RN prepared at the Associates or even Diploma level, despite there being a plethora of published literature that has described how technical nurses and professional nurses are inherently different. In many ways, the three types of basic nursing preparation have morphed over time (unfortunately) into "a nurse is a nurse is a nurse."

Returning to Chapter 1, this has complicated the professionalism of nursing practice and nursing as a discipline. In 1998 Christman noted that nurses as a whole remain among the least educated health care professionals at the point of care. In 2000, BSN-prepared nurses represented only approximately 30% of all RNs, with nurses with associate degrees representing around 60% of all RNs (Gosnell, 2002). Almost a decade later from Christman's observation, not much had changed. Nevertheless, in 2007, in California (our largest state), nurses with associate degrees were noted to be 70% of the total nurse workforce (NLN, 2007a). Recent data by Aiken and colleagues (2009) indicates however BSN prepared nurses have increased to 45% of the nursing workforce nationally. While the ANA is no longer actively pushing the BSN as the required minimal entry degree for nursing, it is noted that one current innovation is the "RN +10" movement, which would require registered professional nurses to earn a BSN within 10 years of their initial basic nursing licensure (Dreher, 2008).[27] So where are we left with this endless discussion point: Is nursing a profession?[28] Also, are all nurses *professional nurses*? Can the discipline ever fully mature with so many entry-level issues, both in professional and advanced practice, left in limbo or unresolved? Will these issues further impact nursing science and nursing knowledge development?

---

[27]At the time of this text's printing, this movement appears most active in New York, New Jersey, and Pennsylvania.

[28]Donley and Flaherty have summarized this question in their excellent 2008 paper by stating "If you view the 1965 statement as a call to close hospital schools of nursing and to move all nursing education inside the walls of colleges or universities, then the American Nurses Association was successful in implementing its vision" (p. 22). They summarize saying "If, however, you view the 1965 Position Paper as a mandate for a more educated nurse workforce to enhance patient care, the goal has not been achieved" (p. 22).

A Distinction: Advanced Practice Nursing versus Advanced *Nursing* Practice

Unquestionably, many graduate nursing students, whether pursuing a career goal in *advanced practice* as an NP, nurse midwife, nurse anesthetist, or CNS (all traditional advanced practice roles), are either pursuing the DNP post-masters or as an entry-level degree after completing a BSN. There are also "advanced nursing roles" (different than traditional "advanced practice roles") encompassing the roles of the clinical executive, clinical scientist, and even educator (all "indirect role functions") roles where students are pursuing a practice doctorate (Bryant-Lukosius, DiCenso, Browne, & Pinelli, 2004; Dreher, Donnelly, & Naremore, 2005).[29] A precursor to "advanced nursing roles" may be what the ANA in 1980 affirmed as *specialization*, but specialization and advanced nursing practice are different. "Specialization involves concentration in a selected clinical area within the field of nursing" (Hamric, Spross, & Hanson, 1996, p. 43), but does not assume necessarily the requirement for an advanced degree. Cronenwett (1995) indicates that in 1980, during discussions of the first ANA social policy document, there was no language proposed to define advanced practice! However, in the revision of the social policy document published in 1995, advanced practice nursing was finally characterized and was defined as clinical practice that included specialization, expansion, and advancement (Lyon, 1996). From the ANA 1995 *Nursing's Social Policy Statement*, "*Expansion*[30] refers to the acquisition of new practice knowledge and skills, including knowledge and skills legitimizing role autonomy within the areas of practice that overlap the traditional boundaries of medical practice" (p. 14). However, "*Advancement*[31] involves both specialization and expansion and is characterized by the integration of theoretical, research-based, and practical knowledge that occurs as a part of graduate education in nursing" (p. 14).

In 2003, the Drexel doctoral nursing faculty explored this tension (or the technical language) between advanced practice nursing and advanced nursing practice when we were developing our own practice doctorate model and having discussions about who would be included: What population of nurses should properly undertake a practice doctorate? Certainly the AACN was struggling with this differentiation too in their *Draft Position Statement on the Practice Doctorate in Nursing* (January, 2004b), which stated that ". . . others have broadened the definition of advanced nursing practice to include both direct clinical practice and areas of practice that support clinical practice" (p. 7), but they had not yet arrived at including the clinical executive role in the DNP degree. However, 9 months later, the AACN adopted the *Position Statement on the Practice Doctorate in Nursing* (October 2004a) where three new recommendations were added including "Recommendation 10: The practice doctorate be the graduate degree for advanced nursing practice preparation, including *but not limited to* [italics ours] the four current APN roles: clinical nurse specialist, nurse anesthetist, nurse midwife, and nurse practitioner" (p. 13). Again, while not made explicit, the language

---

[29]A point of clarity, although emphasized elsewhere—the AACN only recognizes the practitioner and clinical executive role for advanced practice. No other. The NLN does not make this differentiation.

[30]My italics.

[31]My italics.

was created, and ultimately the AACN made the decision to include the clinical executive role, termed the "Aggregate/Systems/Organizational Focus" (p. 1) and the "Advanced Practice Nursing Focus" (p. 1) or practitioner role[32] as appropriate for the DNP degree in *The Essentials of Doctoral Education for Advanced Nursing Practice* document which has become the template for all DNP programs' accreditation (AACN, 2006).

At the time, the presumed inclusion of the executive role with the practitioner role under the rubric advanced *nursing* practice (AACN, 2004a, p. 13) was controversial (Mundinger, 2005).[33] Dean Mary Mundinger (Columbia University School of Nursing) has even indicated that it was the inclusion of the nondirect care role in the DNP degree that led to the need to develop the Diplomate in Comprehensive Care exam[34] (the new and controversial DNP certification exam) by the American Board of Comprehensive Care as "a national standard that distinguishes DNPs who have an advanced clinical knowledge from those who have an emphasis in research, administration or systems management" (Croasdale, 2008, p. 1). Others have alternatively argued, if the *practice of nursing administration* can be considered *advanced nursing practice* or even *advanced practice nursing*, why is the *practice of nursing education* excluded and not acceptable by the AACN as an appropriate role track for DNP degree programs too (Butler, 2009; Wittmann-Price, Waite, & Woda, in press)? Certainly the NLN (2007b) has recently affirmed academic nursing education "as a specialty area of practice and an advanced practice role within professional nursing" (p. 1). So which organization (AACN or NLN) is correct or most consistent and coherent on this issue of the domain of advanced practice nursing with regard to the DNP degree? The Drexel doctoral nursing faculty working group therefore first defined *clinical nursing practice* as

> ... the dynamic implementation of either professional or advanced nursing research-guided interventions, tasks, and responsibilities using competencies (knowledge, skills and attitudes) that support critical thinking and sound decision-making, ensure quality patient/client outcomes, uphold safety, and support the optimal promotion of health of diverse individuals, families, and communities.
>
> —*Dreher et al., 2005, p. 28*

and broadened the definition of *advanced nursing practice* as follows: "Advanced nursing practice is the professional work of a Registered Nurse with a Master's degree in nursing who has advanced nursing knowledge that can be applied directly or indirectly in the provision of nursing care" (Dreher et al., 2005, p. 29). Our interpretation was that all masters-prepared nursing education leads to advanced nursing practice, but we left the precise domain of advanced *practice* nursing to the four primary specialty areas which is also consistent with the kind of state regulation across the

---

[32]*Practitioner* here is defined as a traditional advanced practice nurse—NP, CNM, CRNA, or CNS.

[33]Pragmatically, that had to be done since no one recognizes the clinical executive role as advanced *practice* nursing in the same way we recognize the four traditional APRN roles as advanced practice nurses.

[34]For more information on the DNP exam, see Landro, 2008; Mundinger, 2007; and Stanik-Hutt, 2008.

country which defines *who is an advanced practice nurse* (Gaffney, 2001). It is also consistent with the 2008 National Council of State Boards of Nursing (NCSBN) *Consensus Model for APRN Regulation: Licensure, Accreditation, Certification & Education* which underwent vigorous debate by the nursing profession. The evolution of the Clinical Nurse Leader (CNL) role (first introduced by the AACN in 2004), which is considered *advanced nursing* but technically not considered a traditional advanced practice role, appears to be further confirmation of this distinction between advanced nursing and advanced practice (Lundy & Huch, 2009). The AACN describes the CNL as a "designer/manager/coordinator" (2007, p. 25). Today, the CNL role continues to be controversial, although there is some evidence that the role has been effective, especially as it has been implemented in the Veteran's Administration hospital system (Donley & Flaherty, 2008; NACNS, 2004; Nelson, 2010, Ott et al., 2009).

However, to further complicate the definition and landscape of advanced nursing, the CNL role has also been described as an "advanced generalist role" and a "generalist clinician with a masters degree" (Drenkard & Cohen, 2004; Karshmer, Seed, & Torkelson, 2009; Lundy & Huch, 2009). Our view is that the introduction of the CNL role and degree as another advanced nursing role is not necessarily unusual or extraordinary. It is a sign that the nursing profession continues to experiment with innovation that may improve nursing's disciplinary contribution to a nation's improved health. Nurse executives have been nominally open to pilot projects with the CNL role with mixed success (Goudreau, 2008; Sherman, 2008). However, introducing a masters degree preparing a CNL for *generalist* advanced nursing practice seems incredibly confusing and not coherent with the current paradigm of nursing practice.[35]

We thought we would try to diagram this complex hierarchal of nursing practice as follows in Figure 2.2.

In the epigram for this chapter Robinson (1946) is quoted as writing, "The untrained nurse is as old as the human race; the trained nurse is a recent discovery" (p. ix). For this reason, the most prevalent type of nursing care (care, not practice) is the universal nursing care provided across the globe by untrained caregivers. This is nursing with a small "n," as in "the nursing mother" or "he nursed his wife back to health" etc. The next level of Nursing Practice is "trained" and is denoted by a capital "N" and would refer to the basic or technical nurse, which includes any level of educational nursing preparation below the baccalaureate degree (Licensed Practical Nurse, Licensed Vocation Nurse [LPN, LVN], and diploma, or associate degree preparation for the RN). The rest of the pyramid is self-explanatory and builds vertically to represent the professional RN with a BSN, followed by the CNL with a masters degree,

---

[35]It is not the purpose of this text to lay out all the pros and cons for the CNL role, as our goal is more to describe the theoretical and practical landscape of practice disciplines in general and nursing practice specifically. We should note, however, that CNSs have been the most vocal opponents of the CNL role as the national organization has published at least three White Papers expressing concerns over the encroachment of the CNL into the CNS role. There are also concerns by some in the profession that this generalist advanced practice role has been introduced to eventually replace the BSN as entry-level into nursing. The AACN in 2004 addressed this issue and expressed their support for the BSN (AACN, 2008).

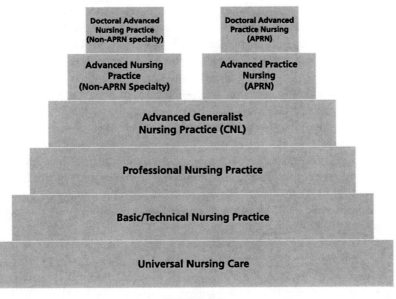

FIGURE 2.2
The complexity of nursing practice

followed by the masters-prepared APRN on one side and the masters-prepared non-APRN (educator, administrator, etc.) on the other. The top of the pyramid represents the doctoral-prepared APRN and non-APRN.

Valuing *Direct* and *Indirect* Nursing Functions and Roles Differently

We believe much of this confusion over the definitions of advanced nursing and advanced practice has been partly the result of a dichotomy in nursing, where members of the profession have historically valued the *direct* and *indirect* roles of nursing differently. These terms, as used in the nursing literature, also have both macro- and microinterpretations.

Some of the seminal work in this area (at the microlevel of conceptualization) was led by McCloskey and Bulechek in the 1990s as part of the Iowa Intervention Project. In 1992 they first described nursing interventions as being mostly direct care functions and stated, "A nursing intervention is any direct care treatment that a nurse performs on behalf of a client. These treatments include *nurse-initiated treatments* resulting from nursing diagnoses, *physician-initiated treatments* resulting from medical diagnoses, and performance of the *daily essential functions* for the client {who} cannot do these" (1992, p. 21). They defined *indirect care* nursing interventions as "treatments performed away from the patient but on behalf of a patient or group of patients" (1996, p. 42), but this definition did not necessarily include indirect care interventions that were administrative in nature. Much of the groundbreaking work of the Iowa nursing scholars over the classification of nursing interventions (and later over the classification of nursing outcomes) beginning in the 1990s was very related to Snyder's earlier work to define just what are *independent nursing interventions* (1985)?

Why is this important? In many ways, this period in nursing's history exemplified a time when the domains of professional nursing practice were first being clarified for the public and for other health professionals who worked with nurses (at all levels). With the publication of the 1980 ANA definition of nursing as "the diagnosis and treatment of human response to actual and potential health problems" (p. 9), nursing began to better establish the domain of professional nursing practice which was critical to the developing discipline. For the first time there was finally a codified recognition (and admission!) that nurses actually *diagnose and treat*.[36] In 2003, the definition of nursing was again modified as "The protection, promotion, and optimization of health and abilities; prevention of illness and injury; alleviation of suffering through the diagnosis and treatment of human response; and advocacy in the care of individuals, families, communities, and populations" (ANA, 2003, p. 6). Burkhart and Sommer (2007) have described this new definition as progress and recognition of nursing's contemporary complex, but holistic role in providing primary, secondary, and tertiary prevention strategies for individuals, families, groups, and populations.

At a macrolevel, direct care and indirect care have been more analogous to direct practice (the clinician or the practitioner) and indirect care with the administrator, academic, or researcher (Doughty, 2000; Flanagan & Jones, 2009; Matteo & Young, 2001; Thomas, 2009). We do not dispute this description technically, only that we find this a disappointing simplification of the focus of nursing (both professional and advanced) that has been perpetuated over time.[37] What this simplified conceptualization (those who *practice* versus those who do not) has done is actually create great discord among all types of nurses, for example:

> ... bedside nurses minimizing the value of nurse managers, ADN or Diploma educated nurses resenting the BSN prepared nurse, MSN prepared nursing faculty resenting PhD prepared faculty, graduate nursing faculty looking down on undergraduate nursing faculty, critical care nurses feeling superior to med-surg nurses, nurse practitioner faculty feeling superior to undergraduate nursing faculty, nurse anesthesia faculty feeling superior to nurse practitioner faculty, labor and delivery nurses looking down on post-partum nurses, hospital based nurses minimizing the complexity of the work of

---

[36]The influence of the nursing diagnosis movement and the work of the National Conference Group (founded in 1973) and the North American Nursing Diagnoses Association (NANDA, founded in 1982) cannot be overestimated, even if nursing has now had a long, tortured history over its direct application in day to day bedside clinical practice. Nevertheless, this movement gave nursing a common language and a contemporary taxonomy (in many ways building on the earlier work of Henderson and Abdullah), that nursing could use, if nothing more, then to begin to cost out nursing services. In our view one of the great tragedies of nursing has been its inability to quantify the work of the professional nurse and properly assign a cost for nursing services. To this day, the cost of nursing care remains in the hospitalized patient's room rate; it doesn't matter if a patient has a higher (requiring more nursing labor) or lower acuity (requiring less) on any given unit, the cost of nursing care is the same (Chiang, 2009; Dochterman et al., 2001).

[37]This language is so prevalent that even some DNP programs have chosen to label their DNP clinical/practitioner tracks the "Direct Track" and their clinical executive tracks the "Indirect Track." We do not want to offend these programs that have chosen these descriptors or labels, but at minimum they do not sound inviting. These programs also, if unintentionally, seem to have boxed the domain of advanced nursing education into either *direct* (black?) or *indirect* (white?) functions. Isn't much of advanced nursing a synergy of direct *and* indirect dynamic shades of gray?

home care nurses, chief nursing officers ridiculing the need for a doctorate, tenure track faculty feeling superior to non-tenure track faculty, tenured faculty marginalizing non-tenured faculty, PhD prepared faculty minimizing the need to maintain some sense of current clinical practice, non-BSN nurses resentful they need to return to school, nurse managers resentful they need a BSN or MSN ...

The scenarios could go on forever and we are sure you could add lots more. We are not, of course, taking a stand nor affirming that in all circumstances the above generalizations are true, but they have likely been true too often. We suspect the inability of nurses (basic or technical, professional and advanced, soon to be MSN versus DNP educated, and PhD faculty versus DNP faculty) to value each other has led the profession to this inability to arrive at consensus on a variety of issues. This in turn hampers the development of the discipline at all levels. With some 2.4 million nurses constituting the largest health profession by far (e.g., there are more RNs than MDs), we have never translated our numbers into proportional influence, power, or leverage at the highest levels of health policy (Dall, Chen, Seifert, Maddox, & Hogan, 2009). We ought to move from rigid distinctions of direct and indirect care or responsibility and prestige and embrace the reality that without contributions to the nursing profession by—practitioners at all levels; scholars (nurses with graduate preparation and educated to contribute to the evidence base of nursing); nurse scientists (at the forefront of knowledge development); nurse managers and executives (charged with the efficient delivery of nursing and health care); nursing professors (responsible for the producing all kinds of safe and competent nurses from LPN to PhD and post-doc); and everyone else (including consultants, clinical scientists in clinical trials research, and nurses in every diverse job position from nurse coroner to legislator, etc.)—our discipline will never fulfill its potential.

Beyond the MSN: Doctoral Advanced Nursing Practice

While DNP graduates are not the first doctoral-prepared nurses to be engaged in advanced practice,[38] they are fast becoming the first critical mass of nurses *distinctly prepared* to engage what has been defined recently as *doctoral advanced nursing practice* (Dreher & Montgomery, 2009). According to Dreher and Montgomery, it is folly to call the practice of *both* masters-prepared (MSN) graduates and doctoral-prepared (DNP/ DrNP) graduates *advanced practice nursing*. By indicating that one can engage in advanced practice nursing with either a masters or a doctoral degree, it begs the question "why get a doctorate" (and spend all the extra time and all that extra expense)?

---

[38]First, the first ND graduates *were not* advanced practice nurses despite their earned doctorate. In the early 1990s, Case Western Reserve University changed their ND to post-masters RNs only (personal communication former Dean, Dr. Joyce Fitzpatrick November 2009). Therefore, these graduates were later prepared for *doctoral advanced nursing practice*. However, their education was very different conceptually from today's DNP curriculum. The ND programs/schools never created a critical mass of graduates to study. Second, there have long been PhD prepared nurses in advanced practice, but their doctoral curriculum was research oriented, not practice oriented. It remains controversial whether these nurses truly engage in doctoral advanced nursing practice, but they cannot sit for the DNP Diplomate exam.

Since the advent of the DNP degree, the nursing discipline appears to have struggled with what to label this new type of practice where the graduate student is educated *beyond the MSN*. Various scholars have labeled it:

* *Advanced practice nursing* (AACN, 2006);
* *Doctoral level training in clinical practice* (Kuehn, 2009);
* *Doctoral nursing practice*—the title of a new journal *Clinical Scholars Review: The Journal of Doctoral Nursing Practice* first published in 2008; and
* *Advanced, advanced practice nursing.*[39]

Our critique of the first label advanced practice nursing is that it doesn't indicate any difference from MSN-prepared advanced practice. In 2006, National Organization of Nurse Practitioner Faculties (NONPF) published their *Practice Doctorate Nurse Practitioner Entry-Level Competencies* and stated "The practice doctorate for the nurse practitioner (NP) includes *additional* [our italics] competencies that are to be combined with the existing Domains and Core Competencies of [MSN] Nurse Practitioner Practice" (p. 1). To us, this is a clear indication that this type of practice at least *should be different* and thus be differentiated somehow. The second label of doctoral level training in clinical practice or clinical nursing seems divorced somehow from the word *advanced*. The title of this role, described in *JAMA* in 2009 (Kuehn), also seems to primarily reflect the Columbia DNP (first a DrNP) degree model where the graduate is prepared to practice multisite care with a primary and comprehensive care focus and includes a one-year full-time residency. We are not aware of any other DNP program in the country that has adopted a one-year full-time residency.[40] The third label doctoral nursing practice is not actually precise enough and could mean the practice of any nurse with any type of doctorate, unless it is defined as the clinical practice of a nurse with a practice nursing doctorate. Again, doctoral nursing practice (versus doctoral advanced practice) could technically encompass the nonclinical roles of the executive or even the educator (at least according to the NLN); thus we believe there needs to be a more fine-tuned differentiation among roles when defining this new type of practice. Finally, we only mention the label advanced, advanced practice nursing as it was mentioned (perhaps even jokingly) from the podium of a major conference. Dreher and Montgomery (2009) propose that doctoral advanced practice nursing provides the best technical description of the practice of a certified advanced practice nurse *who has a practice doctorate.* Dreher and Montgomery have recently written that unless there is differentiation between the practice of the MSN and DNP/DrNP graduate, "... then there really is no inherent extra value to obtaining the doctor of nursing practice degree except perhaps to gain an extra title and look a

---

[39]This was suggested, or at least hypothesized, by a speaker at a recent DNP conference during an oral paper presentation, and we wish to maintain the speaker's confidentiality among peers. We mention it, however, as symbolic of the struggle to define this new type of practice.

[40]We are not making an evaluative statement regarding this program. We also do not believe just because other programs have not adopted the residency model that it is not a good idea. To the contrary, as often said, "innovation can be very lonely."

lot more like the other 'health care' doctoral prepared professionals" (p. 2). Their description of this type of new practice is also in line with the 2006 NONPF *Practice Doctorate Nurse Practitioner Entry Level Competencies* by further stating, "We certainly see real advantages for APRNs who complete this degree as there is curricular content and specialized knowledge *beyond the MSN* that gives DNP/DrNP graduates additional, enhanced skills" (p. 2).

We would similarly (and consistently) also suggest that the nonclinical, practice doctorate nursing of the clinical executive, educator, and others be described conversely as *doctoral advanced nursing practice* (DANP) (see Figure 2.2) leaving *doctoral advanced practice nursing* (DAPN or DAPRN) for the certified traditional APRN (CRNA, CRNP, CNM, and CNS). We predict that until there is more consensus on the titling of this new type of practice, there will continue to be exhaustive debates about both the MSN and DNP graduate practicing the same advanced practice. In many ways, the DNP graduate working alongside the MSN graduate (e.g., they are both family NPs) will experience what physical therapy has gone through with their gradual transition to the Doctor of Physical Therapy (DPT) degree (Threlkeld, Jensen, & Royeen, 1999). Doctoral-prepared physical therapists with the DPT often work alongside masters-prepared physical therapists with the MPT degree, and they likely do the very same work and experience workplace tension (Salzman, 2010).

SUMMARY: NURSING AS A PROFESSIONAL PRACTICE DISCIPLINE

In this chapter we have tried to create an overview of the landscape of nursing as a practice discipline. We do not claim our approach is by any means exhaustive, as tomes have been written about nursing practice and nursing as a practice discipline. We have tried to focus on the evolution of nursing practice, led by doctoral level scholars, that has led us from the first early doctorates in our profession in the 1920s and 1930s, to the first critical mass of doctoral programs in the 1960s, and finally to the decade of 2001–2010 in which the DNP degree has exploded on the scene. The heyday of our historical nursing theories by Martha Rogers, Dorothea Orem, Imogene King, and many others is past us as some nursing scholars have admitted (Cody, 2000; Dekeyser & Medoff-Cooper, 2001; Timpson, 1996). Further, an honest examination of the state of nursing theory in our baccalaureate and masters nursing programs also reflects this. But the complexity of the practice environment recently described by Redman (2009) is now fertile ground for what we must call the experiment of the DNP degree. We suspect the plethora of DNP (and maybe even more DrNP programs) programs and graduates may reorient nursing to its roots as a practice discipline. Will this come at the expense of theoretical nursing and pose a threat to nursing's continued trajectory to establishing an even more scientific basis for practice as Meleis and Dracup have suggested (2005)? Who knows? Time will tell. O'Shea has written:

> Nursing as a practice discipline and as an academic discipline has come a long way in a relatively short time. The challenges include continuing to contribute to the evolution of the discipline, educating the public about what nursing is and what it can be, attracting

bright young men and women who want to make a difference in the lives of others, and ultimately improving the health of people everywhere.[41]

—*O'Shea, 2001, p. 1*

We, nevertheless predict that knowledge development by the DNP graduate may take a less formal, but still important form. Smith Glasgow and Dreher (2010) promote the idea that professional doctoral graduates (like the DNP) indeed can be the pioneers of Mode 2 knowledge development in nursing which is the knowledge of application and practice. One scholar has even boldly boasted that the professional doctorate graduate may be better prepared for the knowledge economy than the PhD graduate (Fink, 2006). Chapter 16 will explore this argument and further suggest that the production of *practice knowledge* is the best description of the domain of scholarship for the DNP graduate. However, before the DNP student can participate in the important enterprise of the production of science (or the generation of knowledge) that will help define our practice discipline and add to our evidence base, the student will need some grounding in philosophy of science. As we conclude this chapter, anticipating nursing's new dialogue about the DNP degree and the nature of doctoral nursing education, we will explore our next central question: How much philosophy of science does a DNP student (or student in any practice discipline) and a PhD in Nursing student need? It should be an interesting discussion.

CRITICAL THINKING QUESTIONS

1. How important do you believe nursing theory is to nursing practice? Give examples with your answer.
2. Read a nursing article from the *American Journal of Nursing* from 1910. How would you describe the state of nursing science represented?
3. Read a nursing article from *Nursing Research* from 1960. How would you describe the state of nursing science represented?
4. Describe some of the conversations nursing faculty were having with members of other disciplines (e.g., history, psychology, chemistry etc.) in the 1960s when they were trying to convince their colleagues that nursing should be permitted to offer the PhD?
5. Can nursing absolutely be described as a profession, as long as nurses with associate degrees predominate? Please elaborate.
6. What do you perceive are the central tensions between viewing nursing as an academic discipline versus nursing as a practice discipline?
7. Debate the following: Resolved, "MSN practice and DNP practice should both be described as *advanced practice nursing* and educational preparation should not dictate a change in this established definition." Make a case for this resolution and make a case that they should indeed be defined differently.
8. As a future graduate with a doctoral degree, describe the ways that you have a responsibility to advance the nursing discipline or not?

---

[41]Reprinted with the permission of author Helen O'Shea, RN, PhD, Professor Emerita, Nell Hodgson Woodruff School of Nursing, Emory University, Atlanta, Georgia.

9. How do you view the current tension between those termed practicing *direct care* (clinicians/practitioners) and those charged to practicing *indirectly* (managers and educators)?
10. Does the discipline of nursing need more consensus, need to instead embrace its diversity, or perhaps seek solutions that do both? Please be specific.

REFERENCES

Aiken, L. H. (2003). Workforce policy perspectives on advanced practice nursing. In M. Mezey, D. McGivern, & E. Sullivan-Marx (Eds.), *Nurses, nurse practitioners: Evolution to advanced practice* (4th ed.) (pp. 431–442). New York, NY: Springer.

Aiken, L., Cheung, R., & Olds, D. (2009). Education policy initiatives to address the nurse shortage in the United States. *Health Affairs, 28*(4), w646–w656.

Aiken, L., Clarke, S. P., Cheung, R. B., Sloane, D. M., & Silber, J. H. (2003). Educational of hospital nurses and surgical patient mortality. *The Journal of the American Medical Association, 290,* 1617–1623.

American Association of Colleges of Nursing. (2004a). *AACN position statement on the practice doctorate in nursing. October 2004.* Retrieved on 4/12/2010, from http://www.aacn.nche.edu/DNP/pdf/DNP.pdf

American Association of Colleges of Nursing. (2004b). *AACN draft position statementon the practice doctorate in nursing January 2004.* Washington, DC: Author.

American Association of Colleges of Nursing. (2006). *Essentials of doctoral education for advanced nursing practice.* Retrieved on 4/12/2010, from http://www.aacn.nche.edu/DNP/pdf/Essentials.pdf

American Association of Colleges of Nursing. (2007). *White Paper on the role of the clinical nurse leader.* Retrieved on 4/12/2010, from http://www.aacn.nche.edu/Publications/WhitePapers/ClinicalNurseLeader07.pdf

American Association of Colleges of Nursing. (2008). *CNL frequently asked questions.* Retrieved on 4/12/2010, from http://www.aacn.nche.edu/cnl/faq.htm

American Association of Colleges of Nursing. (2009). *Institutions offering Doctoral Programs in Nursing and degrees conferred.* Retrieved on 2/17/2010, from http://www.aacn.nche.edu/IDS/pdf/DOC.pdf 17

American Association of History of Nursing. (2008). *Nursing history calendar.* Retrieved on 2/12/2010, from http://www.aahn.org/nursinghistorycalendar.html

American Nurses Association. (1980). *Nursing's social policy statement.* Washington, DC: Author.

American Nurses Association. (1995). *Nursing's social policy statement.* Washington, DC: Author.

American Nurses Association. (2003). *Nursing scope and standards of practice.* Washington, DC: Author.

American College of Nurse Midwives. (2007). *Midwifery education and the doctor of nursing practice.* Retrieved on 4/12/2010, from http://www.midwife.org/siteFiles/position/Midwifery_ Ed_and_DNP_7_09.pdf

American College of Nurse Midwives. (2009). *Midwifery education and the doctor of nursing practice.* Retrieved from http://www.midwife.org/siteFiles/position/Midwifery_Ed_ and_DNP_7_09.pdf

American Organization of Nurse Executives. (2007). *Consideration of the doctorate of nursing practice.* Retrieved from www.acnm.org/siteFiles/position/Midwifery_Ed_and_DNP_7_09.pdf

Apold, S. (2008). The doctor of nursing practice: Looking back, moving forward. *The Journal for Nurse Practitioners, 4*(2), 101–107.

Bellack, J. (2002). A matter of degree. *Journal of Nursing Education, 41*(5), 191–192.

Breakiron, M. (1995). A salute to the nurses of World War II. *The Association of Perioperative Registered Nurses, 62*(5), 710–722.

Bryant-Lukosius, D., DiCenso, A., Browne, G., & Pinelli, J. (2004). Advanced practice nursing roles: Development, implementation and evaluation. *Journal of Advanced Nursing, 48*(5), 519–529.

Burkhart, L., & Sommer, S. (2007). Integrating preventive care and nursing standard terminologies in nursing education: A case study. *Journal of Professional Nursing, 23*(4), 208–213.

Butler, K. (2009). The DNP graduate as educator. In L. Chism (Ed.), *The Doctor of Nursing Practice: A guidebook for role development and professional issues* (pp. 169–193). Sudbury, MA: Jones and Bartlett.

Carter, M. (1996). The evolution of doctoral education in nursing. In L. C. Andrist, P. K. Nicholas, & K. A. Wolf (Eds.), *History of nursing ideas* (pp. 383–392). London, UK: Jones and Bartlett.

Chiang, B. (2009). Estimating nursing costs—A methodological review. *International Journal of Nursing Studies, 46*(5), 716–722.

Chinn, P. (2008). The discipline of nursing. *Advances in Nursing Science, 31*(1), 1.

Christman, L. (1998). Who is a nurse? *Image: Journal of Nursing Scholarship, 30*(3), 211–214.

Cody, W. (2000). Paradigm shift or paradigm drift: A meditation on commitment and transcendence. *Nursing Science Quarterly, 13*(2), 93–102.

Coghlan, D. (2007). Insider action research doctorates: Generating actionable knowledge. *Higher Education, 54*(2), 293–306.

Croasdale, M. (2008). Medical testing board to introduce doctor of nursing certification. Retrieved on 4/12/2010, from http://www.ama-assn.org/amednews/2008/06/16/prl10616.htm

Cronenwett, L. R. (1995). Molding the future of advanced practice nursing. *Nursing Outlook, 43*(3), 112–118.

Dall, T. M., Chen, Y. J., Seifert, R. F., Maddox, P. J., & Hogan, P. F. (2009). The economic value of professional nursing. *Medical Care, 47*(1), 7–104.

Dekeyser, F. G., & Medoff-Cooper, B. (2001). A non-theorist's perspective on nursing theory: Issues of the 1990s. *Research and Theory for Nursing Practice, 15*(4), 329–341.

DeMarco, R. F., Pulcini, J., Haggerty, L. A., & Tang, T. (2009). Doctorate in nursing practice: A survey of Massachusetts nurses. *Journal of Professional Nursing, 25*(2), 75–80.

Dickoff, J., James, P., & Wiedenbach, E. (1968a). Theory in a practice discipline: Part I. Practice-oriented theory. *Nursing Research, 17*(5), 415–435.

Dickoff, J., James, P., & Wiedenbach, E. (1968b). Theory in a practice discipline: Part II. Practice-oriented research. *Nursing Research, 17*(6), 387–480.

Dochterman, J. M., Bulechek, G., Heal, B., Ahrens, D., Androwich, I., & Clark, M. (2001). Determining cost of nursing interventions: A beginning. *Nursing Economics, 19*(4), 146–160.

Donahue, M. P. (1996). *Nursing, the finest art: An illustrated history* (2nd ed.). St. Louis, MO: Mosby.

Donaldson, S. K., & Crowley, D. (1978). The discipline of nursing. *Nursing Outlook, 26*(2), 113–120.

Donley, R., & Flaherty, M. J. (2008). Revisiting the American nurses association's first position on education for nurses: A comparative analysis of the first and second position statements on the education of nurses. *The Online Journal of Issues in Nursing, 13*(2). Retrieved 4/12/2010 from http://www.nursingworld.org/MainMenuCategories/ANAMarketplace/ANA-Periodicals/OJIN/TableofContents/vol132008/No2May08/ArticlePreviousTopic/EntryIntoPracticeUpdate.aspx

Doughty, D. (2000). Integrating advanced practice and WOC nursing education. *Journal of Wound, Ostomy and Continence Nursing, 27*(1), 65–68.

Dreher, H. M. (2005). The doctor of nursing practice: Has this train left the station? If so, just where is it going? *The Pennsylvania Nurse, 60,* 17, 19.

Dreher, H. M. (2008). Innovation in nursing education: Preparing for the future of nursing practice. *Holistic Nursing Practice, 22*(2), 77–80.

Dreher, H. M. (2009a). *The Doctor of Nursing Practice Degree in the U.S — History & politics, problems & progress.* International Conference on Professional Doctorates (ICPD), Sponsored by the UK Council for Graduate Education, London, England, UK, November 9–10, 2009.

Dreher, H. M. (2009b). Education for advanced practice: The question: Is the PhD or DNP the right degree model for future advanced practice nurses? In L. Joel (Ed.), *Advanced practice nursing: Essentials for role development* (2nd ed., pp. 58–71). Philadelphia, PA: FA Davis.

Dreher, H. M., Donnelly, G., & Naremore, R. (2005). Reflections on the DNP and an alternate practice doctorate model: The Drexel DrNP. *Online Journal of Issues in Nursing, 11*(1). Retrieved from www.nursingworld.org/ojin/topic28/tpc28_7.htm

Dreher, H. M., Smith Glasgow, M. E., Gonzalez, E., Suplee, P., Falkenstein, K., & Rundio, A. (2005). *Doctor of Nursing Practice Degree (DrNP) proposal to the Pennsylvania Department of Education.* Unpublished manuscript.

Dreher, H. M., & Montgomery, K. E. (2009). Let's call it "doctoral" advanced practice nursing. *The Journal of Continuing Nursing Education, 40*(12), 530–531.

Drenkard, K., & Cohen, E. (2004). Clinical nurse leader: Moving toward the future. *The Journal of Nursing Administration, 34*(6), 257–260.

Emerson, R., & Records, K. (2005). Nursing: Profession in peril? *Journal of Professional Nursing, 21*(1), 9–15.

Fang, D., Tracy, C., & Bednash, P. (2010). *2009–2010 Enrollments and graduations in baccalaureate and graduate programs in nursing.* Washington, DC: American Association of Colleges of Nursing.

Fink, D. (2006). The professional doctorate: Its relativity to the Ph.D. and relevance for the knowledge economy. *International Journal of Doctoral Studies, 3,* 35–44.

Fitzpatrick, J. (2003). The case for the clinical doctorate in nursing. *Reflections on Nursing Leadership, 29*(1), 8–9, 37.

Fitzpatrick, J. (2008). *The doctor of nursing practice and clinical nurse leader: Essentials of program development and implementation for clinical practice.* New York, NY: Springer Publishing.

Flanagan, J., & Jones, D. (2009). Evaluation of the advanced practice nurse: Cost efficiency, accomplishment, trends and future development. In L. Joel (Ed.) *Advanced practice nurses: Essentials for role development* (2nd ed.) (pp. 390–402). Philadelphia, PA: F.A. Davis.

Flaumenhaft, E., & Flaumenhaft, C. (1989). American nursing and the road not taken. *Journal of the History of Medicine and Allied Sciences, 44*(1), 2–89.

Florczak, K. (2010). Research and the doctor of nursing practice: A cause for consternation. *Nursing Science Quarterly, 23*(1), 13–17.

Fulton, J., & Lyon, B. (2005). The need for some sense making: Doctor of nursing practice. *Online Journal of Issues in Nursing, 10*(3), 4. Retrieved on 9/4/2010, from www.nursingworld. org/MainMenuCategories/ANAMarketplace/ANAPeriodicals/OJIN/TableofContents/ Volume102005/No3Sept05/tpc28_316027.aspx

Fulton, J., & Lyon, B. (2006). Reply by Jan Fulton and Brenda Lyon on "The need for some sense…" *Online Journal of Issues in Nursing.* Retrieved from http://www.nursingworld. org/MainMenuCategories/ANAMarketplace/ANAPeriodicals/OJIN/LetterstotheEditor/ ReplytoLoriEllis.aspx

Gaffney, T. (2001). Regulation of nursing practice. *ANA continuing education: The nursing risk management series.* Retrieved on 2/24/2010, from https://nursingworld.org/mods/ archive/mod310/cerm102.htm

Gortner, S. (1986). Impact of the division of nursing in research development in the USA. In S. M. Stinson, & J. C. Kerr (Eds.), *International issues in nursing research* (pp. 113–130). Milton Park, UK: Taylor & Francis.

Gortner, S. (1991). Historical development of doctoral programs: Shaping our expectations. *Journal of Professional Nursing, 7*(1), 45–53.

Gosnell, D. (2002). The 1965 entry into practice proposal—is it relevant today? *Online Journal of Issues Nursing, 7*(2). Retrieved on 12/6/2009, from www.nursingworld.org/ojin.

Goudreau, K. (2008). Confusion, concern, or complimentary function: The overlapping roles of the clinical nurse specialist and the clinical nurse leader. *Nursing Administration Quarterly, 32*(4), 301–307.

Haase, P. (1990). *The origins and rise of associate degree education.* Durham, NC: Duke University Press.

Habermas, J. (1971). *Toward a rational society: Student protest, science, and politics* (J. Shapiro, Trans.), Boston, MA: Beacon Press.

Hamric, A. B., Spross, J. A., & Hanson, C. M. (1996). *Advanced nursing practice: An integrative approach.* Philadelphia, PA: W.B. Saunders.

Hawkins, R., & Nezat, G. (2009). Doctoral education: Which degree to pursue? *American Association of Nurse Anesthetists Journal, 77*(2), 92–96.

Hongcai, W. (2007). Education: A discipline or a field? *Frontiers of Education in China, 2*(1), 1673–3533.

Honig, J., & Smolowitz, J. (2009). Clinical doctorate at Columbia University school of nursing: Lessons learned. *Clinical Scholars Review, 2*(2), 51–59.

Horrocks, S., Anderson, E., & Salisbury, C. (2002). Systematic review of whether nurse practitioners working in primary care can provide equivalent care to doctors. *British Medical Journal, 324*(7341), 819–823.

Karshmer, J., Seed, M., & Torkelson, D. (2009). The clinical nurse leader: How will the role affect psychiatric nursing? *Journal of Psychosocial Nursing & Mental Health Services, 47*(10), 8–9.

Kramer, L. W. (2010). Evaluation and early recognition of systemic inflammatory response syndrome in critical care patients. *Dimensions of Critical Care Nursing, 29*(1), 20–28.

Kuehn, B. (2009). Doctoral-level programs prepare nurses for expanded roles in care and research. *Journal of the American Medical Association, 302*(19), 2075–2078.

Landro, L. (2008). Making room for 'Dr. Nurse.' *The Wall Street Journal Digital Network.* Retrieved on 4/1/2010, from http://online.wsj.com/article/SB120710036831882059.html?mod=WSJBlog

Leininger, M. L. (1976). Doctoral programs for nurses: Trends, questions, and projected plans. *Nursing Research, 25*(3), 201–210.

Lenz, E. R. (2005). The practice doctorate in nursing: An idea whose time has come. *Online Journal of Issues in Nursing. 10*(3), 2. Retrieved on 9/4/2010, from www.nursingworld.org/MainMenuCategories/ANAMarketplace/ANAPeriodicals/OJIN/TableofContents/Volume102005/No3sept05/tpc28_116025.aspx

Lohr, K. N., & Steinwachs, D. M. (2002) Health services research: An evolving definition of the field. *Health Services Research, 37*(1), 15–17.

Lundy, K. S., & Huch, M. H. (2009). Advanced nursing practice in the community. In K. S. Lundy, & S. Janes (Eds.), *Community health nursing: Caring for the public's health* (pp. 1060–1074). Sudbury, MA: Jones and Bartlett.

Lyon, B. (1996). Defining advanced practice nursing role diversity is essential in meeting nursing's social mandate. *Clinical Nurse Specialist, 10*(6), 263, 264.

Matteo, M. A., & Young, E. B. (2001). Determining indirect caregivers' contribution to patient care. *Journal of Nursing Administration, 31*(3), 109–112.

Mantzoukas, S. (2007). A review of evidence-based practice, nursing research and reflection: Leveling the hierarchy. *Journal of Clinical Nursing, 17*(2), 214–223.

Mawdsley, S. (2005). Nursing theories and their relevance to contemporary infection control practice. *Journal of Infection Prevention, 6*(3), 26–29.

McCaugherty, D. (2006). The theory–practice gap in nurse education: Its causes and possible solutions. Findings from an action research study. *Journal of Advanced Nursing, 16*(9), 1055–1061.

McCloskey, J. C., & Bulechek, G. M. (1992). *Nursing Interventions Classification (NIC)*. Saint Louis, MO: Mosby.

McCloskey, J. C., & Bulechek, G. M. (1996). *Nursing Interventions Classification (NIC)* (2nd ed.). Saint Louis, MO: Mosby.

McNeil, P. (2010). The nursing faculty shortage: Adding to the U.S. nursing shortage. *Nursing PhD.org.* Retrieved on 9/9/2010, from http://nursingphd.org/articles/shortage.php

Meleis, A., & Dracup, K. (2005). The case against the DNP: History, timing, substance, and marginalization. *Online Journal of Issues in Nursing, 10*(3), 3. Retrieved on 9/4/2010, from www.nursingworld.org/MainMenuCategories/ANAMarketplace/ANAPeriodicals/ OJIN/TableofContents/Volume102005/No3Sept05/tpc28_216026.aspx

Melnyk, B. M., & Fineout-Overholt, E. (2005). *Evidence-based practice in nursing & healthcare: A guide to best practice.* Philadelphia, PA: Lippincott Williams & Wilkins.

Mundinger, M. (2005). Who's who in nursing: Bringing clarity to the doctor of nursing practice. *Nursing Outlook, 53*(4), 173–176.

Mundinger, M. (2007). Who will be your doctor? Retrieved on 10/7/2009, from http://www. forbes.com/2007/11/27/nurses-doctors-practice-oped-cx_mom_1128nurses. html?partner=alerts

Mundinger, M. O., Kane, R. L., Lenz, E. R., Totten, A. M., Tsai, W., Cleary, et al. (2000). Primary care outcomes in patients treated by nurse practitioners or physicians: A randomized trial. *JAMA, 283*(1), 59–68.

National Association of Clinical Nurse Specialists. (2004). *NACNS position statement on the clinical nurse leader.* Retrieved on 8/24/2009, from www.nacns.org/positionstatement.pdf

National Association of Clinical Nurse Specialists. (2005). *White paper on the nursing practice doctorate.* Retrieved on 4/12/2010, from http://www.nacns.org/LinkClick.aspx?filetick-et=xHLMMgMYJ98% 3D&tabid=138

National Association of Clinical Nurse Specialists. (2009). *Position statement on the nursing practice doctorate.* Retrieved on 9/4/2010, from http://www.nacns.org/LinkClick.aspx?fileticket= TOZlongI258%3d&tabid=116

National Council on State Boards of Nursing. (2008). *Consensus model for APRN regulation: Licensure, accreditation, certification & education.* Retrieved on 4/12/2010, from http://www.aacn. nche.edu/Education/pdf/APRNReport.pdf

National League for Nursing. (2007a). California community college system approves NLN's pre-admission examination—Seventy percent of state's RNs, its largest group of health care providers, graduate from community college nursing programs. Retrieved on 12/6/ 2009, from http://www.nln.org/newsreleases/exam_release_112007.htm

National League for Nursing. (2007b). *The Certified Nurse Educator[CM] (CNE) examination.* Retrieved on 9/4/2010, from http://www.nln.org/facultycertification/index.htm.

National Organization of Nurse Practitioner Faculties. (2006). *Practice doctorate nurse practitioner entry level competencies.* Retrieved April 12, 2010, from http://www.nonpf.com/ associations/10789/files/DNP%20NP%20competenciesApril2006.pdf

Nelson, M. (2002). Education for professional nursing practice: Looking backward into the future. *Online Journal of Issues in Nursing.* 7(3), 4. Retrieved on 9/4/2010, from http://www.nursingworld.org/MainMenuCategories/ANAMarketplace/ANAPeriodicals/OJIN/TableofContents/Volume72002/No2May2002/EducationforProfessionalNursing-Practice.aspx

Nelson, R. (2010). The clinical nurse leader. *American Journal of Nursing, 110*(1), 22–23.

Nurse Practitioner Roundtable. (2008). *Nurse practitioner DNP education, certification and titling: A unified statement.* Washington, DC: Author.

Nursing Research. (1962). Research reporter. *Nursing Research, 11*(3), 181–182.

O'Shea, H. (2001). The state of the discipline in nursing: Science, technology, and culture have stirred rapid change. *The academic exchange: An online place for scholarly conversation at Emory. 4*(2), Retrieved on 4/18/2010, from http://www.emory.edu/ACAD_EXCHANGE/2001/octnov/oshea.html

Ott, K. M., Haddock, K. S., Fox, S. E., Shinn, J. K., Walters, S. E., Hardin, J. W. et al. (2009). The clinical nurse leader: Impact on practice outcomes in the veteran's health administration. *Nursing Economics, 27*(6), 363–383.

Redman, R. W. (2009). Complexity in practice environments. *Research and Theory for Nursing Practice, 23*(4): 253–255.

Robb, I. H. A. (1893) *Nursing: Its principles and practice for hospital and private use.* Cleveland, OH: E. C. Koecklert.

Robb, W. J. W. (2005). PhD, DNSc, ND: The ABCs of nursing doctoral degrees. *Dimensions of Critical Care Nursing, 24*(2), 89–96.

Robinson, V. (1946). White caps: The story of nursing. Philadelphia, PA: Lippincott.

Sakalys, J. A., & Watson, J. (1986). Professional education: Post-baccalaureate education for professional nursing. *Journal of Professional Nursing, 2*(2), 91–97.

Salzman, A. (2010). The DPT degree: Our destiny or a cosmetic change? *Advance for Physical Therapy & PT Assistants, 14*(4), 55.

Schmidt, K. (2001). A sharper image: Nurses strive to garner more—and more accurate—media coverage. *Nurseweek.com.* Retrieved on 2/15/2010, from http://www.nurseweek.com/news/features/01-12/mediaimage.html

Shaw-Weeks, C. (1885). *A textbook of nursing for the use of training schools, families, and private students.* New York, NY: D. Appleton.

Sheehy, S. (2007). US military nurses in wartime: Reluctant heroes, always there. *Journal of Emergency Nursing, 33*(6), 555–563.

Sheriff, S., & Chaney, S. (2007). Should DNP programs follow the same rigorous coursework as PhD Programs? *The Journal for Nurse Practitioners, 3*(10), 704–705.

Sherman, R. (2008). Factors influencing organizational participation in the clinical nurse leader. *Nursing Economics, 26*(4), 236–249.

Silver, H. K., Ford, L. C., & Steanly, S. (1967). A program to increase health care for children. *Pediatrics, 39*(5), 756–760.

Shever, L. L., Titler, M. G., Kerr, P., Qin, R., Kim, T., & Picone, D. (2008). The effect of high nursing surveillance on hospital cost. *Journal of Nursing Scholarship, 40*(2), 161–169.

Smith Glasgow, M. E., & Dreher, H. M. (2010). The future of oncology nursing science: Who will generate the knowledge? *Oncology Nursing Forum, 37*(4), 393–396.

Snyder, M. (1985). *Independent nursing interventions.* New York, NY: John Wiley and Sons.

Spetz, J. (2005). The cost and cost-effectiveness of nursing services in health care. *Nursing Outlook, 53*(6), 305–309.

Stanik-Hutt, J. (2008). Debunking the need to certify the DNP degree. *The Journal for Nurse Practitioners, 4*(10), 739.

Stevens, S. (1990). Sale of the century: Images of nursing in the Movietonews during World War II. *Advances in Nursing Science, 12*(4), 44–52.

Stew, G. (in press). Enhancing the doctoral advanced practice role with reflective practice. In H. M. Dreher, & M. E. Smith Glasgow, *Role development in Doctoral Advanced Nursing Practice*, New York, NY: Springer.

Sussman, D. (1999). *Nursing 1910 style: Camaraderie, housekeeping, and a life of service*. Retrieved on 2/12/2010, from http://www.nurseweek.com/features/99-12/workhist.html

Thomas, P. (2009). Case management delivery models: The impact of indirect care givers on organizational outcomes. *Journal of Nursing Administration, 39*(1), 30–37.

Thompson, D. R. (2009). Is nursing viable as an academic discipline? *Nursing Education Today, 29*(7), 694–697.

Threlkeld, A. J., Jensen, G. M., & Royeen, C. B. (1999). The clinical doctorate: A framework for analysis in physical therapist education. *Physical Therapy, 79*(6), 567–581.

Timpson, J. (1996). Nursing theory: Everything the artist spits is art? *Journal of Advanced Nursing, 23*(5), 1030–1036.

Tomes, M. (1978). 'Little world of our own': The Pennsylvania hospital training school for nurses, 1895–1907. *Journal of the History of Medicine and Allied Sciences, 33*(4), 507–530.

Veeser, P. I., Stegbauer, C. C., & Russell, C. K. (1999). Developing a clinical doctorate to prepare nurses for advanced practice at the University of Tennessee, Memphis. *Journal of Nursing Scholarship, 31*(1), 39–41.

Vogel, W., & Gobel, B. (2006). The doctorate of nursing practice. Synopsis of literature and practicing advanced practice nurse concerns. *Oncology nursing society nurse practitioner special interest group newsletter*. Retrieved on 2/21/2010, from http://onsopcontent.ons.org/Publications/SIG Newsletters/np/np17.2.html

Walker, L. (1900). How to prepare nurses for the duties of the alumnae. In N. Birnbach, & S. Lewenson (Eds.), *First Words. Selected addresses from the National League for Nursing 1894–1933* (pp. 203–207). New York, NY: NLN Press.

Wittmann-Price, R., Waite, R., & Woda, D. (in press). The role of the educator. In H. M. Dreher, & M. E. Smith Glasgow, *Role development for doctoral advanced nursing practice*. New York, NY: Springer.

Witte, F. (1934). Opportunities in graduate education for men nurses. *The American Journal of Nursing, 34*(2), 133–135.

Wuest, J. (1994). Professionalism and the evolution of nursing as a discipline: A feminist perspective. *Journal of Professional Nursing, 10*(6), 357–367.

3

Philosophy of Science in a Practice Discipline

It is my contention that the present misuse of science by nurses, and its attendant consequences, will persist unless and until philosophy, as a mode of inquiry, is allowed to take its rightful place in the nurse's world, for it is only by philosophizing that we can ascertain the kind of nursing question that is (and those that are not) amenable to scientific study.

J. K. KIKUCHI[1]

INTRODUCTION

This chapter begins with the question: "How much philosophy of science does a practice discipline student need?" We will then quickly move on to: "How much does a doctoral nursing student need, and centrally how much does a doctor of nursing practice student need?" What we hope to quickly accomplish is (1) repudiate any suggestion that disciplines where practice is more the focus have less reliance on the principal concepts in philosophy of science; (2) dispel any notion that doctor of nursing practice students do not need substantive content on philosophy of science (because of its practice focus or because these students are not educated to be chiefly researchers or scientists); and (3) quell any weak argument by naysayers or skeptics who proclaim this content is more appropriate for PhD students.

In reality, there would not even be textbooks of content for use in doctoral nursing curricula if the ideas presented on the pages of each chapter in each text were not first derived from the methods that lead to knowledge generation. From Thomas Kuhn's (1962) discussions of paradigm shifts to contemporary discussion of the praxis of interpretive inquiry, nursing scholars have advanced our science and practice based on its reliance on philosophy of science and the evolutionary scientific method. Even if the doctor of nursing practice student, at minimum, is going to

---

[1]Kikuchi, J. F. (1992). Nursing questions that science cannot answer. In J. F. Kikuchi & H. Simmons (Eds.), *Philosophic inquiry in nursing* (pp. 26–37). Chicago, IL: Sage Publications, Inc. Reprinted with permission by Sage.

evaluate and disseminate evidence,[2] then nursing academicians will be doing their students a great disservice if the importance of such topics, for example, induction, deduction, experimental testing, observation, concept analysis, theory construction, and inference to the best explanation, is not adequately addressed. And if practice knowledge development is the ultimate goal of the doctor of nursing practice student and graduate (a thesis of the last chapter), then these topics become critically germane. Section II discusses the philosophy of science topics above; Section III discusses practice knowledge development as an emerging nursing epistemology. In this chapter we address the issues outlined in the first paragraph above, first from a nursing perspective (H. M. D.) and then from a philosopher's perspective (M. D. D.).

A NURSING PERSPECTIVE

Philosophy of Science in a Practice Discipline

Let us pose the most rudimentary, basic question here. First, do professional members of any practice discipline—education, medicine, nursing, physical therapy, psychology, public health, or social work—need education in philosophy of science? To best answer this question, it is useful to understand some of the central questions that philosophy of science poses:

1. What is science?
2. How does science differ from religion and pseudoscience?
3. How do misperceptions (a semi-truth or falsehood) become established as common belief and perpetuated as scientific fact?
4. What are empirical data? What are models? What are theories?
5. How do the real world, empirical data, models, concepts, and theories relate to each other?
6. What is deductive reasoning? What is inductive reasoning? What is the proper place and function of each in producing evidence and good science?
7. How does probability impact induction?
8. Is there a male bias in reasoning? Is there a feminist method?
9. How does one arrive at scientific truth? Is truth possible? What is causation? How does one establish a causal relation?
10. What is explanation in science?
11. How is scientific belief impacted by the realism versus antirealism debate?
12. What methods of inquiry embrace scientific reductionism or holism? Can either of these be shown to be superior or more appropriate to scientific study?
13. What is a paradigm? How do paradigms shift?
14. What is a hypothesis? How is it tested? How is it verified? Falsified?
15. Is natural science more objective than social science?

---

[2]Again, we anticipate that the profession is going to revisit the urgent issue of whether doctor of nursing practice graduates should generate new knowledge for the discipline or not.

As an exercise, we suggest you now take these 15 questions (which constitute the framework of philosophy of science, but by no means are comprehensive) and ask yourself: How would each question be relevant for study when pursuing a doctorate in a practice discipline or, more precisely, a health professions practice discipline? *Practice inquiry*[3] has been recently proposed as a set of small-group, practice-based learning (PBL) methods designed to help internal medicine clinicians better manage *clinical uncertainty* using a case-based approach (Sommers, Morgan, Johnson, & Yatabe, 2007). In describing the skill set requisite for practitioners and clinicians to undertake analyses of complex patient problems, they state:

> Although contexts for coping with uncertainty have changed, most physicians would support Light's 1979 observation that "regardless how technically developed a professional field is, it will define the treatment of problematic cases as its true work." Social constructivist learning theorists, medical educators, and primary care researchers identify the problematic patient case as a powerful professional learning opportunity. Whether and how one decides to take on these problems in the "swampy lowlands" of practice become, according to Guest, decisions about "deliberate practice." Practitioners develop expertise when they move from their comfort zones to examine problems "at the upper limit of the complexity they can handle;" they learn, and iteratively gain mastery through cycles of reflecting on practice, obtaining feedback, and adjusting performance.[4]
> —*Sommers et al., 2007, p. 246*

We attest that this statement applies to all practitioners involved in clinical care and certainly not just physicians. Similarly, scientific inquiry in social work practice has a rich history (Choi, Choi, & Kim, 2009; Lewis & Bolzan, 2007; Thyer, 2010). Social work scholars have long advocated the integration of scientific thought and research into clinical social work practice (Orcutt, Flowers, & Seinfeld, 1990). It is doubtful whether there is a valid argument that other practice disciplines should operate differently or educate their new practitioners without this emphasis. In Anderson's (2010) recent paper on reexamining the distinction between research and practice, he states that this attempt at distinction really misrepresents the aim of clinical inquiry. He indicates that clinical research and clinical practice "are not sharply distinct but intimately intertwined" (Anderson, 2010, p. 46). We also do not see the fine distinctions between scientific inquiry and clinical inquiry. Scientific inquiry and clinical inquiry are both analogous to critical inquiry, which has been defined as an open cycle of questioning based on empirical data and is a combination of deliberation and action (Karlik, 2010). We suggest that critical inquiry is essential to any practice discipline that seeks the best evidence, the best interventions, and the best practices.[5] Knowledge

---

[3]Practice inquiry has also been reinterpreted differently in nursing by scholars at the University of Washington School of Nursing, and this will be discussed at length in Chapter 16.

[4]Sommers, L. S., Morgan, L., Johnson, L., & Yatabe, K. Practice inquiry: Clinical uncertainty as a focus for small-group learning and practice improvement. *Journal of General Internal Medicine*, 22(2), 246–252. Reprinted with permission by Springer.

[5]Perhaps one interesting indicator of the scholarly interest in the application of philosophy of science to practice is the founding of the Society for Philosophy of Science in Practice (SPSP) in 2006. This new organization aims to create an interdisciplinary community of scholars who approach philosophy of science emphasizing scientific practice and practical uses of scientific knowledge beyond mere esoteric analytical discussions. Their website is http://www.gw.utwente.nl/spsp/

cannot be properly evaluated or advanced without an understanding of the principles of philosophy of science that underlie this discourse and that support all types of practice-oriented decision-making.

Philosophy of Science in the Discipline of Nursing

There should be no debate that philosophy of science belongs in the curricula of graduate students pursuing a doctor of philosophy degree (PhD) (DiBartolo, 1998).[6] One of the curricular issues that PhD in Nursing/Nursing Science programs often face is who should teach this content? Should it be PhD-educated nurses who have an intellectual interest in philosophy of science, who have taken advanced coursework, or who are philosophers of science, trained in the analytic methods of philosophy with either specialization or competency in philosophy of science?[7] At minimum, the research training of any graduate student in any discipline must begin with rigorous training in the *scientific method*. Commonly but wrongly attributed to Roger Bacon[8] and other eminent 18th-century European scholars, one of the earliest records of the techniques of scientific investigation is attributed to Al-Biruni,[9] a Persian genius who conducted precise experiments on laws of gravitation, momentum, and motion (O'Connor, Robertson, & Edmund, 1999).[10]

The emergence of nursing as a discipline in the 1960s (discussed in Chapter 2) largely corresponded to the drive to prepare more doctoral-prepared nurse scientists outside (with formation of the Nurse Scientist Training Program in 1961) and ultimately inside the discipline with rapid establishment of numerous doctoral nursing programs (Gortner, 2000). In 1962, Thomas Kuhn published *The Structure of Scientific Revolutions*, and its impact on philosophy of science and even nursing has been profound. While for many disciplines, practically, it signaled an abrupt break with logical positivism (which predominated American philosophy between the two world wars), for nursing just emerging as a discipline, the influence of logical positivism persisted (Monti & Tingen, 1999; Whall, 1989). Logical positivism (to be discussed in detail in Chapter 6) had its roots with a group of scholars who in 1907 formed the

---

[6]We should note that we are confining our comments to philosophy of science and not philosophy *in general* (which is a much larger discussion and which of course subsumes this content).

[7]Again, there is a similar discussion in doctoral nursing education with regard to the teaching of ethics, particularly (but not exclusively) at the graduate level. Should it be taught by doctoral-prepared nursing faculty with an interest in ethics or only by those with some formal credential (e.g., Master of Bioethics degree—MBE, PhD in Philosophy, or at least a post-master's certificate in ethics) in the discipline?

[8]The historical record is complicated, but historians likely give Bacon (b. 1214 in Somerset, England, d. 1294 in Oxford, England) credit for being at the nexus of a late medieval, but not quite modern, scientist who promoted some of the earliest uses of the scientific method rather than inventing it (Hackett, 1997).

[9]b. 978 in what is now Uzbekistan, d. 1048 in what is now Afghanistan.

[10]Al-Biruni is also credited with performing the most precise measurement of the specific gravity of precious stones and metals, mathematical calculation of the earth's radius, mathematical determination of the earth's solar orbit, and measurement of the height of mountains by seconds and degrees (O'Connor et al., 1999).

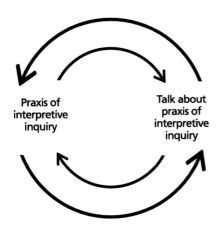

Praxis of interpretive inquiry

Talk about praxis of interpretive inquiry

FIGURE 3.1
Praxis of interpretive inquiry. (Adapted from work
of Wolff-Michael Roth, 2001)

"Vienna Circle" and their branch of philosophy held in high regard facts, empirical data, and experiments as the basis of science (Rodgers, 2004). At the time of Kuhn's book and for the decade thereafter, discussion of *what is the nursing paradigm* of the time became a preoccupation for nursing scholars of the day. Further, part of nursing's struggle to create a respectable disciplinary identity has been rooted in its ability to "look like the other scientific disciplines" and we think this has shaped nursing in both positive and negative ways. Logical positivism and later empiricism seem to have induced a type of rigid orthodoxy (even preoccupation) with quantitative inquiry and measurement in nursing. This has further complicated the debate about whether nursing is more science than *art* or *practice*. Empiricism, defined as both a scientific term (empirical knowledge) and a philosophical school (logical empiricism—which generally indicates that all scientific claims must be evaluated solely on their empirical evidence), has thus maintained a stranglehold on nursing knowledge development (Giuliano, 2003; Parrini, Salmon, & Salmon, 2003; Silva & Rothbart, 1984).

It has been difficult, at least in the U.S. nursing scientific community, for qualitative approaches and nursing knowledge emerging from a competing interpretive paradigm[11] to be regarded equally. In Figure 3.1, we have provided a diagram of this *praxis of interpretive inquiry*. It illustrates that praxis employs "talk" about interpretive inquiry and "doing" interpretive inquiry (Roth, 2001). According to Jun (2006), ". . . practice may take place without an individual employing any type of critical consciousness" (Jun, 2006, p. 136). But while the bidirectional arrows indicate that praxis (and practice) imply action, praxis is more transformative (to some, even having moral significance) (Joachim, 1951; Lobkowicz, 1967). Thus, the praxis of qualitative or interpretive inquiry may indeed have particular appeal to nurse investigators with a strong holistic disciplinary orientation.

---

[11]The interpretive paradigm is largely associated with qualitative methods of inquiry and with an ontology that embraces multiple realities that are not quantitatively generalizable (White, 2006, p. 141). Qualitative inquiry seems to have a much larger following in the United Kingdom, Ireland, Australia, and New Zealand. Further, since 2005, our DrNP program has had a 2-week mandatory study abroad program in London or Dublin, and both students and faculty have been very surprised that among British and Irish nursing faculty and graduate nursing students, qualitative methods actually appear more predominant.

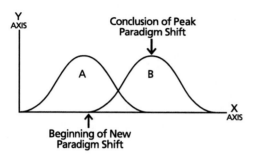

FIGURE 3.2
Paradigm shift: moving from one
paradigm to the next

However, even the contemporary evidence-based research movement appears to have marginalized qualitative research findings. The highly regarded Cochrane Criteria operationally minimizes the contribution that qualitative studies provide to the highest levels of evidence, and this has led to criticism of its validity (Morse, 2006a, 2006b). But, how to best conduct and classify qualitative systematic reviews is controversial (Booth, 2001). A quantitative analysis of qualitative studies in clinical journals for the 2000 publishing year found that only 9% of clinical articles used qualitative methods, and most were published in nursing journals with low impact factors (McKibbon & Gadd, 2004). Recently however, Guba and Lincoln (2005), authors of the classic *Naturalistic Inquiry* (Lincoln & Guba, 1985), which fundamentally helped shepherd qualitative inquiry in the 1980s beyond the confines of mostly anthropology and sociology to nursing and other fields, have declared that there has been a *paradigm shift* toward more interpretive, postmodern, and critical theory (and away from the predominant quantitative/positivist paradigm). We illustrate this paradigm shift in Figure 3.2 where the shift from a largely quantitative/positivist paradigm (A) has not been overtaken by a qualitative/interpretive paradigm (B). Perhaps you can have a classroom discussion about the current state of these two competing paradigms in nursing science and research.

It is likely, however, that as the maturation of nursing as a discipline continues, contemporary scholars (and graduate students!) will further embrace the realization that some nursing phenomena simply cannot be easily measured quantitatively and that interpretive approaches are perhaps more valid (Carr, 1994). Also, as many have suggested, attention to more rigorous methods of qualitative data analysis will be essential for this kind of research to be funded and integrated more readily into emerging discussions surrounding the nature of nursing knowledge, evidence-based practice, and practice-based evidence[12] (Caelli, Ray, & Mill, 2003; Sandelowski, 1986; Sharts-Hopko, 2002; Thorne, 2006).

As we return to our earlier statement that there should be no debate that philosophy of science belongs in PhD curricula, there should be increasing realization that some of these questions ought to be included even in baccalaureate nursing programs. Today, all nurses are obligated to maintain currency of practice and to read and evaluate nursing research studies (at least at a basic level). The ability to advocate and

---

[12]Although not a nursing article, we encourage the reading of a very provocative article on *practice-based evidence* by Midgley (2009).

articulate nursing's need for nursing knowledge development means that philosophy of science must be acknowledged as more than a conglomeration of esoteric concepts to which nursing students are exposed. Graduate students certainly have an even greater responsibility toward the evaluation and dissemination of research findings. And if PhD graduates (or at least those educated to be nurse scientists) are going to be the primary knowledge generators of our discipline,[13] then more rigor and attentiveness to philosophy of science is indeed warranted.

Philosophy of Science in the Doctor of Nursing Practice Curriculum

The central question of this chapter is whether doctor of nursing practice degree programs should include philosophy of science content. This point is certainly much debated by current doctor of nursing practice educators, as can be seen by glancing at various doctor of nursing practice curricula plans on websites. Our fairly comprehensive review of current national doctor of nursing practice curricula from published electronic material indicates that a minority of programs require a "stand-alone" course that focuses on basic philosophy of science principles. These programs are represented in Table 3.1 as Curricula A and explicitly emphasize this content.

A larger number of programs are represented in Table 3.1 in Curricula B. These programs appear to embed some of the basic principles of philosophy of science, but without a review of actual course syllabi, it is difficult to discern to what extent the course emphasis is on the actual philosophy of science. We found an even larger number of programs (probably around 25%) where there is either a stand-alone course or a course description outlining the inclusion of explicit content on *nursing epistemology,*[14] but again this is not a nursing epistemology text (excluding Chapter 16, which introduces practice epistemology). Our suspicion, nonetheless, is that many of these doctoral courses that address nursing epistemology or nursing knowledge development must include some introductory content on philosophy of science (e.g., What is evidence? What is explanation? What is deductive, inductive reasoning?) If they do not, then this is worrisome. It seems awfully superficial to skip the philosophical principles of evidence and the scientific method before beginning a discussion of "What do you plan to investigate as part of your final DNP project?" practice dissertation, or whatever the final project is called (Dreher, 2009a). Packard and Polifroni (1999) at least share this concern with regard to the development of our emerging nursing epistemology and state: "The fundamental issues emanating from the philosophy of science must be fully addressed in the critique and analysis of the emerging body of knowledge [in nursing science]" (Packard & Polifroni, 1999, p. 126). The programs that appear in Curricula C are only representative of the majority

---

[13]We hope that DNP graduates become the primary generators of practice-based knowledge development in nursing. However, the discussion of knowledge development in the DNP degree is in its infancy within contemporary U.S. practice doctorate academic circles. This will be discussed in Chapter 16.

[14]A reminder that *epistemology* is the branch of philosophy concerned primarily with the nature of knowledge, its presuppositions and foundations, and its extent and validity.

TABLE 3.1
Examples of Doctor of Nursing Practice Programs and Philosophy of Science Content

Doctor of Nursing Practice Programs[a]		
Curricula A: Philosophy of Science Explicit (Course Focus)	**Curricula B:** Philosophy of Science Implicit (Embedded)	**Curricula C:** Philosophy of Science Absent (Not Implicit)
Barnes-Jewish College— Philosophy of Science required in combined DNP/ PhD program	**Samford University—** Nurs 700: Theory and Philosophy of Nursing Practice	**Columbia University**
Drexel University— Nurs 700: Philosophy of Natural and Social Science: Foundations for Inquiry into the Discipline of Nursing	**St. Catherine University—** Nurs 8500: Underpinnings of the Discipline of Nursing	**Rush University**
Loyola University of New Orleans— Nurs 900: Philosophy of Science	**Texas Woman's University—** Nurs 6023: Philosophy of Nursing Science	**University of Massachusetts Lowell—** Nurs 33701: Philosophy of Nursing Science offered as elective
Oklahoma City University— Nurs 7103: Philosophy of Science	**University of Arizona—** Nurs 705: Philosophy of Nursing Science[b]	**University of Pittsburgh**
University of Tennessee Health Sciences— Nurs 911: Philosophy of Science	**Vanderbilt University—** Nurs 410: Evidence-Based Practice I: The Nature of Evidence	**University of Virginia**

[a]This list is not comprehensive, but representative of DNP/DrNP curricula across the United States.

[b]Verified with program that Philosophy of Science is embedded in course content and not just Philosophy of Nursing Science.

of programs that do not explicitly indicate in any way that philosophy of science (in some form) is part of their normal DNP curriculum. A couple of schools even indicated that this content *is* in their PhD but *not* in their DNP programs. This *should not* lead to the assumption that Curricula C schools (or other schools that might be classified in this category) do not teach any philosophy of science content, but that its emphasis is unknown.

But let us return to our question: How much philosophy of science should there be in a DNP degree? As the number of DNP students now surpasses the number of PhD students in 2009–2010 (Fang, Tracy, & Bednash, 2010)[15] and with PhD enrollments and graduations in such a flux over the last 15 years (Dreher, 2009b), we strongly predict that there is going to be a larger discussion among nursing scholars about what kind of knowledge is being generated in doctor of nursing practice programs. While we will wait until Chapter 16 to discuss this in more detail, it is evident from our review of DNP programs that there are many where the final project is clearly

---

[15]5,165 (DNP) versus 4,177 (PhD).

empirical in nature. In other words, the DNP graduate is not simply evaluating what is known and translating and disseminating this, but actually *creating new nursing knowledge*. If that is too threatening for DNP purists who honestly believe that only PhD graduates should be building new nursing knowledge,[16] then perhaps there can be more consensus to call it *practice knowledge*. If doctor of nursing practice graduates are going to produce new practice knowledge for the discipline, then the inclusion of philosophy of science content in DNP curricula presents a stronger argument.

The term practice knowledge has not been widely clarified in the nursing discipline and certainly not adopted by DNP programs, at least not yet. Mantzoukas and Jasper (2008) describe five different types of knowledge that nurses use in nursing practice: personal practice knowledge, theoretical knowledge, procedural knowledge, ward cultural knowledge, and reflexive knowledge. Personal practice knowledge is "person-specific, acquired in a moment of interaction with each patient and developed via the dialectical relationship that is created between each patient and nurse" and "is grasped in a conscious moment of encountering and interacting with a specific patient" (Mantzoukas & Jasper, 2008, p. 321). We are describing something different from this. Estabrooks et al. (2005) also describe practice knowledge used by nurses as social interactions, experiential knowledge, documentary sources, and *a priori* knowledge. Again, this type of nursing knowledge is different as it is presented as *user knowledge*. We, however, do not view the doctor of nursing practice graduate as a mere *user* of practice knowledge, but as a *generator* of practice knowledge. Our question is who is best prepared to produce this *new* practice knowledge–knowledge that ultimately becomes *new user knowledge* for use by many different types of nurses in the profession.

Nursing scholars Rolfe and Davies (2009) indicate that in the traditional paradigm, applied science maintains a separation between the generation and application of knowledge. However, with second-generation doctorates (contemporary professional doctorates), this wall of separation is "blurred to the point of meaninglessness" (Rolfe & Davies, 2009, p. 1269). In other words, in our knowledge economy (where we need reliable data to quickly improve health care efficiency and data to indicate the best way to utilize resources to gain the maximum health care product) a "from bench to bedside" slow approach to science is no longer sufficient (Fink, 2006). Nor, we fear, can we have doctoral graduates who are trained to discover and others *to apply* what is discovered. What we really need are knowledge-development methods and strategies that support almost real time discovery with near-immediate translation. To accomplish this, however, the investigator/practitioner will need to be literally in the field and very close to practice. Usher (2002) indicates that "the workplace becomes the site of research" (Usher, 2002, p. 150) for the professional doctorate student.[17] Five solid years into the doctor of nursing practice degree, this is an exciting discussion and it is one we simply must have.

---

[16] Again, we simply cannot support this idea although we respectfully know that there are those who do. However, if nursing scholars and doctoral nursing students cannot debate and disagree, then what is the purpose of doctoral-level critical thinking?

[17] For this reason, the Doctor of Psychology degree (PsyD) mentioned in Chapter 2 describes their graduates as "local scientists" who apply the scientific method to problems in psychology in the field (Murray, 2000, p. 52).

Finally, in 1996, and nearly a decade before the contemporary doctor of nursing practice movement, Reed (1996) wrote that "[Hildegard] Peplau's theory may be one of those nursing theories that seems to lack relevance to today's nursing practice" (Reed, 1996, p. 30). However, Reed's analysis that Peplau was an early pioneer theorist who believed nursing knowledge development began with observations made in the context of practice is a reminder that the practice knowledge described by Peplau in 1952 may yet become fashionable again. We thus conclude that if doctor of nursing practice programs are going to indeed lead the contemporary knowledge economy by producing graduates who will generate practice knowledge, then the question of whether there must be more philosophy of science content in those programs committed to this mission is obvious.

A PHILOSOPHY PERSPECTIVE

All men [and women] by nature desire to know.

—*Aristotle, 1941, p. 689*

Philosophy of Science in a Practice Discipline

Let us begin by revisiting and hopefully extending the analysis of "practice," "discipline," and "practice discipline" from Chapter 1. Most of us likely have some intuitive notion of what is meant by these terms, but a close investigation, especially one founded in philosophical literature, of what we mean when we use them and attribute them to human activities may lead not only to a deeper understanding of the concepts in question themselves, but also to an understanding of the needs of the practitioners of these disciplines, including a possible need for an understanding of the philosophy of science.

Scottish-born philosopher Alasdair MacIntyre (1929–) provides a possibly helpful starting point with his definition of practice:

> Any coherent and complex form of socially established cooperative human activity through which goods internal to that form of activity are realized in the course of trying to achieve those standards of excellence which are appropriate to, and partially definitive of, that form of activity . . . .
>
> —*MacIntyre, 2007, p. 187*

This definition is fairly broad, but it does provide some delimitation of the concept. MacIntyre notes that it may include activities such as football and chess, but exclude tic-tac-toe and the mere skill of throwing a football. It would also include the aforementioned practice disciplines of nursing, medicine, physical therapy, psychology, social work, education, and public health. Some elaboration of this definition, though, may be in order. First, a practice is a human activity, not one performed merely by an individual or by disconnected individuals but one performed *cooperatively* among a group of people. The *complexity* of the activity likely necessitates the cooperative aspect. Complex activities typically require working together. And the cooperative aspect necessitates *coherence*. Little can be achieved if practitioners of different disciplines do not share a fundamental understanding of what one another is doing. Cooperation on the scale implied by "practice" does not happen spontaneously but is the result of activity established in a social context. The practice is a part of society, not the spontaneous action of individuals; it has an established history or tradition. In the first line of this definition, we have already placed "practice" in a deep context, one that transcends the actions or beliefs of any individual but has a place in history and society.

Second, a practice produces "internal goods." MacIntyre divides the goods that result from a practice into "external goods" and "internal goods." The former are "externally and contingently attached" to the practice in question (MacIntyre, 2007, p. 188). They are not goods inherently connected to the activities associated with the practice, but goods that can be attained through alternative means. External goods may include such things as fame, wealth, social status, and power. Internal goods, however, are inherently connected to the activities associated with the practice and can then only be achieved through the practice itself. Internal goods also "can only be identified and recognized by the experience of participating in the practice in question" (MacIntyre, 2007, pp. 188–189). If psychology is a practice, an internal good it produces may be mental health or improvement of mental pathologies. If medicine is a practice, an internal good it produces may be the improvement of individuals' physical health. If public health is a practice, an internal good it produces may be the improvement of the health of society in general. All of these could provide an external good such as wealth or self-fulfillment of the practitioners, but these external goods are not definitive of individual practices or of practice in general.

Third, a practice includes "standards of excellence." These standards are not defined by any individual practitioner, but are an expression of the social aspect of a practice. No individual defines these standards for himself/herself or for others, but these arise from the aggregate, social activity of the practice itself. They are standards that transcend the individual and place the individual in a social context where skill is determined and judged. "To enter into a practice," writes MacIntyre, "is to accept the authority of those standards and the inadequacy of my own performance as judged by them" (MacIntyre, 2007, p. 190). Again, a practice is a social activity established within the history and traditions of a society transcending any individual practitioner. These standards of excellence define not only the practice, but also the appropriate quality and activity of the practice as geared toward achieving the internal goods of the practice.

The concept of "practice" developed in Chapter 1 includes one important aspect not included in or wholly consistent with MacIntyre's concept analyzed here. The assertion in Chapter 1 is that the most distinctive feature of a practice is the interpersonal quality. A practice implies an important, even intimate, interaction between practitioners and those served by the practice—those who benefit from the internal goods of the practice. This further delimitation emphasizes the practical nature of the fields we have in mind and distinguishes them from more theoretical and research-oriented fields that may be socially cooperative and provide internal goods, but lack the practical and moral engagement of activities that are essentially and integrally interpersonal. This further delimitation works for us here by providing us with a class of activities for which the internal goods have direct impact upon individuals in society who benefit. The internal goods of many practices under MacIntyre's concept may at times be somewhat abstract, not connected to interpersonal activity. Under our concept, the internal goods of a practice are concrete and specific.

Let us now take a step back from this. One of the clearest, most important influences in MacIntyre's work here is Aristotle. The English word *practice* (and all the more archaic versions noted in Chapter 1) derives from the ancient Greek word *praxis*, which along with art (*poiesis*)[18] and theory (*theoria*) comprise the three types of knowledge identified by Aristotle. "Art" refers to knowledge of production, making things. "Theory" refers to contemplative knowledge, the knowledge of universals rather than individuals or particulars, the "why's" and causes of things. *Praxis* refers to knowledge regarding action, knowing how to do something, the knowledge of individuals and particulars. So "doing" is not just doing, but a "knowing how" as opposed to the "knowing that" or "knowing why" of theory. The specific activities (skills) of a practice and the standards of excellence attached to those activities are a type of knowledge, a knowledge gained primarily through experience as opposed to academic study. Theory, knowing that or why, is often viewed as transcendent of and superior to *praxis*. But *praxis* is a socially necessary type of knowledge, necessary to achieve the internal goods of a practice, for "[if] . . . a man [or woman] has the theory without the experience, and recognizes the universal but does not know the individual included in this, he [or she] will often fail to cure; for it is the individual that is to be cured" (Aristotle, 1941, p. 690). Yet theory is also necessary. As indicated by Aristotle, theoretical knowledge without practical knowledge (knowledge of experience) is less effective if not ineffective, but practical knowledge without theoretical knowledge is blind or at least near-sighted: "men of experience know that the thing is so, but do not know why, while the others know the 'why' and the cause" (Aristotle, 1941, p. 690). The practitioner with just *praxis* may be able to contribute to society and to her practice in a substantive way. But she lacks the deeper understanding that provides social, epistemic, and moral justification to what she is doing. Her ability to extend her practice and improve upon it is limited. It is the level of theory that allows such progress to occur. With our interpersonal concept of practice, focusing on the direct delivery of internal goods more concretely and specifically, Aristotle's concept of *praxis* is more clearly and directly instantiated.

Let us now move on to the concept of *discipline* before furthering this analysis. Chapter 1 investigated the concept of discipline, noting its essence as a field of study. It further alludes to the social and historical contexts of discipline and standards of evaluation. A close look, especially at King and Brownell's (1966) criteria, will reveal much overlap between discipline and MacIntyre's concept of practice. *Discipline* is narrower and a more formalized activity. As noted in Chapter 1, psychology and nursing existed (possibly as practices) long before they were recognized as disciplines. MacIntyre's practice exemplars of chess and football would not (at least at present) be accepted as disciplines (but also not as practices as we are using the term), although perhaps a more general category they fit into might be. The recognition of an activity as a discipline is largely a social recognition that imbues it with status. It is a field we

---

[18]Do not be confused by modern meanings. The meaning of "art" here is not that of esoteric creation of unique beauty or any other modern use of the word. The English word "art" is derived from the Latin word "ars," which is a translation of the ancient Greek word "poiesis." Poiesis merely refers to human production in general, not only the production of what we might call "art" today. The confusion is furthered when we realize that our word "poetry" is derived from the Greek word "poiesis."

socially recognize as worthy of focused study, a field that can generate new and valuable knowledge. The conceptual overlap of *practice* and *discipline* allows for the coherent combination of the two into *practice discipline*. A practice discipline then would be a socially established cooperative human activity geared toward the achievement of internal goods through the excellence of practice (delivered interpersonally), which is deemed worthy of focused (academic) study, possible of generating new knowledge. This new knowledge, knowledge of the *why* and the cause, presumably would reflect back on practice itself, bringing together *theoria* and *praxis*.

If a practice discipline falls under the heading of "science," then the new knowledge generated will fall under the category of scientific knowledge and be subject to the traditions, standards, and criteria of knowledge acquisition and justification in science. The standards of excellence of the practice will be at least partially subsumed by the standards of science. Practitioners at the most basic level (associate or baccalaureate prepared) of a scientifically oriented practice discipline may be well served with a *praxis*-focused education and knowledge base. Those at the furthest academic level (PhD) undoubtedly need the knowledge of the *why* and the cause. Not only that but they should have knowledge of *why* and cause **of** "the 'why' and the cause"—a second level knowledge of science itself, philosophy of science. Yet again from Aristotle, the man or woman of theory will often fail to cure for lack of knowledge of the particular. Thus, the practice doctorate may provide that link between theory and practice. The generation of new knowledge among practice doctorates will be grounded in the particular at one end, but also needs to be founded in the theoretical at the other. The practice doctorate needs to engage in discourse both with men and women of theory and with men and women of practice. We can presume knowledge of practice in early training and experience. A focus in theory then becomes more of a necessity in doctoral study. The question for the discipline of nursing, especially in light of the doctor of nursing practice degree, is whether Dickoff, James, and Wiedenbach's (1968) musings on "Theory in a Practice Discipline" still have relevance today in modern practice curricula.

Philosophy of Science in the Discipline of Nursing

As a discipline, and as a profession, nursing is still quite young—particularly relative to nursing as a practice. It is not surprising then to find some significant alienation between the discipline of nursing and the practice of nursing. To define and justify itself as a discipline, nursing had to mark out its epistemic territory and identify its own knowledge base. In doing this, it may well have overcompensated toward the theoretical, toward knowledge for its own sake, leading to a gap in nursing between theory and practice. More traditional disciplines (like philosophy) have a long history of theoretical knowledge and study. Despite still having minor intradisciplinary disputes regarding the relationship between theory and practice, that relationship has largely been settled for these more traditional disciplines. So it is not surprising at nursing's relatively young age as a discipline that this dispute is more central and still being negotiated. The emergence of nursing as a discipline has clearly raised philosophical issues regarding the nature of nursing, the methods of nursing research, and the relation of practice and discipline, among others. An appeal to theory at various levels will no doubt figure into the discussions and resolutions of these issues.

Risjord (2010) identifies two types of theory–practice gaps referred to in nursing literature. The first type "arises when the theory is not translated into action" (Risjord, 2010, p. 3). The problem is that the theory and research of nursing scholars are not made practical and meaningful for practicing nurses and nursing students. The problem here is really one of "translation." Either theory and research are not presented to the student in a pedagogical manner in which they can find meaning and utility, or the demands of practice for the practicing nurse leave little time for reeducation and integration of the latest theory and research. The second type of theory–practice gap is more profound. The first presumes that the theory and research of nursing scholars are relevant to practice, but the second type denies this very claim. According to this second type, theory and research in nursing provide no aid or guidance in nursing practice. It has become knowledge for knowledge's sake or knowledge for the sake of something else, but not for the sake of nursing practice. If this is so, then that identifies a serious problem for nursing. Either nursing as a discipline is irrelevant itself to nursing practice, or the way in which nursing research and theory have proceeded has made the discipline of nursing irrelevant to nursing practice. Alternatively, this second type of gap may not be the case, and the appearance of such a gap may be reducible to the first type, which is a mere problem of translation. Whichever of these three alternatives is the case is a matter for nursing itself to determine and resolve.

Risjord (2010) identifies two competing camps attempting to resolve this problem of the theory–practice gap. There are practice theorists who believe practice should guide discipline, that the "first obligation of the professional in nursing is the responsibility for nursing practice or its improvement . . . that contribution to general or specific knowledge . . . is less [nursing's] responsibility than is that for practice" (Ellis, 1968, p. 222; Wald & Leonard, 1964). Nursing's long history as a practice prior to developing into a discipline makes this impulse understandable. There have also been nursing theorists who argue that discipline should lead practice, that the "scientist . . . must be the one upon whom the profession relies" (Schlotfeld, 1960, p. 494). This impulse is also understandable in a young discipline. Attempting to define and justify itself as a legitimate, autonomous discipline, it is understandable that many nursing scholars have argued for the dominance of the theoretical and research arms of nursing. At the same time, such an emphasis risks abstracting new knowledge out of relevance for practice, thereby instantiating that second type of theory–practice gap. Whichever strategy is employed, or some third alternative, a rapprochement of theory and practice in nursing is needed.

Philosophy of Science in the Doctor of Nursing Practice Curriculum

The DNP/DrNP student and practitioner are uniquely placed to effect this rapprochement. The nurse with a PhD may arguably be too far removed from practice. The baccalaureate and master's prepared nurses may not have the requisite advanced study. The practice doctorate nurse is still immersed in practice and yet also prepared through advanced study.

As noted earlier, given the analysis of Aristotle, practice is not just practice, but a form of knowledge as well. Regarding the practice of nursing, this knowledge encompasses the areas of physiology, medicine, psychology, public health, and a variety of other fields, which places nursing knowledge within the context of science. Nursing practice is on some level scientific practice and informed by scientific knowledge—both practical and theoretical. Nursing as a science at present may not be fully and coherently defined, but that is the nature of a new discipline in the area of science. Theorists have been struggling for such definition much the way that Kuhn describes a pre-paradigmatic or immature science (1962), which led to the metaparadigm approach in nursing theory in the 1970s and 1980s. One of the basic incommensurable conflicts (which are indicative of a pre-paradigmatic science) that may preclude the advancement of nursing into a clear scientific paradigm is the dispute between quantitative and qualitative research. It is not clear to us that nursing must choose one of these, that they are in fact incommensurable and irreconcilable. But this is a philosophical question and one regarding the proper methodology of science and the structure of theories. It will hence be worked out in both the theoretical discourse of nursing and the actual research conducted. Practice itself will provide the proof of these research methodologies.

For the practice doctorate nurse to effect this rapprochement, she must be able to engage in discourse and research at all levels. The valuable practice knowledge she has will need to be supplemented and reconciled with new theoretical knowledge. This rapprochement will then bring about the creation of new practice knowledge. Going back to Aristotle, the theorist knows the universal, the practitioner knows the particular, and the practice doctorate can bring these together. The ultimate foundation of this theoretical knowledge is found within the philosophy of science. One might analogize the practitioner to an auto mechanic. An auto mechanic can be perfectly competent without the knowledge of physics that ultimately explains the operation of the internal combustion engine, let alone the philosophy of science that critiques and investigates the claims of the physicist on a deeper level. The engineer who designs automobile engines may well need an understanding of physics, but it is questionable whether an understanding of philosophy of science would be of benefit even to him. Some nurses might reject and even be offended by this auto mechanic analogy—and with good reason. The practice of nursing (as a practice in our understanding), with the interpersonal essence of nursing, raises far more important and significant professional and ethical concerns than the fixing of cars or designing of engines. The interpersonal essence of nursing demands a deep understanding of the knowledge being produced, in order to more legitimately and ethically produce knowledge for practice. The practice doctorate nurse must have not only practice knowledge, but theoretical knowledge regarding the basis of this practice knowledge in order to address the many philosophical questions above that will affect nursing at all levels of practice and study. Otherwise, this rapprochement will not occur or will forever be incomplete.

The practice doctorate nurse will also interact with other doctorally prepared health professionals of various sorts in the interdisciplinary context in which health care occurs today. In order to actively and effectively engage, she must display and be prepared with a commensurate degree of knowledge and study.

Such interaction will further not only health care knowledge and practice, and nursing knowledge and practice, but also the deeper understanding of nursing, science, and nursing science.

SUMMARY

We began this chapter with three goals: (1) to repudiate any suggestion that disciplines where *practice* is the focus will have less reliance on the principal concepts in philosophy of science; (2) to dispel any notion that doctor of nursing practice students do not need substantive content on philosophy of science (because of its practice focus or because these students are not educated to be chiefly researchers or scientists); and (3) to quell any weak argument by naysayers or skeptics who proclaim this content is more appropriate for PhD students. In general, those involved in practice disciplines will be not just *doing* but employing *practice knowledge* (*praxis*). This leads to the question of the development of practice knowledge, a subject still under debate. But of course, the practice doctorate will be uniquely placed to further this investigation into the creation and development of practice knowledge. In support of this, Sommers et al. (2007) argue for the value of scientifically treating problematic cases, bringing together the Aristotelian categories of *theoria* and *praxis*, the universal and the particular. More specifically, in nursing there has been a growing recognition that nursing phenomena cannot be easily measured quantitatively, raising the question of the place and value of qualitative investigation in nursing, and more deeply raising the question of nursing's essence and status as a science or pre-paradigmatic (immature) science. If practice doctorate nurses are going to be generating practice knowledge, some understanding of this philosophical problem will be essential. In terms of DNP curricula, we note that many programs across the country require a final project that is empirical in nature. A full understanding of what these students are doing will necessitate not only methodology and concepts of methodology, but also the concepts that support those concepts. We also recognize that in the contemporary health care environment the slow approach *from bench to bedside* is no longer sufficient, necessitating doctoral graduates neither at the far end of theory nor at the far end of practice, but placed in between to effect a rapprochement.

MacIntyre's (2007) concept of practice brought a deeper understanding of the social and cooperative aspect of practice with standards of excellence geared toward the achievement of specific internal goods. We add to this the further delimiting quality of interpersonal interaction, thereby highlighting the direct, concrete delivery of internal goods and better instantiating the Aristotelian concept of *praxis*. With nursing not only a practice, but a discipline as well, the importance of *theoria* cannot be denied. Yet this has to be a *theoria* that is not alienated from practice, as much nursing literature seems to agree it is. Once again, the practice doctorate is uniquely placed to resolve this alienation, to mend this theory–practice gap. To do this, a full and deep understanding of theory, including questions in the realm of the philosophy of science, will be a necessity. And finally, the interdisciplinary nature of health care today where nursing practice doctorates will by necessity be interacting with a variety of other health professionals and scholars, requires a deep understanding of theory for all doctorally prepared nurses in order to discourse and effectively interact with these others, given the presumption that they will have a similar advanced education.

Chapters 4 through 14 focus exclusively on philosophy and the philosophy of science. Major questions regarding theory, justification, observation, philosophical challenges to the presumptions of science, and the specific problems of the social sciences are presented. Little specific to nursing appears in these chapters. This focus reflects our contention that the nursing scholar, including the practice doctorate, needs to be well founded in the intellectual traditions of inquiry that are the basis of scientific investigation. And again, as the practice doctorate will be operating in an interdisciplinary environment, the student is meant to see the application of these questions to science and health care in general and extend this application themselves to nursing specifically.

CRITICAL THINKING QUESTIONS

1. Discuss your exposure to philosophy of science concepts in your baccalaureate degree and master's degree (if applicable).
2. Choose one of the 15 topics listed at the beginning of this chapter and retrieve an article from a practice discipline other than nursing. Discuss how the topic philosophy of science principles are applicable to the respective discipline. Example:

   Cosgrove, L., & McHugh, M. (2000). Speaking for ourselves: Feminist methods and community psychology. *American Journal of Community Psychology, 28*(6), 815–838.
3. In what ways are *practice inquiry* relevant to the discipline of nursing and your future practice?
4. Discuss whether you believe doctor of nursing practice graduates should produce *practice knowledge.*
5. Debate the following: Resolved, "Doctor of Nursing Practice degree programs which emphasize practice do not need substantive content in philosophy of science." Make a case for and against this resolution.
6. Review MacIntyre's concept of practice and identify some activities that would fit his criteria.
7. Review our amendment to MacIntyre's view and identify activities that would fit our concept of practice but not MacIntyre's.
8. Review our concept of discipline and identify a practice (according to our concept) that is not a discipline. Why is it just a practice and not a discipline? What keeps it from being a discipline? Might it someday become a discipline as well as a practice?
9. In your experience, do you find a gap between nursing practice and nursing theory/research? In your practice have you found the nursing theory you learned as a student applicable? Is nursing research generally and typically applicable to nursing practice?
10. Consider the idea of a rapprochement between theory/discipline and practice in nursing. Which do you think should be the guiding force in this rapprochement? Theory/discipline or practice?

REFERENCES

Anderson, J. A. (2010). Clinical research in context: Reexamining the distinction between research and practice. *Journal of Medicine and Philosophy, 35*(1), 46–63.

Aristotle, (1941). *Metaphysics* (W. D. Ross, Trans.). In R. McKeon (Ed.), *The basic works of Aristotle* (pp. 689–926). New York, NY: Random House.

Booth, A. (2001). *Cochrane or cock-eyed? How should we conduct systematic reviews of qualitative research?* Paper presented at the Qualitative Evidence-based Practice Conference, Taking a Critical Stance. Coventry University, May 14–16, 2001. Retrieved from http://www.leeds.ac.uk/educol/documents/00001724.htm

Caelli, K., Ray, L., & Mill, J. (2003). "Clear as mud": Toward greater clarity in generic qualitative research. *International Journal of Qualitative Methods, 2*(2), 1–24.

Carr, L. T. (1994). The strengths and weaknesses of quantitative and qualitative research: What method for nursing? *Advances in Nursing Science, 20*(4), 716–721.

Choi, J. S., Choi, S., & Kim, Y. (2009). Improving scientific inquiry for social work in South Korea. *Research on Social Work Practice, 19*(4), 464–471.

DiBartolo, M. C. (1998). Philosophy of science in doctoral nursing education revisited. *Journal of Professional Nursing, 14*(6), 350–360.

Dickoff, J., James, P., & Wiedenbach, E. (1968). Theory in a practice discipline: Part 1. Practice-oriented theory. *Nursing Research, 17*(5), 415–435.

Dreher, H. M. (2009a). *A novel way to approve DNP projects and clinical dissertation topics.* Paper presented at the 2nd National Conference on The Doctor of Nursing Practice: The Dialogue Continues..., Hilton Head Island, South Carolina, March 24–27, 2009.

Dreher, H. M. (2009b). Education for advanced practice: The question: Is the PhD or DNP the right degree model for future advanced practice nurses? In L. Joel (Ed.), *Advanced practice nursing: Essentials for role development* (2nd ed.) (pp. 58–71). Philadelphia, PA: FA Davis.

Ellis, R. (1968). Characteristics of significant theories. *Nursing Research, 17*(3), 217–222.

Estabrooks, C. A., Rutakumwa, W., O'Leary, K. A., Profetto-McGrath, J., Milner, M., Levers, M. J. et al. (2005). Sources of practice knowledge among nurses. *Qualitative Health Research, 15*(4), 460–476.

Fang, D., Tracy, C., & Bednash, G. D. (2010). *2009–2010 Enrollment and graduations in Baccalaureate and Graduate programs in nursing.* Washington, DC: American Association of Colleges of Nursing.

Fink, D. (2006). The professional doctorate: Its relativity to the Ph.D. and relevance for the knowledge economy. *International Journal of Doctoral Studies, 3*, 35–44.

Giuliano, K. K. (2003). Expanding the use of empiricism in nursing: Can we bridge the gap between knowledge and clinical practice? *Nursing Philosophy, 4*(1), 44–52.

Gortner, S. (2000). Knowledge development in nursing: Our historical roots and future opportunities. *Nursing Outlook, 48*(2), 60–67.

Guba, E. G., & Lincoln, Y. S. (2005). Paradigmatic controversies, contradictions, and emerging influences. In N. K. Denzin, & Y. S. Lincoln (Eds.), *The Sage handbook of qualitative research* (3rd ed.) (pp. 191–215). Thousand Oaks, CA: Sage.

Hackett, J. (1997). Roger Bacon. *Stanford Encyclopedia of Philosophy.* Retrieved from http://plato.stanford.edu/entries/roger

Joachim, H. H. (1951). In D. A. Rees (Ed.), *Aristotle: The Nicomachean ethics: A commentary.* Oxford, UK: Clarendon Press.

Jun, J. S. (2006). Understanding action, praxis, and change. In J. S. Jun (Ed.), *The social construction of public administration: Interpretive and critical perspectives* (pp. 123–146). Albany, NY: State University of New York Press.

Karlik, S. J. (2010). Building a teaching module in clinical inquiry for radiology residents. In T. V. Deven (Ed.), *The practice of radiology education: Challenges and trends* (pp. 57–69). New York, NY: Springer.

Kikuchi, J. F. (1992). Nursing questions that science cannot answer. In J. F. Kikuchi, & H. Simmons (Eds.), *Philosophic inquiry in nursing* (pp. 26–37). Chicago, IL: Sage Publications, Inc.

King, A. R., & Brownell, J. A. (1966). *The curriculum and the disciplines of knowledge: A theory of curriculum practice.* Hoboken, NJ: Wiley.

Kuhn, T. (1962). *The structure of scientific revolutions.* Chicago and London: University of Chicago Press.

Lewis, I., & Bolzan, N. (2007). Social work with a twist: Interweaving practice knowledge, student experience and academic theory. *Australian Social Work, 60*(2), 136–146.

Lincoln, Y., & Guba, E. G. (1985). *Naturalist inquiry.* Newbury Park, CA: Sage Publications.

Lobkowicz, N. (1967). *Theory and practice: History of a concept from Aristotle to Marx.* Notre Dame, IN: University of Notre Dame Press.

MacIntyre, A. C. (2007). *After virtue: A study in Moral Theory.* Notre Dame, IN: Notre Dame University Press.

Mantzoukas, S., & Jasper, M. (2008). Types of nursing knowledge used to guide care of hospitalized patients. *Journal of Advanced Nursing, 62*(3), 318.

Midgley, N. (2009). Improvers, adapters and rejecters—The link between evidence-based practice and evidence-based practitioners. *Clinical Child Psychology & Psychiatry, 14,* 323–327.

McKibbon, K. A., & Gadd, C. S. (2004). A quantitative analysis of qualitative studies in clinical journals for the 2000 publishing year. *BMC Medical Informatics and Decision Making, 4,* 11.

Monti, E., & Tingen, M. (1999). Multiple paradigms in nursing. *Advances in Nursing Science, 21*(4), 64–80.

Morse, J. (2006a). It is time to revise the Cochrane criteria. *Qualitative Health Research, 16,* 315–317.

Morse, J. (2006b). The politics of evidence. *Qualitative Health Research, 16*(3), 395–404.

Murray, B. (2000). The degree that almost wasn't: The PsyD comes of age. *The Monitor, 31*(1), 52.

O'Connor, J. J., Robertson, E. F., & Edmund, F. (1999). *Abu Arrayhan Muhammad ibn Ahmad al-Biruni.* MacTutor History of Mathematics archive. University of St Andrews. Retrieved from http://www-history.mcs.st-andrews.ac.uk/Biographies/Al-Biruni.html.

Orcutt, B. A., Flowers, L. C., & Seinfeld, J. (1990). *Science and inquiry in social work practice.* New York, NY: Columbia University Press.

Packard, S., & Polifroni, E. C. (1999). The nature of scientific truth. In E. C. Polifroni, & M. Welch (Eds.), *Perspectives on philosophy of science in nursing: An historical and contemporary anthology* (pp. 126–134). Philadelphia, PA: Lippincott, Williams & Wilkins.

Parrini, P., Salmon, W. C., & Salmon, M. H. (2003). *Logical empiricism: Historical & contemporary perspectives.* Pittsburgh, PA: University of Pittsburgh Press.

Reed, P. (1996). Transforming practice knowledge into nursing knowledge—A revisionist analysis of Peplau. *The Journal of Nursing Scholarship, 28*(1), 29–33.

Risjord, M. (2010). *Nursing knowledge: Science, practice, and philosophy.* Chichester, West Sussex, UK: Wiley–Blackwell.

Rodgers, B. (2004). *Developing nursing knowledge: Philosophical traditions and influences.* Philadelphia, PA: Lippincott, Williams & Wilkins.

Rolfe, G., & Davies, R. (2009). Second generation professional doctorates in nursing. *International Journal of Nursing Studies, 46,* 1265–1273.

Roth, W.-M. (2001). *Interpretive inquiry (ED-B580).* Retrieved from http://www.educ.uvic-ca/faculty/mroth/580/InterpretiveInquiry.html

Sandelowski, M. (1986). The problem of rigor in qualitative research. *Advances in Nursing Science, 8*(3), 27–37.

Schlotfeld, R. M. (1960). Reflections on nursing research. *American Journal of Nursing, 60*(4), 492–494.

Sharts-Hopko, N. (2002). Assessing rigor in qualitative research. *Journal of the Association of Nurses in AIDS Care, 13*(4), 84–86.

Silva, M. C., & Rothbart, D. (1984). An analysis of changing trends in philosophies in science on nursing theory development and testing. *Advances in Nursing Science, 18*(1), 1–13.

Sommers, L. S., Morgan, L., Johnson, L., & Yatabe, K. (2007). Practice inquiry: Clinical uncertainty as a focus for small-group learning and practice improvement. *Journal of General Internal Medicine, 22*(2), 246–252.

Thorne, S. (2006). Reflections on "Helping practitioners understand the contribution of qualitative research to evidence-based practice." *Evidence Based Nursing, 9,* 7–8.

Thyer, B. A. (2010). Twenty years of publishing research on social work practice: Past accomplishments new initiatives. *Research on Social Work Practice, 20,* 5–10.

Usher, R. (2002). A diversity of doctorates: Fitness for the knowledge economy. *Higher Education Research & Development, 21*(2), 143–153.

Wald, F. S., & Leonard, R. C. (1964). Towards development of nursing practice theory. *Nursing Research, 13*(4), 309–313.

Whall, A. (1989). The influence of logical positivism on nursing practice. *Journal of Nursing Scholarship, 21*(4), 243–245.

White, J. (2006). Patterns of knowing: Review, critique, and update. In L. C. Andrist, P. K. Nicholas, & K. A. Wolfe (Eds.), *A history of nursing ideas* (pp. 139–150). Sudbury, MA: Jones and Bartlett Publishers, Inc.

4

Philosophy and Philosophizing

This sense of wonder is the mark of the philosopher.
Philosophy indeed has no other origin ...

PLATO

PHILOSOPHY AND ITS MISCONCEPTIONS

Students often come to a first (or sometimes even second or third) philosophy class with grave misconceptions about philosophy. These misconceptions are largely engendered and fueled by misunderstandings of philosophy active in our culture and ambiguities of the word "philosophy." People commonly misunderstand both the purpose and methodology of philosophy and confuse colloquial uses of the term for the more academic concept and tradition. First, in a society that powerfully values the practical, any academic field is commonly looked upon with suspicion. With philosophy arguably the most "academic" of academic fields, this suspicion is often especially strong. This suspicion of course depends upon a strong distinction between theory and practice: that there is a clear and apparent line between studies and disciplines that have direct practical values and those which are impractical, ivory-tower musings available only to an educated elite whose practical needs are met and thus can afford the time and luxury of the theoretical. Yet such a distinction is often far from clear. Any practice, including those most necessary for daily life, includes underlying theoretical issues. Understanding of such underlying theory can have profound effect upon the direction and purpose of the practice in question, as well as social and moral justifications. The line between theory and practice may be far more blurry than commonly supposed.

A little history of philosophy may also demonstrate the indistinctness of this line between theory and practice. Western philosophy is commonly understood to have begun about 2,500 years ago with the first Western philosopher Thales (ca. 585 B.C.E.) who lived in Miletus—the area where Turkey now is. In these early days of philosophy, the concept if not always the word (actually coined somewhat later in Greece), included not just what philosophers today would consider philosophy but any advanced studies: physics, biology, psychology, mathematics, history, art criticism, political science, and so forth. As these various fields developed distinct bodies of knowledge and distinct methodologies, they separated from philosophy to become independent disciplines. In fact, up until the 18th century the science of physics was known as *natural philosophy*. Until the theories of Darwin, the science of biology was oriented around the insights and theories of Greek philosopher Aristotle. Psychology did not completely separate from philosophy until the mid to late 19th century. These acts of separation left philosophy the most profound, most difficult (possibly unanswerable) questions. Thus, nonphilosophers often hold a second misconception, that philosophy, unlike science or even other humanities fields, is composed of nothing more than opinion that there are no standards for knowledge claims in philosophy. This view is also fed by the ambiguity according to which many people use philosophy as a synonym for policy, principle or belief, which leads to further common misconceptions. For example, a store might promote their business saying, "Our philosophy is that the customer comes first." This of course is a policy and not a use of the word consistent with the traditional academic meaning. Or consider this statement from a book on holistic health: "A holistic philosophy takes a systems perspective in emphasizing that the 'lifestyle choices' a person makes must be understood in the context of his or her genetic propensities, personality, relationships, and the environment" (Robison & Carrier, 2004, p. 72). Here, "philosophy" refers to a belief system or worldview, as such its use is not in the academic sense of "philosophy." Holistic philosophy, as it is defined here, could be the result of philosophical study or an element of a larger philosophical inquiry, but it does not refer to the academic sense of "philosophy" itself. The use of the word "philosophy" as a policy, belief, or even belief system does not imply questions of knowledge claims or critical engagement with those beliefs, which is central to the academic meaning.

Although philosophy deals with the most profound, most difficult, possibly unanswerable questions; that does not mean that there are no answers, no objective criteria for knowledge claims, no right or wrong. Traditionally, philosophy has committed itself to standards of logic and rationality. Beginning with Thales, developing with the *elenchus* of Socrates, the arguments of Plato, and the multidisciplinary study of Aristotle and beyond, any claim posited in a philosophical context must be supported by reasons someone else should accept that claim as true. Philosophy thus developed the study of logic and argumentation employed now in all other academic studies and practices, including most notably science and law. Therefore, it is not the case that just any claim or theory is philosophically meaningful. It must address a philosophical issue in an insightful manner and it must be rationally supported. Of these two criteria, the former needs some development and clarification. That will be the focus of the next section. Before that, however, a caveat regarding the latter criterion is necessary. Although traditionally some form of rational support has been an integral part of philosophical study, even that most essential element of philosophy has come under critical review in recent postmodern philosophy. The very meaning of rationality and its applicability to philosophical study has been questioned by some recent philosophers. Such issues will be raised in later chapters, especially Chapter 14.

PHILOSOPHIZING AND PHILOSOPHICAL ISSUES: LESSONS FROM *EUTHYPHRO*

The safest general characterization of the European philosophical tradition is that it consists of a series of footnotes to Plato.

—*A. N. Whitehead, 1978, p. 39*

Let us begin at a philosophically uncontroversial place: Plato. Specifically, I want to start with Plato's dialogue known as *The Euthyphro*. A dialogue is a form of writing which is similar to a small play: a number of characters discuss a question in a give-and-take manner. This writing form was not uncommon in Plato's day but is rarely seen today, being largely replaced by the dry essay or treatise. These dialogues of Plato usually star his mentor Socrates, who never wrote anything of his own, in discussions with philosophers, sophists, politicians, soldiers, and others. In most of these, Socrates turns out looking good and wise, whereas his interlocutors often (but not always) look foolish.

This particular dialogue begins with Socrates on his way to court to face the charges of impiety and corrupting the youth that will lead to his eventual execution. On his way, he meets his friend Euthyphro, also on his way to court but to charge his own father with murder. Socrates questions whether it is appropriate for a son to charge his father with a crime. Euthyphro asserts quite confidently that he is in the right. He bases this confidence on his self-expressed status as an expert on morality and piety. Upon hearing of this expertise Socrates suggests that Euthyphro's knowledge and learning could help him in defending his own case and engages Euthyphro in a discussion of the very meaning of piety. At this early point, a well-known quality of Socrates is already apparent: irony. It is subtly apparent that Socrates does not accept Euthyphro's expertise at face value—indeed he likely doubts Euthyphro's expertise. Yet, he flatters Euthyphro and entreats him for help. This rhetorical strategy has come to be known as Socratic Irony. Socrates used it to draw people out, to get them talking in order to further discussion. And whether Euthyphro is indeed an expert should come out of an in depth discussion of the concept of piety, not simply his bold assertions.

Already we can see an essential aspect of philosophy and philosophical study. A philosophical issue involves concepts (or ideas) of a general and fundamental nature. The concept here of course is piety. Other fundamental concepts open to philosophical investigation include space, time, knowledge, love, and science. These are concepts we encounter on a daily basis but typically do not give much thought. "There is a sense," writes American philosopher Joseph Margolis (1924–), "in which philosophical questions are both remote and familiar ..." (Margolis, 1968, p. 3). They are familiar in that they often involve concepts we encounter everyday. And regarding concepts such as these, everyone holds some, usually unquestioned, beliefs and assumptions. Given the inquisitive nature of the human mind, each person at some point in her life will question at least some of the concepts. When philosophers pursue such questioning, the questions and the concepts themselves can seem to be remote. A critical stance toward fundamental beliefs and assumptions can alienate these usually familiar concepts from us. What was once familiar and certain becomes alien and uncertain.

A concept (idea) is contained within the human mind. But its existence must transcend any individual mind. First, since we can collectively and coherently discuss and refer to concepts such as space, time, moral correctness, and so forth, such concepts must in some manner exist in minds in general. Second, the source of these concepts, given the collective ownership of them, must come from beyond the individual mind, whether that is the nature or structure of the human mind itself, the natural world, or culture and society. When we philosophically study a concept like time, we are first investigating a concept contained in our heads. But this is also a concept existent on a social level. That is, we have common, social understandings of what such concepts mean. We can investigate the understanding in our own mind, but also expand that investigation to how we understand the concept socially. Beyond this there is the question of whether this concept accurately reflects or represents some independent reality, and if it does, whether our investigation can bring our concept to a more accurate representation of this independent reality.

Philosophical investigation of these concepts often focuses on what exactly they mean. Although we all seem to have general concepts like space, time, and so forth in our minds, we typically have difficulty in providing a coherent definition to such concepts—particularly a definition that will meet general assent. Plato's dialogue *The Euthyphro* is an enlightening text on the philosophical method itself. In this dialogue, Socrates discusses the meaning of "piety" with his friend Euthyphro. Although Euthyphro fancies himself an expert on piety, he seems incapable of providing a clear and coherent definition. Each definition he posits ends up facing some logical problems.

To get to the heart of the issue, to have a fundamental starting point, Socrates asks Euthyphro for a definition of piety. Euthyphro's first answer is that what he is presently doing, prosecuting his father for murder is piety. Socrates gently demurs, explaining that this response does not answer his question. Euthyphro's answer supplies merely an example. What Socrates is requesting is a statement on the essence of the concept: what qualities are essential to the concept of piety, what distinguishes some acts, like prosecuting one's father, as pious from other (impious) acts. Although, philosophers at times utilize examples to strategically investigate a difficult concept. A mere example as Euthyphro proposes is of limited value, but what are known as paradigm and borderline examples can be more useful (see Woodhouse, 2006, pp. 58–59). Paradigm examples are proposed instances of the thing in question of which it is posited that they illustrate the essence of the thing. Paradigm examples may at times be controversial, but generally they appeal to largely accepted intuitions about the concept in question and what counts as a member of that class. Having a paradigmatic example of the concept in question provides for something more concrete to investigate than an admittedly fuzzy concept. By investigating the paradigm example, its main characteristics can be used to comprise a general definition that would be helpful in understanding what are and are not other instances of that concept. For example, in investigating the meaning of "science" many philosophers might use physics as a paradigm example. The characteristics of physics would then be analyzed and formed into a proposed definition to test other possible sciences against. One problem with paradigm examples though is that they may play upon preconceptions and prejudices and thus limit investigation and lead to a form of academic conservatism. Some critics of using physics as a paradigm example of science may claim that it plays upon prejudices of certain philosophers of science (especially logical positivists) and unfairly exclude or at least make questionable many forms of social science.

Borderline examples, rather than putting forth an instance largely accepted as indicative of the concept in question, test the limits of that concept. Uses of borderline examples usually presuppose that we have a basic understanding of the concept but need to understand how far it may extend. Borderline examples may have some of the qualities we normally attribute to the concept in question, but may lack some important qualities or include some that we do not normally associate with the concept. Freudianism may be an interesting borderline example of science. Freudianism seems to conform to our ideas of science as investigating our world of experience—our inner world of experience. Yet, many scientists and philosophers of science find it not empirical enough to fully and unambiguously qualify as a science. By analyzing this example, "certain limits of applicability of ['science'] will be clarified, and the meaning of that concept will be understood to extend to those limits" (Woodhouse, 2006, p. 59).

Euthyphro's second response is more (formally) satisfactory. Euthyphro asserts that piety is what the gods love. This response better satisfies Socrates' formal request for a definition, but whether it is satisfactory as a definition of piety must await critical analysis. Socrates notes that within the Greek pantheon of gods there are many disputes and squabbles, disagreements over right and wrong. Thus, there would be disagreement among the gods about what they each love, meaning that some might love one thing while others hate that thing. Under Euthyphro's most recent definition, any act or thing that is loved by some gods and hated by others would be both pious and impious—which is not a logically tenable conclusion. This form of argumentation has come to be called *reductio ad absurdum* (reduction to absurdity). In this form of argumentation, one takes a claim or argument of another person and demonstrates that it logically leads to an absurdity like a contradiction. Since contradictions cannot be rationally maintained, there must be something wrong with the original claim or argument. In this case the logical consequence of self-contradicting judgments of piety indicates something must be wrong with Euthyphro's definition.

Euthyphro then proposes a second definition, a revision of his first that attempts to take account of Socrates' critical analysis: piety is what *all* the gods love. This qualification of "all" would prevent the logical problem of the first definition. But that of course does not mean that this definition does not have problems of its own. As part of his investigation into this definition, Socrates asks Euthyphro whether what is pious is pious because the gods love it or the gods love it because it is pious. Euthyphro answers the latter. If it were the former, the attribution of piety would depend on no more than the gods' fancy. Euthyphro seems to intuitively recognize this and find it an unacceptable foundation for piety. However, the latter option implies that piety depends on a quality or qualities independent of the gods' love. Thus, while it may be true that the gods love what is pious, that love would not be the essential, defining quality of the pious.

This part of the dialogue illustrates other important aspects of philosophizing. First, beyond the meaning of concepts, philosophical investigation also includes analysis of logical connections among concepts and the beliefs and claims related to them. Generally speaking, two claims can be logically connected in a number of ways.

1. *Logical Implication.* To say that one claim logically implies another means that the truth of one guarantees the truth of the other. For example, the claim that the gods love what is pious because it is pious, not the other way around, implies that the essence of piety is a quality independent of the gods' love.
2. *Logical Incompatibility.* A second logical connection is that of logical incompatibility. Two claims are logically incompatible if they cannot both be true. For example, let us assume Euthyphro's definition that piety is what the gods love. And let us suppose that Zeus loves when people sacrifice goats, but Hera hates this practice. This would mean that goat sacrifice is pious and also that goat sacrifice is impious. The two claims contained in the previous sentence are logically incompatible. It cannot be true that goat sacrifice is both pious and impious.
3. *Logical Contingency.* Additionally, claims that have no logical connection between them are "contingently related," meaning that the truth (or falsity) of each is completely independent of the truth (or falsity) of the other. For example, the claims "A square is a polygon" and "The moon is made of green cheese" are contingent. The truth or falsity of one is wholly independent of the truth or falsity of the other.

This exchange also illustrates the critical nature of philosophy. Now, some caveats are in order at this point. The word "critical" is commonly understood negatively and perceived negatively. Colloquially, it is understood to refer to degrading language, insults, and so forth. Philosophically, however, to be critical means to investigate the limits of any concept or claim. Socrates is clearly employing this critical function of philosophy regarding the concept of piety and Euthyphro's definitions of piety. This "critical" function is also less negative than the colloquial understanding of the word in that by Socrates uncovering logical problems with Euthyphro's definition, we get a little closer to an actual, accurate definition. By cutting away flawed ideas, we get closer to good ideas.

In addition to this critical function of philosophy, philosophy also has a more patently positive function, often called speculative philosophy: "Its business is to take over all aspects of human experience, to reflect upon them, and to try to think out a view of Reality, as a whole which shall do justice to all of them" (Broad, 1968, p. 18). Speculative philosophy presupposes a certain amount of critical philosophy as part of its function. Broad theories of reality are composed as attempts to reach a coherent, holistic understanding of our World and our place in it. Critical philosophy operates within speculative to test these theories and the many elements of them, to cut away what does not make sense and leave what does.

After Socrates' critical analysis of Euthyphro's definitions of piety, Euthyphro becomes obviously frustrated. Socrates asks Euthyphro to stay and take the discussion further, but Euthyphro begs off saying he must go. It is common for students to conclude from this discussion that there is no definition (or at least no single definition) of piety and that this further is the belief of Socrates and/or Plato. Neither of these conclusions, however, is logically implied or supported by the dialogue. If we take Socrates at his word, he wishes to continue the discussion, indicating that he believes a definition is at least possible. Further, the fact that two proposed definitions of piety have failed does not entail that the discovery of a definition is not possible. And given that the lack of a definition is not logically entailed and that it is unlikely that Socrates believes there is no definition, it seems also unlikely that the author, Plato, means to communicate that there is no definition. However, nothing here proves there is a single definition of piety. Thus, as Socrates suggests, more discussion is warranted.

The character Euthyphro is often seen as representative of a dogmatic, anti-philosophical way of thinking. His knowledge claims and his confidence (even arrogance) in his expertise on all things pious are based on his reading of books. He places unquestioning faith in these books and never seems to have critically reflected upon what he learned from them. When his expertise and beliefs are seriously challenged, he retreats rather than engage in self-discovery or truth-seeking.

From Socrates we see a very different attitude, what might be called a philosophical attitude. First, Socrates does not fancy himself an expert—on this or any other subject. Instead, he professes ignorance. Professing ignorance, ironically, from a Socratic viewpoint, is the beginning of wisdom. If you believe you know already, then there is no place to go, nothing to learn. If you recognize your limitations, do not assume expertise, you will be more open to learning, to critical reflection, to entertaining new ideas and not dogmatically holding on to old ones. Second, at the end Socrates seems to wish to continue. He does not fear critical discussion but seeks it. For, what he seems to wish more than being right or being seen as wise and knowledgeable by others is the truth. On the path toward truth, Socrates asserts, one must follow the logic where it leads. This principle suggests truth may be contrary to one's present, even cherished beliefs and desires and that there is a standard of truth (based upon logic and rationality) independent of any individual's subjective emotions, desires, and beliefs. This independent standard is traditionally the standard against which philosophers measure themselves.

One final lesson from *Euthyphro* takes us back to the misconceptions of philosophy. Philosophy is commonly viewed as a solitary practice: the lonely philosopher turned inward in an act of solipsistic contemplation and introspection. It is understandable that people perceive philosophy this way as philosophy itself (especially modern philosophy) has encouraged this perception. But in reality, philosophy is largely a collaborative activity. The Socratic dialogues are premised on the belief that no one person can be assumed to have the truth of any matter, but through critical discussion of many perspectives and divergent thoughts, philosophers are more likely to reach or at least get near to the truth—as Socrates attempts to do with the collaborative help of Euthyphro. Today, it is true that most philosophers work largely alone, writing their own papers, their own books. But at the same time, the large majority of philosophers work in an academic setting as part of the philosophy faculty of a college or university. In addition, even though most philosophers may be alone when writing their papers and books,[1] once these works are presented to the community through publication, they become part of philosophical discourse—an enlarged

---

[1]Philosophers may occasionally collaborate on books and papers, but this type of collaboration is not the norm that it is in the sciences.

version of a Socratic dialogue one might say. Thus, just as no one character in a Socratic dialogue is presumed to have the truth, no one philosophical paper or book today is presumed to have the truth. But each published paper and book is a contribution to the philosophical discourse as a whole, which is aimed at reaching the truth through critical and speculative philosophical discourse.

A LITTLE LOGIC

Logic, traditionally, is the basis of philosophical thought. Logic is also a word often misused and distorted in colloquial discourse but most simply refers to the manner in which *statements* (also called "propositions") are rationally connected. First, then, we have to understand what a statement is. A statement (or proposition) is the thought behind an indicative sentence. An indicative sentence makes a claim that is or could be true or false. For example, "Albany is the capital of New York," "Water boils at 100° C," "The moon is made of green cheese," "I am in Philadelphia" are all indicative sentences. They all are either true or false. This criterion of being true or false typically excludes sentences that are questions or commands. Although, at times sentences that are explicitly questions or commands can imply statements. Rhetorical questions often imply statements. For example, in a debate on abortion one might say, "But abortion is murder and isn't murder wrong?" In this case, the speaker is not literally asking whether murder is wrong. That claim is widely accepted or even true by definition. What they are really saying is "Murder is wrong." Rhetorical questions are often used to sneak in questionable statements without providing needed support. Critical thinkers should recognize when this deceptive technique is used and not use it themselves. Logically, what is of interest about indicative sentences is the meaning behind the sentence (the statement or proposition), not the sentence or words of the sentence, because a statement can be expressed in many different sentences. For example, the statement, "I am in Philadelphia" could also be expressed as "My present location is Philadelphia." Although as a matter of practice this distinction is not always made explicitly, and you will find philosophers and logicians use "sentence" instead of "statement," the conceptual distinction is still always in mind.

Statements are used to construct *arguments*. "Argument" is often used colloquially to refer to a quarrel. Philosophically, it has a more specific definition: a set of statements, one of which is given support or reasons for belief by the others(s). The statement which is "given support" is called the conclusion. The statement(s) supporting are called premises. In an argument, premises are meant to logically lead to the conclusion. Here is a simple argument that Aristotle, the first Western philosopher to systematize logic, used as a heuristic:

> All men are mortal.
> Socrates is a man.
> Therefore, Socrates is mortal.

The first two statements are premises which logically lead to the third statement, the conclusion. In fact, if you just read the premises, the conclusion would likely jump to mind before reading it. This mental process is called making an inference. Upon reading the premises you infer the conclusion. Inferring and implying are often confused processes and words. "Inferring" is a mental process we perform. "Implying" is less a process or activity than a quality of statements. So here we *infer* the conclusion from the premises, but the premises *imply* the conclusion. Or another person can use explicit statements to imply to us something she is not explicitly saying. Here again we would be inferring from their claims. Of course logical implications are not always as clear as this and need to be drawn out through logical analysis.

One further thing to note about statements and arguments is that no statement is in itself a premise or a conclusion. Its status as a premise or conclusion is determined by the argument context, its relationship to the other statements in the argument. The conclusion of the above argument could be a premise of some other argument:

> Socrates is mortal.
> All mortal beings die.
> Therefore, Socrates will die.

This relative quality of statements leads to a problem in argumentation. For any argument to be good, the premises must be true or accepted as true. So each premise might be subject to needing proof, to arguments supporting them. And the premises of these arguments may be subject to needing proof. This process needs to stop somewhere. To prevent an infinite regress of proof, ultimately premises that are either self-evidently true or commonly accepted as true must be employed. A self-evident truth would be like an axiom in geometry or a self-defining statement. It is so clearly true that no one could dispute it. A commonly accepted truth may not be self-evidently true but is a basic element of most people's background knowledge. To prove such a statement would be a waste of time. Founding arguments on premises like these provides solid, common ground for investigation of an issue.

Generally speaking, two types of argumentation or reasoning are recognized: *deductive* and *inductive.* In deductive reasoning, one claims to argue to a certainty, that the conclusion is necessitated by the premises. The two arguments above are deductive. But this leaves the question of whether they are *good* deductive arguments. Deductive arguments are evaluated on the basis of two qualities. The first is **validity**. The word "valid" is colloquially used as a vague synonym for good, but in deductive logic it has a specific meaning. To say that an argument is valid is to say that the conclusion *is* necessitated by the premises. In other words, if the premises are true, then the conclusion must also be true. Consider Aristotle's argument above. If the two premises are accepted as true, the conclusion must also be true. If you think closely about it, you will realize that there is no way you can deny the conclusion (say it is false) but accept the premises (say they are all true). This leads to another way of thinking about validity: in a valid argument it is impossible to deny the conclusion but accept (all) the premises.

Consider this next simple argument:

> All men are over 7 feet tall.
> Socrates is a man.
> Therefore, Socrates is over 7 feet tall.

Many students upon seeing this argument will immediately judge it invalid, because the first premise is clearly false. But it is in fact valid. Consider the definition of validity again: *if* the premises are true *then* the conclusion must be true. There is nothing in this definition about the actual truth of the premises or the conclusion, just what would logically follow *if* the premises were true. And a little thought should demonstrate that if the premises of this last argument were true, so would be the conclusion. That is, if it were true that all men were over 7 feet tall and that Socrates was a man, then it would of necessity be true that Socrates is over 7 feet tall. Validity then is not about the actual truth of the claims involved but the logical connection between them. The other quality of deductive arguments is *soundness*. For an argument to be sound it must (a) be valid and (b) have all true (or at least accepted as true) premises. Being valid and having true premises then guarantees that the conclusion will be true and will be accepted as true by any rational person.

In inductive reasoning one claims to argue to a probability, that the conclusion follows with a degree of probability from the premises. For example,

> Most philosophers have a pro-choice view on abortion.
> Don Marquis is a philosopher.
> Therefore, Don Marquis is pro-choice.

Given that most philosophers think this way and that Don Marquis is a philosopher, it is likely that Don Marquis is pro-choice. It is likely, but it does not necessarily follow. And thus even in a good inductive argument there is a possibility that the conclusion is false even when all the premises are true. And in this case the conclusion does turn out to be false. The evaluation of inductive arguments is quite loose compared to that of deductive arguments. Inductive arguments are judged as weak or strong depending upon the probability of the truth of the conclusion based on the premises. Validity as a quality of deductive argument is absolute. An argument is either valid or invalid. There is no in between, no gray area. Inductive arguments admit of degrees of strength, and hence, a weaker inductive argument may be made stronger. But a deductive argument that is invalid will forever be invalid.

Two of the most common types of inductive arguments, and argument types especially relevant to the study of science, are generalizations and casual arguments. In generalizations, one asserts a quality of a sample of a population and infers that that quality applies to the whole of a population. A generalization could be as simple as not trusting Ford cars because one has had the experience of a few unreliable Ford cars or as complex as a statistical generalization. In a causal argument one infers from a set of repeated observations that one event causes or brings about a second event. As noted, these types of arguments are especially relevant to the study of science and the process and problems of these argument types will be addressed in later chapters.

There is one further type of reasoning but one that is not always recognized as a distinct type of reasoning. American philosopher Charles Sanders Peirce (1839–1914) identified abductive logic as distinct from both deductive and inductive reasoning. Also called "inference to the best explanation," Peirce identified abductive reasoning as the reasoning process by which initial hypotheses are reached in science—but not tested. The reasoning process is encapsulated in the statement, "If A were true, C would be a matter of course" (Peirce, 1955, p. 152), where C is some observed fact or event and A is a proposed explanation for C. Abductive reasoning is exemplified in the medical school aphorism, "When you hear hoof beats, think horses, not zebras." The best explanation for the sound of hoof beats in our part of the world is horses, as we do not have many zebras in our environment. So, even though it is logically and physically possible that the hoof beats you here are caused by zebras, zebras are not the best explanation. Given that abductive reasoning is employed in hypothesis construction and hypotheses, by their nature, are in need of testing, abductive reasoning is not a very strong form of reasoning. Yet it is, arguably, a form of reasoning we all use successfully in our everyday lives.

With some basics and fundamentals of philosophy in mind then we can begin our studies of science as a philosophical issue hopefully a little better prepared.

CRITICAL THINKING QUESTIONS

1. What misconceptions of philosophy did you have before reading this chapter?
2. Many sciences today were once considered branches of philosophy. What makes these sciences today and no longer philosophy?
3. How would you describe Euthyphro's character? How does that contrast with Socrates' character?
4. Socrates claimed to be ignorant. Was this true? Was he being sincere in saying this? Why might he make such a claim?
5. Euthyphro bases his expertise on having read all the books on piety, on the gods and dictums of right and wrong. In our culture we value learning from books. So what is wrong with Euthyphro's claims to expertise?
6. From this brief introduction to philosophy, what value can you find for nursing in studying philosophy?
7. How might you go about defining "nursing" in the manner Euthyphro and Socrates attempt to define piety?
8. Consider the statement "All nurses are college graduates." Which of the following statements are incompatible with this statement? Answers to 8, 9, and 10 are at the bottom of the page.[2]
    (a) No nurses are college graduates.
    (b) Some nurses are college graduates.
    (c) Some nurses are not college graduates.
9. Consider the statement "All nurses are college graduates." Which of the following statements are logically implied by this statement?
    (a) All college graduates are nurses.
    (b) Some nurses are college graduates.
    (c) Some college graduates are nurses.
    (d) Some college graduates are not nurses.

---

[2]8. a, c. 9. b, c. 10. a.

10. If all coodles are stroodles and all poodles are coodles, then which of the following statements follows logically?
    (a) All poodles are stroodles.
    (b) All stroodles are poodles.

REFERENCES

Broad, C. D. (1968). Critical and speculative philosophy. In J. Margolis (Ed.), *An introduction to philosophical inquiry: Contemporary and classical sources* (pp. 9–21). New York: Alfred A. Knopf.

Margolis, J. (1968). Introduction. In J. Margolis (Ed.), *An introduction to philosophical inquiry: Contemporary and classical sources* (pp. 1–8). New York: Alfred A. Knopf.

Peirce, C. S. (1955). Abduction and induction. In J. Buchler (Ed.), *Philosophical writings of Peirce* (pp. 150–156). New York, NY: Dover.

Plato (2003). *Theatetus* (F. M. Cornford, Trans.). In *Plato's theory of knowledge: The Theatetus and the Sophist* (pp. 15–163). Mineola, NY: Dover.

Robison, J., & Carrier, K. (2004). *The spirit and science of holistic health: More than broccoli, jogging, and bottled water . . . more than yoga, herbs, and meditation.* Bloomington, IN: Authorhouse.

Whitehead, A. N. (1978). *Process and reality.* New York, NY: The Free Press.

Woodhouse, M. B. (2006). *A preface to philosophy.* Belmont, CA: Wadsworth.

5

The Scientific Revolution

*History, if viewed as a repository for more than anecdote or chronology, could produce
a decisive transformation in the image of science by which we are now possessed.*

THOMAS KUHN

WHAT IS SCIENCE? HOW ABOUT *WHEN* IS SCIENCE?

When "science" actually began is itself a question of some historical and philosophical
significance and debate. One view, sometimes called the "continuist" view holds that
science has developed over millennia stretching back to ancient Greece. Continuists
look to the earliest Western philosophers in the 6th century B.C.E. as the beginning of
science (Lindberg, 2007). Thales (ca. 624–546 B.C.E.), who is traditionally identified
as the first Western philosopher, was interested in the question of the basic structure
of the universe. He theorized that everything was in fact a form of water. As
unusual as that claim may sound to our ears, the basic concept is common in theoretical physics today. Theoretical physicists search for that (particle, energy, etc.) which is
most basic, that composes everything else, that all else can be explained through. The
philosophers who followed Thales (often called pre-Socratic philosophers) pursued
much the same question reaching different answers. Anaximenes (ca. 585–525 B.C.E.)
argued that the most basic element, of which all else was made, was air. He explained
that air took different shapes and forms due to the relative contraction and expansion
of the particles of air. Heraclitus (535–475 B.C.E.) maintained that fire was most basic,
though his meaning was largely metaphoric. The philosophers Leucippus (500–450
B.C.E.) and Democritus (460–370 B.C.E.) composed in part an ancient school of philosophy known as atomism, which held that everything was composed of tiny, irreducible bits of matter called atoms (literally, indivisible). By far the most "scientific" of the
philosophers of the ancient world was Aristotle (384–322 B.C.E.). His famous teacher,
Plato (428–347 B.C.E.), was much more interested in ideal metaphysical worlds, and
Plato's teacher, Socrates (460–399 B.C.E.), was more interested in morality and the
human soul. Aristotle studied and categorized plants and animals, theorized on the
motion of matter, and composed the original laws of logic from which warranted
knowledge could be drawn. Aristotle's physical laws dominated the study of the
natural world until superseded by the mechanistic physics of Newton 2000 years

later. His zoological and botanical categories structured the biological sciences until Darwin revolutionized that field in the 19th century. His logical system defined logic until the development of propositional logic in the late 19th and early 20th centuries by Gottlob Frege (1848–1925), Bertrand Russell (1872–1970), and Alfred North Whitehead (1861–1947).

An opposing view, a discontinuist view, identifies science as a modern development part of a larger cultural movement called the Enlightenment (Lindberg, 2007). In this view, "science" marks a change from the past, from ways of thinking identified with the ancient world, the Middle Ages and the Renaissance. The Enlightenment itself is typically identified as marking a conceptual and cultural change. Most historical eras are named later by historians looking back. The Enlightenment is rare in that it is a historical era that named itself. If you think about it, that seems to reveal a bit of hubris. The implication is that *we* are "enlightened." Those in the past were merely living in darkness and ignorance. As amusing or half-joking as that characterization may seem to be, there is more than a hint of truth to it. The Enlightenment is traditionally understood as a time in which old ways of thinking were shed. Tradition, ritual, superstition, and even religion to an extent were rejected as standards or guarantors of knowledge. Instead, the Enlightenment view advocated rationality, empirical observation, and personal autonomy and judgment in asserting and certifying knowledge claims. Whether one accepts the continuist or the discontinuist view, the Enlightenment marks an important moment in the development of human society and knowledge in the West. Under the continuist view, the advancements in science were especially productive during this period. Under the discontinuist view, the Enlightenment brought a "scientific revolution" that fundamentally changed the way in which we understand the world, the way in which we look at and investigate the world. One possible way around this conflict is to refer to the science that followed the scientific revolution as "modern science." From either perspective, the scientific revolution seems an important era in understanding the nature and development of what we know as science today.

MODERN SCIENCE

Temporally speaking, the term "scientific revolution" refers primarily to the 17th century; although some proto-revolutionary events can be identified in the 16th century and many of the changes did not fully coalesce until the 18th or even 19th century. Even people of this period noted a radical difference or even break in thought, as indicated by the use of the word "new" in the titles of many works: Francis Bacon's *New Organon* (1620), Johannes Kepler's *A New Astronomy* (1609), Galileo Galilei's *Two New Sciences* (1638). It may also be worth noting that the word "science," as we use it today, was not coined until the 19th century. So from a linguistic point of view, there was no such thing as science until the 1800s, until well into this new way of thinking. Prior to this coinage, much of what we would call "science" today was called natural philosophy. Also, much of what we would call science today (specific fields like demography, statistics, information science, etc.) did not exist at all.

To see the causes of the Scientific Revolution, we must look to the wider cultural changes that took place during the Renaissance (roughly 14th to 16th centuries). The

Renaissance was a period of great discovery made possible by the invention of the magnetic compass. Two other influential inventions of this period were gunpowder and the movable-type printing press (Henry, 2002). These technological advances influenced the religious changes of the Reformation and changes in economic and political structures—the development from feudalism and aristocracy to a burgeoning of capitalism and democracy. These cultural changes together can be seen as establishing an increasing sense of personal and social identity, which led intellectuals to an increasing concern with history and interest in locating oneself as an intellectual heir to Ancient Rome and Greece. Thus, the Renaissance "man" was working "his" way out of the overarching rule of the Church and the self-effacement and self-renunciation of a strict Christian worldview. The intellectual side of this working out manifested itself in the development of what was called *studia humanitas,* a group of studies that, influenced by the long-neglected Greeks and Romans, celebrated the achievements and potentialities of mankind (Henry, 2002). Humanists, as these new intellectuals came to be called, emphasized the importance of the active life lived for the public good, which they held as superior to the contemplative life indicative of the outlook of the Scholastics—the leading school of thought of the late Middle Ages. The Scholastics (or Schoolmen as they were sometimes also called) expressed an almost religious devotion to the work of Aristotle. The Humanists questioned the authority of Aristotle and recognized the importance and contributions of other Greek philosophers. This questioning of Aristotle and recognition of other ancient intellects led further to a renewed interest in mathematics and magic (Henry, 2002). And authority as a form of knowledge came to be seen as misleading and unreliable, leading to an increasing emphasis on discovering truth for oneself. A dramatic example of this questioning authority and thinking for oneself is when physician Paracelsus (1493–1541)—sometimes referred to as the Copernicus of medicine—threw Avicenna's *Canon* (the accepted book of medicine of the time) into the fire to protest the unquestioned acceptance of this book. A broader example would be the Reformation. What Luther championed was individual and direct relationships to God, as opposed to the model of the Catholic Church in which one's relationship to God was mediated by the hierarchical structure of the Church (Davis & Winship, 2002). In Luther's view of Christianity, every person is an authority on religion, not just priests and above. This idea is reflected in the early Protestant encouragement of "regular people" to read the Bible.

Although the Reformation was a questioning of the Church, religion was not critically questioned much itself. Rather, the view of religion expanded in many ways to include more often a consideration of this world. It became common, for example, to refer to nature as "God's other book." This is a notion clearly similar to the view of nature held in the Scientific Revolution and in the Enlightenment in general. Copernicus, Newton, Galileo, and most other great intellects of the Scientific Revolution saw science as almost a divine study, in that by studying the universe one may commune with God's creation and even come closer to God. These changes ultimately set the stage for the development of a new experiential or empiricist approach to the understanding of the physical world.

The development and establishment of what is usually taken to be the characteristic methodology of science (the scientific method) has always been regarded as constitutive of the Scientific Revolution. The two main elements of this scientific method are the use of mathematics and measurement to give precise determinations of how the world and its parts work, and the use of observation, experience, and, where necessary, artificially constructed experiments, to gain understanding of nature.

Mathematization

The mathematization of nature indicates a fundamental change in all concepts of the physical world, introducing a Platonic or Pythagorean way of looking at the world, replacing the Aristotelian metaphysics of medieval natural philosophy. Certainly, the Medieval world knew of and studied mathematics. However, the conception of mathematics in the middle ages and in the Renaissance was one that saw mathematics as an isolated, insular study. This mathematical view is now known as instrumentalism: mathematics is an interesting study of its own, but it has no connection or relation to the real world or anything deeper and more significant. The Scientific Revolution developed a "realist" view of mathematics in which it is believed that mathematical analysis reveals deeper truths about the world. If a calculation works, it must work because the broader theory from which it springs must also be true and reflect a truth about the world. This realist view can be seen in the work of Copernicus. No matter how contrary to natural philosophy the motion of the earth may seem, Copernicus insisted, it must be true because the mathematics demands it. This was revolutionary. Johannes Kepler too assumed a connection between mathematics and reality in his discovery that the orbits of the planets comprised ellipses not circles. No one could directly observe the orbits of the planets. It had been accepted since the time Aristotle said that the planets moved in circular orbits, as the circle was considered the most perfect and divine two-dimensional shape. The Scholastics accepted this claim and its "reasoning" from Aristotle without question. Kepler saw that the claim did not fit the numbers and reached the (still accepted) elliptical conclusion that did fit the numbers. Descartes, in his *Discourse on Method* (1637), developed a new metaphysics which provided the basis of a new, more mathematical system of physics. Newton's *Principia Mathematica Philosophiae Naturalis* (1687) can be seen as the culminating point in the mathematization of the world picture. It was even believed by some scientists of the time that a mathematical view, given its precision, rigor, and possible mirroring of nature, "could also improve works on politics, morals, literary criticism, even public speaking . . ." (Hankins, 1985, p. 2).

Experimentation

One of the characterizing features of the Scientific Revolution is the replacement of the self-evident "experience" which formed the basis of scholastic natural philosophy with a notion of knowledge demonstrated by experiments specifically designed for the purpose. This new approach to observation emphasized measurement and quantification. Previous natural philosophy, influenced by an Aristotelian worldview, was concerned with qualities rather than quantities. For example, the nature of specific things was determined in part by the "natural" location in space. Those things naturally of earth were qualitatively different from celestial bodies (planets, stars, etc.) or even those things naturally existing in the sky (clouds, atmosphere, etc.). The Scientific Revolution emphasized, rather, quantities: objects are defined by the many ways in which they can be objectively measured. Qualitative descriptions came to be seen as subjective and unreliable from an epistemological and scientific point of view. This emphasis on measurement moved forward the integration of observation and mathematics in science and led to the invention of more precise and sophisticated instruments for objective, mathematical observation in the 16th and 17th centuries: the telescope, the microscope, the barometer, the air-pump, the thermometer.

It may sound strange to contemporary ears, but alchemy and magic were both significant influences on the development of experimentation in modern science. Keep in mind that alchemy had always been experimental in nature. The underlying assumptions many alchemists were working with may have been mistaken and even unfounded, but their methodology was always experimental. As for magic, what magic means in this context is not merely supernatural, but also refers to aspects of nature. The medieval and renaissance understanding of the term "magic" was the study of occult forces. Again, "occult" is a term that in modern usage has taken on merely supernatural meanings, but what "occult" referred to was the power of natural things to move or affect other natural things at a distance. The most obvious example of this is magnetism. A magnet can draw metal to itself and cause it to move without appearing to touch it. Based on the belief that certain things have hidden, occult powers, natural magicians needed knowledge of physical bodies and how they act upon one another. During the Scientific Revolution, the naturalistic elements of magic were separated from other aspects of magic. Our understanding of magic today is what is left over with those naturalistic aspects removed. For us magic deals with the supernatural. For natural magicians, only God could bring about supernatural events. The natural elements of magic were absorbed into natural philosophy. The use of magic to affect the natural world also closely connected magic to technology in the middle ages and renaissance.

In the most general terms, the Scientific Revolution introduced a completely different worldview, replacing a medieval/renaissance teleological world with a modern mechanistic world. The medieval worldview, again influenced by Aristotle, was one in which (a) space is differentiated, (b) all natural objects have animate qualities, and (c) phenomena are explained in relation to purposes, ends or goals (*telic*). The idea that space is differentiated has been referred to earlier. Those things naturally of the earth are qualitatively and essentially different from those things of the air or of the heavens. Following this differentiation of space is the attribution of seemingly animate qualities to natural objects. The reason solid objects fall to the earth is that they have in them a "desire" (what Aristotle called *entelechy*, literally "to have one's end within") to be in their natural place. The natural place for solid (earth-bound or earth-based) objects is the earth, the center of the universe. Smoke and steam dissipate in the air because that is what their entelechy draws them to do, to be with air itself. Flames flicker to the sky because they wish to be with the fire in the heavens. Even two drops of water brought near each other will reach out to one another. The general physical principle here is "like attracts like." Finally, then, movement is explained in this worldview in terms of ends or purposes, what is called a teleological view from the Greek *telos* for end, purpose or goal. Things act to achieve goals. Heavy objects fall to achieve their end of reclaiming their natural place on the earth. The same can be said from above regarding the movement of smoke, steam, fire, and water.

The modern worldview, however, is oriented around a mechanical philosophy, not an animate and teleological one. Phenomena are explained in terms of the mathematical discipline of mechanics: shape, size, quantity, and motion. Events (the actions and movements of physical objects) are explained in terms of physical causes through contact with other physical objects. Thus, occult properties (magnetism, light, gravity) would similarly have to be explained by mechanical principles: the motion and interaction of particles too small to be seen. This leads to another claim of mechanical philosophy: material bodies are composed of invisibly small atoms or corpuscles. The mechanical philosophy of Descartes was the most influential. He defined matter solely in terms of extension (that is, matter is defined merely as that which extends in, or takes up, space), allowing him to claim that physics could be based upon the geometrical analysis of extended bodies in motion. He thus relates the whole of the material world to one of his most well-known mathematical creations: analytic geometry. This extreme emphasis on mathematics, however, also reveals a more rationalist than empiricist orientation in his thinking. Descartes' system was based less on empirical experiment than on the mathematical certainty of an axiomatic structure with supposedly indubitable foundations and careful deduction of phenomena from these foundations. Rather than careful, mathematically precise observation, a Cartesian "experiment" tended to look like a report of what must happen, assuming that Descartes' reasoning is correct.

Mechanical philosophy in England was much more empirically based, as can be seen in the work of Robert Boyle and of Isaac Newton. Mechanical philosophy in England also differed from that on the continent by commonly attributing active powers to particles of matter, whereas Descartes and other philosophers of the continent tended to view matter as completely inert. In the view of Descartes the only active agents were *non-material* minds or souls which acted upon inert matter. But in England it was widely believed that particles of matter may be endowed with active principles which might account for occult phenomena such as magnetism, gravity, and chemical properties, but which could still be dealt with in natural philosophy by means of experimental demonstration. Mechanical philosophy in its widest sense viewed the universe as a giant clock, which worked in a regular, fixed manner due to its organized mechanical structure. But this mechanistic view was thoroughgoing and worked down to other levels of study including the vital processes of living creatures (e.g., the nervous system, respiration, and circulation), leading to a new concept of living creatures as *bêtes-machines*, which would always act in accordance with the laws of mechanics.

Religion and Culture

It is common today to see religion and science as in conflict. During the Scientific Revolution there was some conflict, but the two were not always in conflict. Certainly the most well-known conflict between religion and science was the Catholic Church's condemnation of Copernicus and Galileo. The actual history of the Church's attitude toward Copernicus and the Church's dealings with and relationship with Galileo is quite complex and cannot be simply reduced to an issue of knowledge versus ignorance (Blackwell, 2002). One of the major goals and motivations of early modern scientists (including Keller, Gasse, Newton, Boyle, and Descartes) was to show how God interacted with the mechanical world (Osler, 2002). Some saw the universe as a huge clock and God as the clockmaker. Thus, studying science became a means of studying God's creation and by extension coming closer to God. Some even tried to use their studies to defeat atheism leading to the rise of natural theology and deism: a rational approach to religion and spirituality that saw God in the beautiful order and regularity of the universe.

The Scientific Revolution coincided with the beginnings of modern capitalism. So, it seems impossible to dismiss the economic factors that played an important role in the rise of science. Some also argue that some important political developments were influenced by both the evolving method of doing science and on new scientific beliefs (Henry, 2002). New political arrangements had to be justified in terms of the arrangement of nature if they were to be seen as natural and feasible. This emphasis on nature can be seen in the political philosophies of Thomas Hobbes, John Locke, Jean-Jacques Rousseau and others. Hobbes' major political work *Leviathan* makes a biological metaphor to build a theory of the state. More explicitly, political philosopher James Harrington's (1611–1677) *Oceana* drew heavily upon William Harvey's (1578–1657) discoveries of the functioning of the heart and the circulatory system to construct his view of the proper political state—justified largely because of its mirroring of human physiology (Cohen, 1994).

CONCLUSION

The scientific revolution is a complex phenomenon in itself and part of a larger complex social change in the West. No one year or even century can be pointed to as the beginning of what we know as modern science. The development of modern science occurred over centuries with an extended transition period in which old and new ideas existed together, in which studies we might call irrational and superstitious (alchemy, magic, numerology) were practiced by the great heroes of early modern science. More broadly, the Enlightenment effected social, cultural, and political changes that still affect us today. The fundamental presuppositions of many of these changes have been challenged during the past century, yet science remains our prime method of understanding and investigating the world geared toward (mostly) making life better.

CRITICAL THINKING QUESTIONS

1. Does "science" begin with the Scientific Revolution or at some time before?
2. In what ways are Enlightenment views and values still active and effective on our contemporary society?
3. In what ways are Enlightenment views and values challenged today?
4. What examples of mathematizing our world and our experience can you point to?
5. What value is there in mathematizing those aspects of our world?
6. What drawbacks may there be to such mathematization?

7. What makes an experiment more than mere experience? What function does this serve for science?
8. The mechanistic worldview introduced in the Scientific Revolution arguably led to great advances in knowledge and technology, but what possible drawbacks might there be to replacing a teleological worldview with a mechanistic one?
9. Are religion and science necessarily in conflict or can they co-exist?
10. Is it possible to be a theist (Christian or otherwise) and still accept the Darwinian theory of biological evolution?

REFERENCES

Blackwell, R. J. (2002). Galileo Galilei. In G. B. Ferngren (Ed.), *Science and religion: A historical introduction* (pp. 105–116). Baltimore, MD: The Johns Hopkins University Press.

Cohen, I. B. (1994). Harrington and Harvey: A theory of the state based on the new physiology. *Journal of the History of Ideas, 55*(2), 187–210.

Davis, E. B., & Winship, M. P. (2002). Early modern Protestantism. In G. B. Ferngren (Ed.), *Science and religion: A historical introduction* (pp. 117–129). Baltimore, MD: The Johns Hopkins University Press.

Hankins, T. L. (1985). *Science and the enlightenment.* Cambridge, UK: Cambridge University Press.

Henry, J. (2002). *The scientific revolution and the origins of modern science.* Hampshire, UK: Palgrave.

Kuhn, T. S. (1996). *The structure of scientific revolutions.* Chicago, IL: The University of Chicago Press.

Lindberg, D. C. (2007). *The beginnings of western science: The European scientific tradition in philosophical, religious, and institutional context, prehistory to A.D. 1450.* Chicago, IL: The University of Chicago Press.

Osler, M. J. (2002). Mechanical philosophy. In G. B. Ferngren (Ed.), *Science and religion: A historical introduction* (pp. 143–152). Baltimore, MD: The Johns Hopkins University Press.

6

One Hundred Years of the Philosophy of Science: A Historical Overview

We may best hope to understand the nature and conditions of real knowledge, by studying the nature and conditions of the most certain and stable portions of knowledge which we already possess . . . to learn the best methods of discovering truth, by examining how truths . . . have really been discovered.

WILLIAM WHEWELL

INTRODUCTION

The purpose of this chapter is to provide a historical overview of the philosophy of science prior to delving more deeply into specific questions, problems, and issues. Philosophy is a type of discourse. It grows and changes through the communication of ideas between thinkers. An idea is put forth. This idea inspires thought elsewhere and that idea is built upon or criticized with the ultimate goal of reaching some notion of truth or at least more in-depth knowledge. Then this new idea or criticism inspires thought elsewhere and the discussion continues. In order to have a clear and comprehensive understanding of any specific issue or idea, the historical context of how this issue developed, the myriad answers posited, becoming aware of the complex discourse surrounding it is necessary. Without this background knowledge understanding will always be incomplete and superficial.

Although one can find elements of the philosophy of science throughout most of the 2500 years of Western philosophy, as a coherent, clearly identifiable branch of philosophy, it is relatively new. Certainly, some of Aristotle's work may be interpreted as work in the philosophy of science. And the modern era saw much reflection in the study of philosophy in what was occurring as part of the scientific revolution, in the work of René Descartes, David Hume, Thomas Hobbes, and others. And in the 19th century, the work of philosophers such as William Whewell (1794–1866) Charles Sanders Peirce, and John Stuart Mill (1806–1873) may be seen as stage-setting for the emergence of this new branch of philosophy. But the philosophy of science, as a coherent, clearly identifiable branch of philosophy, *is* largely a 20th (and now 21st) century phenomenon. There is a certain understanding of philosophy which holds that a subject becomes a philosophical issue or area of study when it becomes a "problem." This conception of philosophy implies then that during the late 19th and early 20th centuries science was becoming a problem. But what do we mean by "problem" in this context? During the early modern period (late 16th to late 18th centuries) science may be considered something of a problem as it was undergoing such profound changes. This is why we see a reflection of these changes and the philosophical questions they raised in the philosophy of the time. However, as a "problem" it did not rise to such a level as to engender a new branch of philosophy. Rather, it affected the existing branches of philosophy (especially epistemology) in profound ways. Science was a new and powerful tool. It was growing to become the most trusted method of knowledge acquisition. In this way, science was not a problem but—especially from the perspective of the optimistic, even utopian, modern mind— a boon, an unquestioned value, the ultimate expression of humanity's rational and manipulative powers.

The late 19th and early 20th centuries saw changes in both science and philosophical outlooks that made science more problematic. The introduction of quantum mechanics and relativity theory challenged some of the most cherished scientific beliefs of the previous centuries and the presumptions underlying them. For example, the thesis of quantum mechanics that at the subatomic level such basic principles as Newton's Laws of Motion did not apply challenged the belief in the universality of all scientific conclusions and the logic by which they were reached. In addition, as science became increasingly focused on forces and entities not directly observable, the commitment to pure empirical observation and experimentation became more difficult to justify. And in the 19th century the work of philosophers such as Karl Marx, Gottfried Hegel, Søren Kierkegaard, Friedrich Nietzsche, and others began to challenge the modern, utopian mindset. From each side then (the side of science and the side of philosophy) the simple, unchallenged view of science as a pure unalloyed study and value was beginning to falter. In other words, science was beginning to become a "problem." Hence, science was in need of a deeper study, more profound justification and a philosophical critique outlining its strengths and its limitations. In answer to these needs arose the first major school in the philosophy of science: Logical Positivism.

LOGICAL POSITIVISM

Logical positivism arose between the world wars primarily among a group of Austrian intellectuals (philosophers, scientists, and mathematicians) known as the Vienna Circle, which included philosophers Moritz Schlick (1882–1936), Otto Neurath (1882–1945), and Rudolph Carnap (1891–1970). The most general and fundamental thesis of the logical positivists was a strict and new interpretation of empiricism, which included a clear and sometimes virulent rejection and repudiation of metaphysics. In addition, they held common theses regarding science, most notably linguistic theses based upon the analytic–synthetic distinction and verifiability theory of meaning.

Empiricism

In its most general sense, empiricism defines a broad epistemological view in which knowledge is attained, affirmed, and even defined by sensory perception. In this broad sense, empirical views can be found throughout the history of philosophy. The term can also be used to refer to more localized and specified epistemological views, such as those of the logical positivists or the British empiricists. This epistemological view is typically contrasted to that known as rationalism. Rationalists hold that knowledge is attained and affirmed not by sensory perception but by the internal operations of the human mind. In addition, rationalists tend to hold that the human mind contains at birth certain innate ideas: beliefs, statements, or principles that are empirically unprovable but generally accepted as intuitively true. Examples from noted rationalists of innate ideas include the existence of God, the existence of one's self, and the noncontradiction principle, as well as other basic logical and mathematical truths. Rationalists also typically hold that sensory perception does not provide real knowledge because sensory perception is often susceptible to illusion and error, and knowledge is classically understood as both true and lasting. However, much of what we perceive is often not true (e.g., the "bent" pencil in the glass of water) and often not lasting (e.g., even the oldest of mountains we see will one day erode and be no more; even the stars in the sky will one day blink out). Real knowledge (e.g., logical and mathematical truths), according to rationalists, is true and will always be true. Empiricists tend to find this view of knowledge and these "truths" of rationalists somewhat empty and circular. Sure, one may rationally intuit that one and one is two, but until one affirms that that mental function has a relationship to the physical world, it is purely formal and of no use-value. Sure, one may rationally intuit his own existence, but how does this aid him in living in this world, or even understanding the world beyond his own mind?

The logical positivists were especially influenced by the school of empiricism known as British Empiricism. This was a school of philosophy from the 17th and 18th centuries. The primary figures in this school were from the British Isles, hence the name: John Locke (Britain, 1632–1704), George Berkeley (Ireland, 1685–1753), and David Hume (Scotland, 1711–1776). These philosophers were only very loosely connected under the heading of British Empiricism. In detail there were many differences in their thinking. However, most generally it can be said that they all agreed that the primary (if not sole) source of knowledge was sensory perception. They denied the concept of innate ideas. John Locke famously expressed this rejection by declaring the mind a blank slate or *tabula rasa* at birth; all knowledge would then be imprinted on the mind through sensory experience. Also, they tended to see knowledge as reducible to "ideas" or sense data. The word "idea" here is a technical term in the school of British Empiricism. It refers to discrete and specifiable contents of the mind. That is, the concept of, say, "table," is an idea. The memory of a specific table is also an idea. So are the constituent sensory qualities of that table: its color, its shape, its hardness, and the sound produced when knocking upon it. The collection of all these ideas comprises the knowledge contained in our minds. Since there are no innate ideas, these ideas can all be traced back to sense perceptions which enter our minds as discrete sense data, that is, discrete bits of sensory information. According to John Locke, we generate general and abstract ideas like "table" by comparing various specific tables seen, felt, and so forth and abstracting the similar qualities between them.

The British Empiricists interestingly seemed to become more strictly empirical over time. John Locke was willing to accept the existence of some empirically controversial ideas such as God and material substance (the matter that underlies our sense perceptions). George Berkeley argued against the existence of physical matter. These arguments of Berkeley have been infamously lampooned, but they raise an important question regarding a strict adherence to empirical principles. Strictly speaking, all we can "know" are the direct sensory impressions we experience. We do not have direct experience of a substrate of physical matter underlying those sense impressions. Consider the movie *The Matrix* (Andy & Larry Wachowski, 1999). Part of the story of this movie is that people are living an illusion. Presumably, they live lives similar to ours with similar experiences and similar vibrancy of sense impressions. In other words, their world seems just as real to them as ours does to us. However, it isn't. The reality is that people are being kept in pods as sort of batteries for the computers really in charge of the world. The world of sense impressions they experience is in fact a kind of virtual reality piped directly into their brains/minds. So there is no substrate of physical matter underlying these impressions. There is no way to prove that we are not in a similar position, that is, that there *is* a material substrate underlying our experience of the "physical" world. This question raises certain metaphysical problems for any strict empiricist. Berkeley simply accepted the nonexistence of the physical world and maintained that reality was "ideal," i.e., composed of nonphysical or immaterial entities such as ideas, souls, and God. And rather than from a physical substrate, the sense impressions we receive come directly from God. This may seem a rather farfetched view, but there is a spiritual beauty to it. Rather than God having created the universe at one point in the far past, God is continually creating the universe by continually providing the sense impressions that comprise our world. There may also be a theological ulterior motive to Berkeley's position. Throughout the modern era and the scientific revolution, modern science (the subject of which was primarily matter) was in some ways supplanting God in providing explanations for phenomena. To Berkeley, an Anglican Bishop, this may have seemed like an eclipsing of God. By removing matter from the equation and asserting God as the source of all our sense impressions, Berkeley perhaps meant to place God at the center of our conceptual universe again. Now, Berkeley did not deny the knowledge, authority, laws, and advances of science. He merely maintained that the subject of science was not matter but the ideas that come from God. The laws science discovers are real laws but not about matter but about the ideas provided by God. Those ideas describe the structure God gives to our ideal world. So, Berkeley was not really denying reality or the reality of what we know, as some mistakenly assume. He was merely denying that our knowledge was knowledge of, or based upon, physical matter. In fact, this knowledge comes directly from God. It's difficult to get more real than that. Being the last of these British Empiricists, David Hume was arguably the most empirically strict. He recognized the difficulty of proving the existence of matter and remained somewhat agnostic on that question. Regarding the idea of God, Hume was an uncompromising atheist, as we have no direct empirical evidence for God's existence. He even questioned the epistemological authority of causality as a force for which we have no direct empirical experience. We will address that issue in some detail in Chapter 8.

British Empiricism is typically contrasted to the contemporaneous school of philosophy known as Continental Rationalism. The "continental" in the name of this school refers to the fact that this school of philosophy originated in continental Europe as opposed to the British Isles. The three primary philosophers in this school are René Descartes (France, 1596–1650), Baruch Spinoza (The Netherlands, 1632–1677), and Gottfried Leibniz (Germany, 1646–1716). As noted earlier, rationalists tend to hold that real knowledge is a pure product of the mind, based on innate ideas and the mental functions of logic and mathematics. This school of rationalism has been especially criticized for indulgence of metaphysical speculation. From an empiricist point of view, without being grounded in sensory perception, the musings of rationalists have nothing to hold them down, allowing rationalists to posit entities (e.g., Leibniz's monads) that seem to spring directly from the mind with no existential substantiation beyond the mere possibility of their existence. Immanuel Kant (1724–1804) attempted to reconcile the two schools, recognizing the strengths and weaknesses of the two positions, noting that, "though all our knowledge begins with experience, it does not follow that it all arises out of experience" (Kant, 1781/1965, p. 41) and "Thoughts without content are empty, intuitions without concepts are blind" (Kant, 1781/1965, p. 93). Kant argued that although there may not be innate ideas as the Continental Rationalists understood them, there were certain *a priori* innate structures in the human mind that bring comprehensible form to direct sensory experience. Thus, without content (sensory experience) we have an empty mind with a basic structure ready to accept sense impressions, like an empty computer, but no actual knowledge. Without these basic, innate structures, sensory experience is incomprehensible, without form, such as the "blooming, buzzing confusion" of a newborn baby's experience of the world (James, 2007, p. 488). Kant's success in reconciling these schools has been a matter of philosophical debate for the last couple hundred years.

Just as the logical positivists were influenced by empiricism (especially British Empiricism), they also defined themselves against the school of rationalism and the speculative metaphysics to which it gave rise. They expressed a commitment to knowledge based in sensory experience and observation. This attitude reflects also the admiration for science they typically espoused. They seemed to study and critique science out of a love for it and admiration for scientists of their day, like Alfred Einstein. Even more than the metaphysical flights of the Continental Rationalists they reviled the obscurantist (in their view) metaphysical writings of Gottfried Hegel (1770–1831), the most influential post-Kantian German philosopher in the 19th century. They found his writing purposefully obscure, contrary to basic logic and replete with meaningless metaphysical speculation, regarding such mysterious concepts as the Absolute.

Positivism

Another important influence on the logical positivists was the French philosopher Auguste Comte (1798–1857), whose philosophy was known as positivism, the obvious inspiration for half of the term "logical positivism." Comte was also a sociologist, in fact one of the founders of that science. The idea that he is most known for and which was likely most influential on the logical positivists was his law of three phases. He proposed that societies evolve through three identifiable and progressive stages. The first stage, the theological, is one in which a society refers all explanations of phenomena to God or some similar religious concept. The second stage, the metaphysical, is marked by a turn to rational thinking but without a foundation in observation and empirical research. The third stage, the scientific, is the highest stage and marked by a commitment to rational and empirical investigation. This third stage, also in his writings, takes on a utopian character. It is through scientific thinking (not theological or metaphysical) that the human race and human society will be perfected and human goods will be fulfilled. It would be the logical positivists' contention, then, that we are finally (and fortunately) in this final stage of development.

Central Ideas

Logical positivists' views about science and knowledge are based upon a general theory of language formulated around two principles: the analytic–synthetic distinction and the verifiability theory of knowledge. According to the analytic–synthetic distinction statements can be divided into those which are analytic and those which are synthetic. Analytic statements are true or false based merely on their meaning, regardless of how the world really is. One example of an analytic statement is "All bachelors are unmarried." This statement is true because the quality of being unmarried is included within the meaning or definition of "bachelor." Thus, it is also said that analytic statements are true by definition. Another way to describe analytic statements is to say that the predicate (in this case being unmarried) is included in the subject (bachelors). Many philosophers (including the logical positivists) believe that mathematical statements are analytic statements. For example, to say that one and one is two is to say, analytically, that the predicate "two" is included in the subject "one and one." This is what makes mathematics so certain and absolute. The truth of these statements is dependent merely upon the meaning of the terms involved and the logical relationship asserted. Synthetic statements, on the other hand, are true or false based upon both meaning and the states of the world. An example of a synthetic statement would be "All bachelors are short." Synthetic statements are "synthetic" in the sense of bringing disparate elements together. The concept of "shortness" is not included in the concept of "bachelor." Thus, the two are separate, distinct, and brought together ("synthesized") in the statement above. The truth of the statement is dependent upon the meaning of "bachelors," the meaning of "short," the logical relationship asserted between the two, and a state of the world. If the world is such that each and every bachelor is short, then the statement is true. If even one bachelor is not short, then the statement is false.

Logical positivists hold that only synthetic statements can make meaningful claims about the world. That is, there are epistemological implications to these two types of statements. Analytic statements are typically accepted as expressing what is called *a priori* knowledge. "*A priori*" refers to knowledge that is attained without or prior to sensory experience. This is the type of knowledge that rationalists tend to accept and affirm as real knowledge, because it is necessarily true. This necessary truth is expressed through analytic statements due to the predicate being part of the subject. However, that aspect of analytic statements and *a priori* knowledge demonstrates their limitation. Such knowledge is somewhat incestuous. Analytic statements only tell us about the ways in which we use symbols, like "bachelor" and "unmarried." They do not give us information about the world itself. Their truth, meaning, and affirmation are completely contained within the mind. Synthetic statements, on the other hand, assert facts about the world outside the mind. In order to truthfully assert that "all bachelors are short," we must look to the world and attain information through sensory experience. This type of knowledge is called *a posteriori* knowledge: knowledge attained due to or after sensory experience. Being dependent upon sensory experience, synthetic statements, and *a posteriori* knowledge do not have the certainty of analytic statements and *a priori* knowledge, but they are, according to logical positivists, more meaningful. Thus, according to logical positivists, analytic statements, having no concrete information about the world, are empty; while synthetic statements are filled with content and meaningful in that sense.

The verifiability theory of meaning holds that the meaning of a (synthetic) statement is determined, and even defined, by its verification. For example, the meaning of the statement, "Water boils at 100° Celsius at sea level" is dependent upon the experiments that could be done to verify this claim. The only real verification for logical positivism is empirical observation. If a statement cannot be verified through empirical observation, it has no meaning. Although one does not have to in fact test a claim to make it meaningful, there must simply exist, at least *in principle*, a means of verifying its truth. Consider the hypothetical case of Planet X. Planet X is a planet in our solar system that has not yet been discovered. The reason it has not been discovered is that it shares its orbit with Earth's orbit in such a way that the sun is always between the Earth and Planet X. The statement "Planet X exists" *is* verifiable in principle but not at the present time, in practice. If we had a powerful enough spaceship, we could fly around the sun and verify this claim. So the statement "Planet X exists" is a meaningful statement, even though we cannot verify it (or refute it) at this time.

The logical positivists used the verifiability theory of meaning to criticize, even attack, much contemporary and past philosophy. Their aforementioned disagreement with speculative metaphysics was often framed around this principle. Claims about substances beyond sensory experience or metaphysical concepts such as forms, monads, and immaterial minds were judged, under the verifiability theory of meaning, meaningless. They were also highly critical of religious claims and much ethical and aesthetic discourse. All traffic in claims about forces and entities that are empirically unverifiable: claims about God, souls, afterlife, good, evil, and beautiful. They were also critical of psychology and not interested in psychological or historical analyses of science. The psychological state of a scientist when making a discovery was, for the positivists, irrelevant. A discovery is a discovery regardless of a scientist's mental state. The history of science was likewise irrelevant to their studies. For historians such a story might be of interest, but in trying to understand what science itself is, the history behind it is not relevant. For logical positivists science existed as a pure study, not affected by the whims of speculative metaphysics, religion, history, or psychology. Science was reducible to nothing more than logic and empirical observation.

The logical positivists, in their day, were seen as radical and revolutionary. They were asserting a fresh, new, and empirically strict approach to philosophy. These days they are often seen as old and stuffy. That which was new and revolutionary quickly becomes the status quo, the new institution. By the 1950s, cracks were beginning to emerge in their framework. Even in the 1940s the movement underwent changes, even a change of name as it came to call itself logical *empiricism*. In the literature of philosophy of science the terms "logical positivism" and "logical empiricism" are not treated in consistent manners. Some writers will use the terms interchangeably. Some will use one or another to refer to the whole movement. And some will use the former to refer to the earlier theorists (roughly writing before WWII) and the latter term to refer to the latter writings (roughly following WWII until the 1960s). Although with this strategy it must be noted that the differences are subtle and often difficult to keep clear when surveying the literature. Logical empiricists—for example, Carl Hempel (1905–1997)—tended to focus more on questions of methodology and were particularly concerned with establishing a theory of inductive logic. Inductive logic holds a central place in scientific investigation, yet it is by its nature an uncertain form of logic. Logical empiricists wanted to strengthen inductive logic in order to strengthen the force and certainty of scientific conclusions. The logical empiricists also furthered another study of the logical positivists: the distinction between observational and theoretical language. Theoretical language refers to terms that have no direct observational reference, such as atom, gravity, neutron, or electron. Given the strict empirical orientation of logical positivists/empiricists, 20th century science's continual use of such terms referring to entities that are not or even *cannot* be directly observed presented a problem. The distinction between logical positivism and logical empiricism is not a clear one. If there is a real conceptual difference, it is subtle and one of degrees rather than kind.

The first major challenge to logical positivism/empiricism came from the American philosopher W.V.O. Quine (1908–2000) in his 1951 paper "Two Dogmas of Empiricism" published in the *Philosophical Review*. The two dogmas to which the title refers are the analytic/synthetic distinction, "a belief in some fundamental cleavage between truths which are *analytic* ... and truths which are *synthetic*," and reductionism, "the belief that each meaningful statement is equivalent to some logical construct upon terms which refer to immediate experience" (Quine, 1951/2000, p. 115). These two "dogmas" relate directly to the two primary linguistic principles of logical positivism/empiricism: the analytic–synthetic distinction and what he called "reductionism" is an expression of the verifiability theory of meaning. Part of that theory is that we verify claims through direct and immediate experience. Regarding verifiability, Quine argued that it is impossible to verify (test) any single claim by itself. For example, the testing of any single claim is going to assume the truth of many other implicit claims: such as the claim that one's testing apparatus is accurate. For example, in testing the claim that water boils at 100°C at sea level, one has to assume that a working thermometer is used and a working altimeter as well. In other words, if one gets a negative result in testing this claim, the claim itself might not be false, but one of the attendant assumptions might be false, such as the assumption of the accuracy of the instruments. He argued for a more holistic approach to knowledge which asserts knowledge composed not of distinct, isolatable principles but an inter-connected "web of belief." If you change or cut one strand (belief) that will have an effect on other strands throughout the web.

Regarding the analytic/synthetic distinction, Quine asserted that the concept of analyticity is dependent upon the concept of synonymy: that of the subject and predi-cate, one is defining of the other. Yet, synonymy itself cannot be defined without some reference to analyticity. Thus we fall into a circular argument. Quine ultimately con-cludes, regarding this distinction, that "truth in general depends on both language and extralinguistic fact . . . for all its a priori reasonableness, a boundary between ana-lytic and synthetic statements simply has not been drawn . . ."—and with an obvious dig at the logical positivists—"That there is such a distinction to be drawn at all is an unempirical dogma of empiricists, a metaphysical article of faith" (Quine, 1951/2000, p. 123). The reason Quine's blurring of this distinction is so devastating to logical posi-tivism/empiricism is that those philosophers relied upon the certainty and analyticity of logical and mathematical statements as a foundation for scientific method. Thus again an approach that is less analytic and more holistic is affirmed by Quine.

Logical empiricism had to take Quine's critique into account. The analytic–synthetic distinction was not rejected but became questionable. The verifiability theory of meaning had to be amended to make room for a more holistic interpretation (Godfrey-Smith, 2003). These changes, however, only postponed the inevitable decline of logical empiricism. By the late 1970s, the school was effectively no more (Godfrey-Smith, 2003). Its decline was brought about by factors already noted, plus others: (1) the breakdown of the logical positivist theory of language, (2) pressure from holist arguments, (3) a failure to develop a stronger theory of inductive logic, (4) a new recognition outside the school of the relevance of history and psychology to the philosopher of science, (5) the aforementioned problem regarding the theoretical/observational language distinction that created a problem for the thesis of scientific realism (Godfrey-Smith, 2003).

KARL POPPER : Demarcation (Science vs. Non-Science)

Perhaps the most influential and even important figure in the philosophy of science was Austrian philosopher Karl Popper (1902–1994). He was respected by philoso-phers and scientists alike and knighted by Queen Elizabeth II in 1965. Although he was Viennese and friendly with the philosophers of the Viennese Circle, he was not part of that circle and never identified himself as a logical positivist or logical empiri-cist. Indeed, he presented serious criticisms of that school of philosophy. With the rise of Nazism in Austria, he left for Britain and took a position at the London School of Economics.

The issue for which Popper is best known is the problem of demarcation, which is the problem of how we define a distinction between that which is science and that which is not—that is, how we demarcate science from nonscience. Given the epistemic authority bestowed upon science, this question is important for distinguishing which fields of study are worthy of that sense of authority. Popper himself was concerned with the validation of such theories as Freudianism, Marxism, and Adlerism. He found that the problem with these theories is that any evidence, even what would appear to be evidence against the theory, could be interpreted as confirming evidence. This problem is in part a result of the verifiability principle of the confirmation of scientific claims: scientific claims can be verified by instances of verifying evidence. Yet any piece of evidence could be used to verify several different scientific claims or principles. Also, due to the limitations of inductive logic, no number of observation instances will definitely confirm a scientific claim. There will always be the possibility of a disconfirming instance in the future. Suppose a meteorologist proposes a theory that washing a car causes rain. To prove this theory, the meteorologist washes a car and waits for rain. If it does in fact rain, then that would be a confirming instance of the theory. Such a theory, of course, is ludicrous. But the fact that it can be so easily "confirmed" indicates that this form of positive confirmation is too loose to be rigorously scientific. Popper proposed something of a negative test for the demarcation of science. A claim is scientific if and only if it may be possible to be refuted by evidence in the future. This is called the falsifiability thesis. Students often find this a confusing thesis upon first hearing it, but some interpretation is necessary. Popper is not making the counterintuitive assertion that a claim is scientific if it *is* refuted, but that there is possibly or *in potentia* a method to refute it. The problem he found with Freudianism was that no evidence would act as disconfirming evidence for this theory. No matter what evidence presented, the Freudian will reinterpret it to make it confirm the theory. Whereas the physicist who claims that "for every action there is an equal and opposite reaction" will be disproven by an instance of an action *not* producing an equal and opposite reaction. To return to the example used in logical positivism, the claim that Planet X exists is not only confirmable or verifiable under the logical positivist view but falsifiable according to the Popperian view. If we had a powerful enough ship we could fly around the sun to disconfirm the existence of Planet X. Thus, according to Popper, what demarcates science and nonscience is this falsifiability principle. All scientific claims and theories are falsifiable. Claims and theories that are not falsifiable are not scientific. Such a criterion would exclude from science—as the logical positivists did as well—claims of a religious or metaphysical nature and claims generated from certain pseudosciences such as astrology and parapsychology.

The falsifiability principle not only provides a criterion for demarcating science, it also has implications for epistemology and the nature of scientific theories. If a theory can never be positively confirmed but only potentially disconfirmed, then we can never attain 100% epistemic certainty about any theory. Further, theories must always exist in a state of uncertainty and continual testability. A theory that has not been falsified is nothing more than that, a theory that has not been falsified. It is not and never will be a "true" theory. This implication might seem to reduce the confidence we can have in scientific claims. That may be true. However, the best we can do is work with and provisionally accept those theories not yet disproven but keep an open mind to their possible fallibility.

THOMAS KUHN

As influential and admired as Popper was, Thomas Kuhn was likely far more revolutionary, which fits given his study of revolution in the history of science. Thomas Kuhn's most important work was his 1962 book *The Structure of Scientific Revolutions*, in which he challenged much of the foundations of previous philosophy of science— particularly as represented by the logical positivists/empiricists and Karl Popper. Kuhn's analysis brings the effect of history, society, culture, and psychology as relevant aspects to the study of the philosophy of science. No longer is science simply a pure, insular, eminently rational method of investigation. It is a cultural practice developed through history, influenced *in se* by forces outside the pure logical/observational concept of science.

The most controversial and influential concepts developed by Kuhn in *Structure* are those of the "paradigm" and the attendant concept of the "paradigm shift." In fact, one might blame, at least in part, Kuhn for the overuse and nauseating trivializing of those terms in the last 40 years. It may be difficult to locate one unequivocal definition of "paradigm" in Kuhn's book, but generally he seems to be referring to a set of preconceived beliefs about the world, methodology for gathering information and analyzing data, and simple scientific dispositions all that comprise a "given" understanding or conception of science at a given moment in history. Contrary to Popper and most of Kuhn's other predecessors then, science does not exist as simply this pure form of investigation. The basic fundamental and foundational (generally unquestioned) beliefs and methods of scientists at any point in time are (1) a result of historical events, (2) adopted nonrationally rather than through rational inquiry, and (3) acted upon largely out of habit and disposition rather than conscious intention.

Kuhn calls the type of science conducted within a paradigm "normal science," which he describes as a form of puzzle solving. Within the strictures of the paradigm a question (puzzle) is investigated and a solution is attempted from within the presuppositions and methodology of the given paradigm. For example, a liquid, believed to be water, is found not to boil at 100 °C at sea level. To solve this puzzle, the present paradigm would dictate that the scientist first look for some form of contamination in the "water." The scientist does not immediately jump to the conclusion that the boiling point of water at sea level is a variable property. Such a conclusion does not fit within the present paradigm. Thus, paradigmatic thinking directs what hypotheses are reasonable possibilities as well. The unquestioned, nonrationally accepted nature of much of the paradigm also challenges some important elements of Popper's normative concept of science. Popper's falsifiability thesis implies that a scientist should adopt an attitude of continual skepticism toward any theory or underlying scientific belief. Kuhn's "paradigmatic" view suggests, however, that scientists must have a nonrational attachment to the paradigm in which they work. Otherwise, they would have no foundation from which to start and direct their work.

At certain points within a paradigm puzzles fail to be solved. These failures are called anomalies. Much of the time anomalies are dismissed, in part to preserve the paradigm. However, after a number of anomalies occurs what Kuhn calls a "crisis" may be reached. This crisis will trigger a paradigm shift. A new paradigm that better allows for or explains the anomalous results will be adopted. This new paradigm will reign until a new crisis point is reached and another paradigm shift occurs.

PHILOSOPHY OF SCIENCE AFTER KUHN

Following the publication of Kuhn's *Structure of Scientific Revolutions*, one sees a marked shift in the philosophy of science. Relative to much that preceded him (especially of course the logical positivists/empiricists and Karl Popper), Kuhn raised challenges regarding the nature, purpose, and logical underpinnings of science and scientific investigation. After Kuhn, history, psychology, society, and culture were relevant and meaningful topics. After Kuhn, the epistemic status of science was far more dubitable, raising the specter of relativism. It seemed that every philosopher of science after Kuhn had to deal with his ideas in one way or another. Some were critical and attempted to reaffirm the older ideas of the pre-Kuhnian philosophers of science. Some found great inspiration in Kuhn and took some of his themes even further. We will first discuss three important philosophers who immediately addressed Kuhn and his ideas in different ways before moving on to larger movements that arose in the decades after Kuhn's book.

Imre Lakatos (1922–1974) was a Hungarian born philosopher and a member of the Nazi resistance in Hungary during WWII. He became an established scholar before his departure from Hungary upon the Soviet invasion. He ended up in England where he earned a doctorate in philosophy from the University of Cambridge and later took a post at the London School of Economics where he worked with and was influenced by Karl Popper.

Due to his somewhat Popperian views, Lakatos found Kuhn's ideas dangerous to science. In his interpretation, Kuhn presents a view of scientific change that is irrational. Changes do not occur due to a reasoned deliberation based on what will work and explain the world better but due merely to "mob psychology" (Lakatos, 1970, p. 178). The "danger" of change based on mob psychology is that it would hinder not only scientific progress but would seem to nullify the very concept of scientific progress at all. If science does not change based on rational principles, then there would be no control, no forward motion that would guarantee that the science of today is better than the science of yesterday. If that were the case, what would be the point of making changes? Indeed, what would be the point of science at all? However, he also recognized the force and relevance of Kuhn's historical arguments. He could not deny (as the logical positivists could) that history has an effect on not only the practice but even the nature of science. Thus, his goal came to be to recognize the force of history on science but also retain a sense of rationality.

In pursuit of this goal, he developed a concept he called the "research program." This concept is very close to Kuhn's "paradigm," although it might be better described as his concept of scientific theory as he allows for several research programs to be at work in any specific field of science. Where it differs is that change from research program to research program occurs rationally, not due to mob psychology. There are two formal parts to any research program: a hard core and a protective belt. The hard core contains the most fundamental and necessary principles, beliefs, and concepts of the research program. During the history of the research program, this does not change. The protective belt contains less fundamental and often contingent principles and beliefs regarding specific applications of the theory. It is in the protective belt that most change occurs. He agreed with Kuhn that science will face anomalies and have to react to them. How a research program reacts is by changing in the protective belt in order to "protect" the theory and keep it viable. As a research program changes, it can either progress or degenerate. If the program progresses, it will explain and predict phenomena better. If the program degenerates, it will begin to lose its explanatory and predictive power. Regarding degenerating programs, Lakatos agreed with Kuhn that scientists tend to protect them. This tendency is in direct contradiction to Popper's view of science that scientists do (or at least should) reject a failing theory. According to Lakatos, not only do scientists often protect a failing theory (by perhaps manipulating the protective belt in rationally improper ways) but scientists *should* protect a failing theory or program, given that some theories in the past have seemed to have failed but been redeemed later. However, no answer is to be had for how long or to what extent a program should be protected before it is reasonable to give it up.

Larry Laudan (1941–) is an American philosopher who, similarly to Lakatos, was influenced by Kuhn's historicist interpretations of science but disturbed by the irrational nature of Kuhn's theory of change—or at least Laudan's interpretation of Kuhn's theory as irrational. As Lakatos described the Kuhnian view as mob psychology, Laudan described Kuhn's theory of scientific change as "political and propagandistic" (Laudan, 1977, p. 4). Thus, Laudan defined for himself a similar goal of taking into account the influence of history on science while retaining a central place for rationality. Laudan developed a concept similar to Lakatos's research programs that he called "research traditions." Perhaps the primary difference was that Laudan's research traditions are more conceptually fluid. He allows for change within the hard core and allows for concepts and theories to move from one (possibly abandoned) research tradition to another.

Paul Feyeraband (1924–1994) was an Austrian born philosopher, who took a vastly different conceptual path than Lakatos and Laudan in the wake of Kuhn's *Structure*. He fought in WWII for Germany and after the war studied sociology, physics, and philosophy in Austria, Germany, and England, eventually ending up at the London School of Economics where he studied under (and was influenced in his early work by) Karl Popper. He held a number of teaching posts, the longest one being at the University of California at Berkeley.

In 1975 Feyerabend published his most famous book, *Against Method*, which came to be probably the most controversial book in the history of the philosophy of science. In this book, he argued for what he called "epistemological anarchism." What he meant by this is suggested in the title: assuming some system of scientific methodology merely constrains the scientist and limits the scope and creativity of scientific investigation. To be creative, the scientist needs to eschew rules and embrace the freedom of thought without limits. The point is to break science and scientists free from rules and enhance creativity, new ideas, and new research projects. What is controversial is that such anarchism would seem to raise the specter of epistemic relativism: there are no objective standards for knowledge; all knowledge claims are equally valid.

THE SOCIOLOGY OF SCIENCE

The study of the sociology of science pre-dates Kuhn's important work, but this study was largely ignored by philosophers of science before *Structure*. In the 1960s and 1970s the sociology of science became a clearer influence on the philosophy of science, likely due to Kuhn's influence in widening the scope of what is relevant to the philosophy of science. An important early figure in the sociology of science was Robert Merton (1910–2003), who theorized that the culture of science conformed to four normative principles: universalism, communism, disinterestedness, and organized skepticism. The principle of universalism holds that the personality and background of a scientist is irrelevant to the quality or value of his/her ideas. This principle can be found in the views of the logical positivists/empiricists and Popper. The principle of communism is that the products of scientific investigation belong to the culture of science, not to any specific scientist. Perhaps this principle is best illustrated by Jonas Salk's refusal to patent his polio vaccine, comparing such an act to patenting the sun. The principle of disinterestedness removes personal bias and desire of any particular scientist from scientific investigation in order to ensure objectivity and the benefit of humanity. This principle is a basic ideal of Enlightenment thinking. The principle of organized skepticism refers to the imperative in science to continually question one's own and others' work and results in order to better ensure true and accurate scientific knowledge. This principle reflects Popper's falsifiability principle and contention that all scientific claims remain forever fallible and open to revision or refutation. Merton's theory appears to be more normative than descriptive, but what he describes is a view of science as a pure intellectual pursuit, unaffected by the vagaries of culture (at least nonscientific culture), psychology, and history and directed by rational rules of observation and logic.

Perhaps the most influential school of sociology of science on the philosophy of science was what was called the Strong Program. This was a school of sociology that arose in the 1970s at the University of Edinburgh in Scotland, led by Barry Barnes and David Bloor. The formative idea underlying the Strong Program is what Bloor and Barnes called the "symmetry principle." The symmetry principle holds that all beliefs and belief statements should be treated the same, understood through the same explanatory methods, regardless of whether we believe them to be true or false. This principle has several consequences or implications. First, it places scientific claims on the same level as nonscientific claims. Scientific claims, under the symmetry principle, are not special due to the supposed rigorous methodology lying behind them. They are placed on the same level as folk beliefs, popular knowledge, or even old wives' tales. Second, the principle further questions the epistemic purity of scientific belief by noting—like many other types of belief—that scientific beliefs are affected or even engendered by the particularities of the scientists who hold them: their political interests, their personal prejudices, and their social positions. Third, this principle suggests a new view of science known as social constructionism (sometimes "social constructivism"). According to the thesis of social constructionism, which would become a powerfully influential idea in sociology, philosophy, and many other areas of study in the 1980s and 1990s, entities that are presumed to have some form of natural existence independent of human perception and conception (what philosophers call "natural kinds") are merely the products of commonly held beliefs within a society. And fourth, this principle appears to lead to a very strong form of epistemic relativism, the thesis that knowledge is not universal or objective but particular and based upon social background and history. Just as in the work of Merton one can see a reflection of logical positivism, the prevailing philosophical view of science at the time, one can see in the strong program a reflection and extension of the ideas introduced in Kuhn's *Structure*.

The Strong Program was highly influential on much of the sociology and philosophy of science to follow. One of the most notable examples of this influence is the book *Laboratory Life: the Construction of Scientific Facts* (1979) by French philosopher/ anthropologist Bruno Latour (1947–) and British sociologist Stephen Woolgar. In preparation for this book, Latour observed work done at the Salk Institute in San Diego with a purposefully naïve, even ignorant, eye, to observe much as an anthropologist might observe a foreign culture. During the period of observation at the Salk Institute the scientists there "discovered" the chemical structure of a human growth hormone. This "discovery" won a Nobel Prize for Roger Guilleman and Andrew V. Schally. What Latour and Woolgar observed was not the kind of sensational, earth-shattering investigation you might expect of Nobel Prize-winning work but very mundane even dull activities, rhetorical negotiations, and power plays. They describe the laboratory almost in the sense of a nonhuman machine in which one inputs raw data and the output (the product of mundane activity, rhetorical negotiations, and power plays) is "scientific fact." Part of their conclusion (perhaps presumption) is that scientific facts are not so much discovered as constructed. For the Salk Institute, the product of the work of this period was a Nobel Prize-winning "discovery." For Latour and Woolgar, the product was the actor-network theory, which holds that society and nature are the products, not the causes, of scientific investigation.

FEMINISM AND SCIENCE

As feminism was a powerful social force in this country in the 1960s and 1970s, it is not surprising that it would also affect science and the philosophy of science. As with any other power-laden, authoritative practice in our society, the general feminist complaint has been that science has been defined by men, reflective of masculinist thinking, dismissive of female contributions (or even of the ability or possibility of women to contribute) and that it perpetuates social inequalities between men and women. Feminism in the philosophy of science has reflected feminism in the culture at large, but also has reflected the new ideas in the philosophy of science from the likes of Kuhn, Feyerabend, and the Strong Program. Thus, feminist philosophers of science tend to question the objectivity of scientific belief and the intellectual purity of scientific investigation.

A general feminist criticism of science is that it plays upon and perpetuates the traditional stereotypical dichotomies that identify males with reason and females with emotion, and males with the mind and women with the body. Traditionally (and stereotypically), men have been identified as the thinkers and the doers: the philosophers and the scientists. Women have been identified as less mental and more embodied, more representative of nature. In fact, of course, women have not traditionally been those who have made intellectual advances in science, philosophy, and other advanced studies. But rather than this fact being indicative of the intellectual inferiority of women, feminists point to social reasons that have excluded women from more intellectual pursuits and achievements. Women have been more identified with the private realm, the hearth, and home. The view of women as more embodied and "natural" stems from a monthly menstruation that continually re-embodies women, as well as the natural "function" of child birth. Being viewed as more embodied brings with it also the greater sense of emotionality (as opposed to rationality) of which women are often perceived. And as women are identified with nature, scientists (men) take the same type of domineering attitude toward nature as men have traditionally taken toward women. Nature is a thing to be controlled, manipulated, and (visually) penetrated. Some feminists then argue for a less domineering, more cooperative relationship with nature.

The most controversial area of feminist philosophy of science is likely in the field of epistemology. Sandra Harding (1935–) identifies two threads of epistemological theory in feminist philosophy of science. The first she calls feminist empiricism. From the perspective of feminist empiricism, science and scientific claims have been distorted, have lacked complete objectivity, due to "social biases—sexism and androcentrism . . . in biology and the social sciences" (Harding, 1989/2000, p. 428). The strategy suggested by feminist empiricism is simply to eliminate these biases. If they can be eliminated, then the ideal of objective scientific investigation will be, if not achieved, at least closer. This approach is somewhat conservative, epistemologically speaking. It adheres to, at least in principle, traditional scientific ideals of rationality and objectivity. The second thread, which Harding calls standpoint theory or the feminist standpoint, is more radical.[1] According to this view, knowledge differs due to gendered perspective or experience. Standpoint theorist further argues that the female experience is "a more complete and less distorting kind of social experience," and is thus one that "increases the objectivity of the results of research" (Harding, 1989/2000, p. 430).

---

[1]A note on the word "radical": In colloquial English, this is an often abused term, often used as or assumed to be a synonym for extreme or extremist. While it is true that radicals often do take extreme positions, this is the wrong interpretation for what they are trying to do. Academically, the term is usually used in its more accurate sense. The word "radical" is derived from the Latin *radicitis*, which means "by the roots." Note that the word "radish," a *root* vegetable, shares the same derivation. So a radical is attempting to address a problem by getting to the root of the problem, not merely addressing the obvious or superficial aspects of the problem. Think of weeding a garden. If you merely pull the weeds you see, they will soon come back. The only way to truly and permanently weed a garden is to remove the weeds by their roots.

THE SCIENCE WARS

Whereas post-Kuhnian philosophy of science saw a rise in philosophies critical of traditional ideals of objectivity and rationality, a rise in relativistic, postmodern, and social constructionist views; such a turn was not universally accepted. First, such views were largely rejected by scientists in the natural sciences. Natural scientists tend to be rationalists[2] and realists[3] regarding their work. Second, some philosophers of science maintained also a rationalist, and often realist, view of science, rejecting the more "fashionable" movements of postmodernism, relativism, and social constructionism. Third, even some nonscientists with not only epistemologically but politically and morally conservative commitments rejected (often vociferously) these new movements. For these, the concern was not only the integrity and elevated epistemic status of science but that relativistic views would lead to relativistic morals. The epistemologically conservative scientists and philosophers usually did not share these moral and political concerns. The conflict between these three groups and the movements of postmodernism, relativism, and social constructionism increased in virulence in the 1990s. This conflict is often referred to as the science wars, a subcategory of the culture wars of the 1990s.

The most sensational battle of the science wars was that waged between Alan Sokal and the journal *Social Text*. In 1996 physicist Alan Sokal published a paper, "Transgressing the Boundaries: Toward a Transformative Hermeneutics of Quantum Gravity" in *Social Text*, a journal with a reputation for publishing postmodern work. The following month he published a piece in the more academically conservative journal *Lingua Franca* entitled "Revelation: A Physicist Experiments with Cultural Studies." In this later article he revealed that the *Social Text* piece was a sham, a quodlibet of sorts composed of buzzwords and postmodern terminology strung together in a seemingly but not really coherent fashion. His point was to show that postmodern discourse and study was substantially empty, devoid of any real knowledge or insight, any meaningful, verifiable, or falsifiable claims. His sham was meant to reveal the sham that he believed postmodernism to be. This hoax made quite a stir that was felt not only in the academic world but beyond as well. We recall first hearing of it on the CBS Sunday morning program with Charles Osgood. The editors of *Social Text* responded in defense that they had to send Sokal's article back for revisions several times. However, that does not change the fact that they did indeed publish it. A firestorm of reactions from intellectuals of all stripes defending both sides soon erupted. The original articles plus much of the reaction was collected into a book published by the editors of *Lingua Franca* titled *The Sokal Hoax: The Sham that Shook the Academy*. And Alan Sokal later expanded on his criticisms in a book he coauthored with Belgian physicist/philosopher Jean Bricmont, *Fashionable Nonsense: Postmodern Intellectuals' Abuse of Science*.

---

[2]Meaning a commitment to reason as the justification for knowledge, whether that is through empirical or rationalist methodologies.

[3]Meaning that what they discover exists as natural kinds in an objective, mind-independent reality.

CONCLUSION

The information presented here is meant to be a broad and general overview, to give the reader both a taste of what the philosophy of science is and a historical orientation regarding its development. Philosophy is a form of discourse. It develops through a system of give and take. For a student to try to jump into the middle of this discourse without some holistic understanding of the discourse itself puts the student at a great disadvantage and may even intimidate and discourage the student. The specific issues addressed here are only addressed in the most general sense, intended to provide an introduction and background to these issues. These issues and others will be explored in greater depth in the chapters to come. And hopefully, the student will now have a more solid background to this more in depth analysis.

CRITICAL THINKING QUESTIONS

1. If it's true that a practice or phenomenon becomes of philosophical interest when it becomes a "problem," in what ways has science become a problem?
2. Reflect on nursing philosophy. In what ways has nursing become a problem?
3. Empiricism seems like a straightforward, commonsense view of knowledge and the world, but what unexpected problems can arise with a strict empirical outlook?
4. Can you ever be sure your existence is not like that of the characters in *The Matrix*?
5. Are we born with innate ideas, as Descartes and the other Continental Rationalists held, or with a mind like a blank slate, as Locke and the other British Empiricists held?
6. What is positive about "positivism"? That is, why do you think it's given that name?
7. What is the difference between verifiability and falsifiability?
8. What is a paradigm? What competing paradigms can you find in medicine or health care?
9. How does Kuhn's theory of scientific change challenge the Enlightenment foundation and presuppositions of science?
10. What relevance does the sociology of science and scientists have to the philosophical study of science? Is science something more than the study of logic and empirical experimentation?

REFERENCES

Godfrey-Smith, P. (2003). *Theory and reality: An introduction to the philosophy of science.* Chicago, IL: University of Chicago Press.

Harding, S. (2000). Feminist justificatory strategies. In J. McErlean (Ed.), *Philosophies of science: From foundations to contemporary issues* (pp. 427–435). Stamford, CT: Wadsworth. (Original work published 1989.)

James, W. (2007). *The principles of psychology.* New York, NY: Cosimo, Inc.

Kant, I. *Critique of Pure Reason* (N. K. Smith, Trans.). New York, NY: St. Martin's Press, 1965. (Original work published in 1781.)

Lakatos, I. (1970). Falsification and the methodology of scientific research programmes. In I. Lakatos, & A. Musgrave (Eds.), *Criticism and the growth of knowledge* (pp. 91–196). London: Cambridge University Press.

Latour, B., & Woolgar, S. (1986). *Laboratory life: The construction of scientific facts*. Princeton, NJ: Princeton University Press.

Laudan, L. (1977). *Progress and its problems: Toward a theory of scientific growth*. Berkeley, CA: University of California Press.

Quine, W. V. O. (2000). Two dogmas of empiricism. In J. McErlean (Ed.), *Philosophies of science: From foundations to contemporary issues* (pp. 115–128). Belmont, CA: Wadsworth. (Original work published 1951.)

Whewell, W. (1840). *The philosophy of the inductive sciences: Founded upon their history*. Charleston, SC: Forgotten Books.

7

What is Science?
The Problem of Demarcation

*Science is very clearly a conscious artifact of mankind, with well-documented
historical origins, with a definable scope and content, and with recognizable
professional practitioners and exponents.*

JOHN ZIMAN

INTRODUCTION

The need to define "science" transcends mere, neutral classificatory goals. The term and
designation "science" has developed cultural and epistemic meaning and authority. This
authority should not be assigned lightly—though philosophically it should be questioned in itself. Right or wrong, we often use "science" and its cognates as marks or
even totems of authority and power. For example, a new product might be advertised
as "scientifically tested," whether it actually is or not, in order to attribute legitimacy
to it. Debates as to whether such controversial theories as Marxism, Freudianism, Dar-
winism, and Intelligent Design are "scientific" also seem to hinge upon questions of
their legitimacy. By corollary, terms like "pseudoscience" carry a negative cultural
meaning and suggest a denial of authority. Recently, the term "junk science" has also
entered the public discourse on science with similar denotation and connotation.
Although this term is largely attributed not academically to scientific methodologies or
arguments but politically to scientific conclusions one simply does not like. "Science"
is not easily defined. It is not a natural kind but a human practice that has evolved
over time. It is connected to our natural instinct to know, to investigate. Like philosophy,
it too begins with wonder. But where it ends up, its limits and boundaries are not so clear.
Accordingly, attempts to provide a clear demarcation between science and nonscience
have been highly contentious. We will survey several of these in this chapter.

THE PURPOSE(S) OF SCIENCE

One avenue to begin to understand science is to take the Aristotelian advice to look to
purpose. That is, once we identify the goal, aim, or function of science, we may well be
on our way to understanding what science is in its essence. We may also see that

understanding the possible purposes of science gives us a window into distinct theoretical views about science. That is, different theoretical schools will emphasize different purposes to science and these emphasized purposes may be a sign of deeper philosophical commitments and beliefs held by these distinct theoretical schools.

The purposes of science are manifold and each may be taken as merely one among many, while there are some philosophers and philosophies of science which will focus on one of these as indicative or definitive of science itself. Each of these purposes may also be associated with a particular traditional branch of philosophy: epistemology, metaphysics. One simple purpose of science is a *descriptive* purpose: the idea that the purpose of science is to merely describe the way the world is; what particular and general (classes, species, etc.) things there are (or perhaps were) in the world. Some specific sciences, such as natural history or anatomy, might be understood as wholly descriptive. But most sciences would not seem to be exhausted by a mere descriptive purpose. This purpose may be connected to the philosophical branch of metaphysics, especially in regard to the presumptions many sciences make about the world and the acceptance of methodology as realist or instrumentalist.

Some will claim that mere description does not go far enough in understanding science's purpose and hold that science has a further *predictive* purpose: to determine not just the way the world is but in what states and with what things the world will be. The predictive function of science allows us to manipulate nature and apply science as technology. If we can accurately predict the results of our actions on nature, we can use our knowledge of nature to our benefit. This predictive purpose is associated with the epistemology of science, as it is directly connected to how we know what will happen, but also secondarily to the metaphysics and ethics of science. To focus on prediction may sometimes imply an abrogation of metaphysical claims through an instrumentalist or pragmatic approach to scientific method. Also, if the predictive function of science allows us to manipulate nature to our benefit, an ethical understanding of what our benefit is would be necessary.

Merely understanding the way the world is or the way the world may be will not be enough for some. For some, science should go further in having an *explanatory* purpose: to explain why events occur or are the way they are, not just that they will occur or that they are the way they are. The explanatory purpose is clearly connected to the epistemology of science, as understanding the why of things and events is clearly a question of knowledge and how that knowledge is attained. Secondarily, the explanatory function may be related to the metaphysics of science, as an explanation may presume an underlying structure of the world.

A somewhat controversial purpose that goes beyond any of these but many argue today is an inescapable part of science is a *prescriptive* purpose: to aid us in determining what we should do, especially in terms of public policy. This purpose is somewhat controversial because traditionally science is seen as value-free or value-neutral. But many today argue that not only is this not true, it is not even possible. Merely choosing a research project or the government funding a particular research goal reflects and expresses a value-system. This function is clearly connected to the ethics of science. This prescriptive purpose appears particularly relevant (and in another way, particularly controversial) in the realm of the social sciences, as the subject of these sciences is humans or humanity.

A final possible purpose is a *justificatory* purpose, which can be seen not as an independent purpose in itself, but as secondary to any one or combination of those above: science should provide a justification for any of its claims, be they descriptive, predictive, explanatory, or prescriptive. This purpose is clearly associated with the epistemology and logic of science. To justify a claim is to know what makes it knowledge and how knowledge claims are connected through logical ties.

Now, most philosophers and philosophies of science will not choose just one of these, as *the* proper function or purpose of science but will accept some combination of those above, while perhaps denying specific ones for important philosophical reasons. Understanding which of these purposes is accepted and how and which are denied and why is one means of coming to understand any particular philosopher or philosophy of science.

LOGICAL POSITIVISM: SCIENCE IS VERIFIABILITY

As indicated in Chapter 6, one of the main tenets of logical positivism was the verifiability principle. This principle can also be identified as the essential feature of science itself according to logical positivists. Recall that the verifiability principle holds that the meaning of a statement is to be found in its verification process. On the surface, to verify a claim means merely to demonstrate its truth. But this is the verifiability principle, not the verification principle. "The meaning of a statement," writes positivist Rudolf Carnap, "lies in the fact that it expresses a (conceivable, not necessarily existing) state of affairs" (1928/1967, p. 325). So the criterion is a hypothetical one: it is not about whether a specific claim is or is not verified but whether it is possible to verify a specific claim. Again, according to Carnap, "One can know that a statement is meaningful even before one knows whether it is true or false" (1928/1967, p. 325). Thus, even a false claim could be considered scientific, in at least a formal sense. Taken broadly the verifiability principle addresses the question of meaning in general, not purely within the domain and practice of science. In their discussions of meaning, the logical positivists commonly directed their criticisms and charges of meaninglessness against metaphysical philosophers. Generally, of course, metaphysics is that branch of philosophy which studies reality and various concepts of reality. More specifically, what they mean by "metaphysics" is philosophy which presumes "knowledge of a reality transcending the world of science and common sense" (Ayer, 1952/2000, p. 28), or "the field of alleged knowledge of the essence of things which transcends the realm of empirically founded, inductive science" (Carnap, 1932/1959, p. 80). The works of Martin Heidegger, Gottfried Hegel and F. H. Bradley are often cited (and even mocked) as examples. Hegelian influenced philosophers were especially prominent in Britain immediately prior to the development of logical positivism. Philosophers like Bertrand Russell and G. E. Moore argued for a less idealist, more concrete and empirical philosophy than what the neo-Hegelians practiced. These philosophers spoke in terms of conceptually vague notions like the "absolute." Religious terms such as "soul," "spirit," and "God" would also fall into this category for the logical positivists. Based upon this "knowledge" beyond science and common sense, metaphysicians would reach what logical positivist A. J. Ayer characterized as "startling conclusions": "time and space are unreal, or that nothing really moves, or that there are not many things in the Universe but only one, or that nothing which we perceive through our senses is real or wholly, or that there is not such thing as matter, or no such things as minds" (Ayer, 1970, p. 64). It did not help also that Hegel and Hegelians often repudiated logic as it is traditionally understood. One of the central concepts of Hegel's philosophy, the dialectic, affirms the meaningfulness of contradictions.

The problem with these metaphysical terms is that they refer to proposed entities that would be "super-empirical" and unable to be deduced from empirical knowledge (Ayer, 1952/2000, p. 28). These metaphysicians often referred to some form of innate knowledge or rational intuition upon which they based their knowledge of such entities. The Russell/Moore/Logical Positivist turn toward strict empiricism illustrated that these claims from rational intuition were without foundation, since no two metaphysicians' rational intuitions seemed completely consistent. What one metaphysician might claim is supported by his rational intuition, another might deny. And there is no independent, objective standard against which to judge the disputed intuitive claims. An empirical standard for knowledge provides, so the logical positivists believed, an independent, objective standard for knowledge claims. By neglecting this empirical standard the metaphysician "produces sentences which fail to conform to the conditions under which alone a sentence can be literally significant" (Ayer, 1952/2000, p. 29). In other words, metaphysicians do not so much produce false claims as they do meaningless or nonsensical claims.

What are these conditions under which a sentence can be significant? According to logical positivists, to be meaningful, a statement must be analytically true, self-contradictory or empirically verifiable. These criteria imply the principle of the analytic–synthetic distinction that was an integral element in the logical positivist philosophy. According to this distinction all statements (assertive sentences) are analytic, self-contradictory, or synthetic. An analytic statement is one in which the predicate is included in the subject. The classic example is "All bachelors are unmarried." What makes this an analytic statement is that the concept of "being unmarried" is included in the concept of "bachelor." Another simple example would be "The red ball is red." Here again, the predicate "red" is included in the subject "red ball." Given that the predicate of an analytic statement is included in its subject, another quality of analytic statements that follows from this is that they are necessarily true. This quality might also be referred to as being analytically true or true by definition. That is, no matter what, a true analytic statement will be true. Its truth does not depend on any matter of fact or state of the world, merely upon the relation of concepts within the statement itself. Since an analytic statement is necessarily true, its negation would be self-contradictory, which is the second type of statement Hempel refers to in his first category. For example, the statement "The red ball is not red" contradicts itself and can under no circumstance be true. The same can be said of the statements "All bachelors are married" and "Some bachelors are married." It is the relation (one of identity or contradiction) among the concepts included in an analytic or self-contradictory statement that makes it cognitively meaningful.

Synthetic statements are empirically verifiable statements. A synthetic statement is one which brings together (synthesizes) two unrelated concepts. This, of course, is in contradistinction to analytic statements in which the predicate is included in the subject. For example, as noted before, whereas "The red ball is red" is an analytic statement, the statement "The ball is red" would be a synthetic statement. There is no necessary or *a priori* relationship between the concept "ball" and the concept "red." The predicate is not included in the subject. Rather, the statement synthesizes two unrelated concepts and asserts a (contingent) relationship between them. This relationship is one that can be verified by empirical observation. In the case of this simple statement, one need only observe the ball in question to verify that it is indeed red. It is also worth noting that the logical positivists intended this standard to be interpreted as "verifiability in principle," and not merely "practical verifiability" (Ayer, 1952/2000, p. 29). A practically verifiable statement would be one that, given current knowledge and technology, it is in fact possible to verify empirically. However, a statement could still be meaningful if it made a claim that was not practically verifiable but was still verifiable in principle. Consider the Planet X hypothesis. This hypothesis is that there is a planet in our solar system that astronomers have so far failed to detect. The reason for this failure is that Planet X shares an orbit with the planet Earth. However, its orbit is such that it is always on the opposite side of the sun. Thus, we can never see this planet from our own. The claim of Planet X's existence is not a practically verifiable claim. However, if we could build a powerful enough spaceship, we could travel around the sun to verify the existence of this planet, or verify its nonexistence. Thus, the claim of Planet X's existence is verifiable in principle, and thus is a meaningful statement given logical positivist criteria.

Statements of a metaphysical sort are not analytic and are not subject to this type of "experiential test"—even hypothetically (in principle). Carnap uses the example of statements referring to "God." As the term "God" refers to an entity "beyond experience" (Carnap, 1932/1959, p. 66), any claim regarding "God" would not be experientially testable. In other words, such a claim would not be verifiable. Any statement that predicates any quality of "God" could not be said to be true or not true. Such a claim would, hence, be not necessarily false but nonsense. Ayer uses as an example a statement from the metaphysical philosopher F. H. Bradley: "the Absolute enters into, but is itself incapable of, evolution and progress" (Ayer, 1952/2000, pp. 29–30). Like metaphysical statements about "God," this metaphysical statement is not verifiable practically or in principle, because, says Ayer, "one cannot conceive of an observation which would enable one to determine whether the Absolute did, or did not, enter into evolution and progress" (1952/2000, p. 30). Thus, like statements about "God," this statement, being neither analytic nor empirically verifiable, is nonsense. Hans Reichenbach used a statement from Hegel as an example: "Reason is substance, as well as infinite power, its own infinite material underlying all the natural and spiritual life; as also the infinite form, that which sets the material in motion" (Reichenbach, 1951, p. 3). Such a statement, Reichenbach claimed, could well inspire a reader to cast the offending book into the fire.[1] Logical positivists even refused to refer to statements such as these as "statements" (given

---

[1] Reichenbach is clearly alluding to one of the positivists' empiricist, anti-metaphysical forbears, David Hume, who famously ended his book, *An Enquiry Concerning Human Understanding*, with these dramatic words: "If we take in our hand any volume; of divinity or school metaphysics, for instance; let us ask; *Does it contain any abstract reasoning concerning quantity or number?* No. *Does it contain any experimental reasoning concerning matter of fact and existence?* No. Commit it then to the flames: for it can contain nothing but sophistry and illusion" (Hume, 1748/1974, p. 430).

that a "statement" should be meaningful, that is, determinable as true or false) and instead referred to them as "pseudostatements" or "pseudopropositions" (Ayer, 1952/ 2000, p. 29; Carnap, 1928/1967, p. 326; Carnap, 1932/1959, pp. 61, 68, 69–78).

Before we can address the question of what this theory of meaning says about science, there is an issue of internal debate among logical positivists that it is worth noting. One can interpret the verifiability principle in two ways, what Ayer refers to as strong and weak verifiability (Ayer, 1952/2000). Strong verifiability requires the truth of a claim to be, in principle at least, *conclusively* verifiable, that is, "conclusively established in experience" (Ayer, 1952/2000, p. 30). Under strong verifiability then, only those statements whose truth could be established absolutely and beyond all doubt could be accepted as meaningful. This interpretation sets a rather high bar for meaningfulness. According to Ayer, Moritz Schlick affirmed this high bar (1952/ 2000). Ayer thought this criterion too restrictive though. Accepting this interpretation would entail rejecting as nonsense many commonly accepted generalities or "general propositions of law" in Ayer's terms (1952/2000, p. 30). For example, the claim "All men are mortal" could not be accepted as meaningful under this interpretation of ver- ifiability. The problem is that general claims such as these are not only commonly and intuitively accepted but quite useful also. One cannot *prove* (in the mathematical or logical sense of the word) that all men are mortal. One can at best prove that all men observed to date have turned out to be mortal. Yet not accepting such a plainly true proposition would seem foolish. Under the strong verifiability principle general claims would be nonsense much the same as claims about "God" or "the Absolute." Moritz Schlick negotiated his way around the problem of recognizing the usefulness of general claims while maintaining their status as nonsense under the strong verifia- bility principle by referring to such claims as "an essentially important type of non- sense" (Ayer, 1952/2000, p. 30).

Ayer favored the weak interpretation of the verifiability principle, describing the strong interpretation as "self-stultifying" (Ayer, 1952/2000, p. 30). He found Schlick's qualification of general laws as *important* nonsense as a hedge: a recognition of a paradox created by this restrictive criterion without actually removing the paradox (Ayer, 1952/2000). According to the weak interpretation, a claim is meaningful only if "it is possible for experience to render it probable" (Ayer, 1952/2000, p. 30). Unlike the strong interpretation, a claim does not have to be provable in an absolute or beyond all doubt sense. It only has to be provable to a degree of probability. Thus, general claims and general laws could be accepted as meaningful under this criterion. One may not be able to prove the truth of a claim like "All men are mortal" to an absolute degree of certainty, but one can prove it to a degree of prob- ability, making it meaningful under the weak verifiability principle. The problem with statements like these is that they do refer to something beyond experience just as metaphysical claims do. The claim "All men are mortal" refers not only to all the men who have died (and thus empirically establishing their mortality), but it refers also to all currently living men whose mortality is yet to be established and to all future men, one of whom it is possible could be born immortal. Schlick, by maintaining these types of statements as nonsense, retained a sense of consistency but at the cost of common sense and an asserted paradox: "important nonsense." Whereas Ayer saved common sense and avoided a paradox, he risked charges of inconsistency.

Although the verifiability principle can be taken as a general principle of meaning, it also establishes an important general criterion for scientific methodology and even the meaning of "science" itself. Since the verifiability principle can be interpreted as a general theory of meaning, it cannot act as a sufficient condition for "science." It, however, does seem a necessary condition. That is, it seems a clear thesis of logical positivism that one cannot have "science" without the verifiability principle as a standard. Otherwise, science would devolve into a morass of pseudostatements and lose meaning, efficaciousness, and authority. "All empirical sciences (natural sciences, psychology, cultural science)," writes Carnap, "acknowledge and carry out in practice the requirement that every statement must have factual content . . . each statement which is to be considered meaningful in any one of these fields . . . either goes directly back to experience . . . or it is at least indirectly connected with experience in such a way that it can be indicated which possible experience would confirm or refute it . . ." (1932/1967, p. 328).

The application of the verifiability principle seems at times normative and at times merely descriptive. This quote from Carnap appears to apply the principle descriptively. He seems to be merely stating the way that science does in fact work, what scientists do in fact do. However, it can also be applied normatively, to ridicule the nonsense of studies outside the realm of science, to establish a proper philosophical method or to establish the proper meaning and practice of science so as to exclude mere pseudosciences. Regarding the second of these, the logical positivists applied this criterion to philosophy, not only cutting away the metaphysical philosophy of the likes of Hegel, Bradley, and Heidegger but establishing a stricter, more empirical approach to philosophy sometimes called by them "scientific philosophy" (Carnap, 1932/1959, p. 77; Reichenbach, 1951), which would focus on the logical analysis of language. Regarding the third of these, if a field of study cannot demonstrate a consistent employment and deployment of meaningful terms, it would then not be science— even if it patently made claims to be so.

The strong versus weak interpretations of the verifiability principle become particularly important in the context of science. General claims and laws are central to science. Reichenbach goes so far as to say that "Generalization . . . is the origin of science" (1951, p. 5). Newton's laws of motion are generalizations. The claim that lead is heavier than gold is a generalization. The claim that a particular therapy is helpful in relieving a particular malady is a generalization. We cannot have science without such generalizations. This is likely the prime reason Schlick qualified these nonsense statements as "important" nonsense. Not only are they central to daily life and common sense, they are central to science. This is likely also why Ayer risked charges of inconsistency.

This centrality of generalization to science also points to the centrality of inductive logic, as it is inductive logic that generates generalizations. And, of course, an inductive argument can establish its conclusion only to a degree of probability. Knowledge, then, is generated by a mixture of empirical observation and logic. Empirical observation itself only provides observations of particular phenomena. In order to generate genuine scientific claims, we have to apply inductive logic to these observations. Thus, we get empirical observation plus logical inference, which is the essence of science for the logical empiricists: empiricism plus logic.

POPPER: SCIENCE IS FALSIFIABILITY

Karl Popper was the first to formally define this issue and coin the term "problem of demarcation" (2002, p. 11). The logical positivists may not have explicitly identified verifiability as a criterion for science, but in their vigorous attacks on metaphysics clearly implied such a criterion. And Popper, in his writings on the question, clearly accepted verifiability as a logical positivist criterion for science. But in accepting verifiability as the logical positivist criterion, he strongly rejected it as the correct criterion. In doing so, he also denied the centrality of inductive logic to science in favor of deductive logic and clearly distinguished the question of meaning from the question of demarcation.

Popper's stated inspiration for embarking on this particular study was the prevalence of a number of theories in the early 20th century. These theories were Einstein's theory of relativity, Marx's theory of history, Freud's psychoanalysis, and Alfred Adler's individual psychology (Popper, 1963/2000, p. 9). Whereas all four of these theories at the time were receiving a lot of attention from some very smart people, to Popper, Einstein's theory seemed different from the other three. To him those three appeared more mythical than scientific, more like astrology than astronomy. He then set out to determine what quality or qualities precisely defined this distinction. The first step in this process is to evaluate the logical positivist answer. He found verifiability inadequate as a criterion for demarcation. It is theoretically illiberal as the "positivists, in their anxiety to annihilate metaphysics, annihilate natural science along with it" (Popper, 2002, p. 13). He makes explicit reference to Schlick and his use of the strong verifiability principle. Recall the problems that principle had with general laws. Under the strong verifiability principle it becomes impossible to verify as seemingly simple a scientific claim as "Arsenic is poisonous." Such a claim depends upon inductive logic, as does the verifiability principle itself. Inductively, it is impossible to *conclusively* prove that arsenic is poisonous. To do so one would have to test every sample of arsenic. One might even have to test every sample on every living being, or at least on every human being if we could delimit the arsenic claim in such a way. Not only did Popper reject the verifiability principle as a criterion of demarcation, he further rejected induction as a form of logic (2002). In this way, he might be said to more consistently follow the ideas of Hume than the logical positivists.

Regarding the theories of Marx, Freud, and Adler, the problem is that they do seem verifiable. These theorists and their followers can point to many confirming instances. Here we get the apparent irony of Popper's position. Confirming or verifying a theory does not really show it to be true. This is due in part to the limits of and Popper's rejection of induction. But there is another related problem as well. Of psychoanalysis and individual psychology specifically, Popper wrote,

> I could not think of any human behavior which could not be interpreted in terms of either theory. It was precisely this fact—that they always fitted, that they were always confirmed—which in the eyes of their admirers constituted the strongest argument in favor of these theories. It began to dawn on me that this apparent strength was in fact their weakness.
>
> —*Popper, 1963/2000, p. 10*

The point was that it seemed to Popper that no matter what apparently discon-firming data might be presented, an adherent of either theory could interpret that data in such a way as to make it a confirming instance of the theory, thus "verifying" the theory. This slipperiness of interpretation negates any rigorous standards the verifia-bility principle might seem to have, making it too "easy" to "verify" a theory. Thus, the apparent strength of these theories—that they seemed to be verified at every turn—turns out to be a weakness. Of Marxism, he said that it makes predictive claims so vague that it would be difficult for them to fail. That is, confirming instances become too promiscuous. But further, of Marxism he claimed that it has faced discon-firming instances in the past. In response Marxists have merely adjusted the theory to accommodate this apparently inconsistent data and "save" the theory. It becomes so easy to "confirm" or "verify" this theory that it seems nothing of any consequence is being verified.

Popper proposed that the principle of verifiability be replaced by the principle of falsifiability, which holds that *"it must be possible for an empirical scientific system to be refuted by experience"* (2002, p. 18). This too is a hypothetical or subjunctive principle. It does not hold that a scientific claim, theory or system *be* refuted or falsified. That would be ridiculous. Rather, the principle holds that any proposed scientific claim, theory, or system must have the possibility of being refuted or falsified by empirical evidence. That is, if the theory were false, there should be a way to empirically and logically demonstrate its falseness. Whereas the verifiability principle relies upon a foundation of inductive logic (which is inherently uncertain, or not even really logic according to Popper [2002, p. 18]), the falsifiability principle relies upon a foundation of deductive logic. Since deductive logic results in conclusions of certainty (not merely probability), science as oriented around the principle of falsifiability would generate knowledge that is certain. Logically, this defines an asymmetry between these two principles. One results in, at best, probable knowledge; the other results in certain knowledge. Logically, the verifiable principle looks like this in practice:

1. Observation 1 confirms Theory 1.
2. O_2 confirms T_1.
3. O_3 confirms T_1.

   . . . .

   ∴ T_1 is (probably) true.

The ellipsis represents an indefinite number of possible observation premises. Given the nature of inductive logic there is no formal rule regarding the adequate or requisite number of premises to justify a conclusion. The falsifiability principle in practice would employ the deductive *modus tollens* argument form:

1. If A then B.
2. Not B.
3. Therefore, not A.

This is a valid, deductive argument form, meaning that for any argument in this form, if the premises are true, then the conclusion will be so also. This particular form will be explained more fully in the following chapter. In the *modus tollens* form falsifiability would look like this.

1. If T_1 is true, then Consequence 1 should follow.
2. C_1 does not follow.
   ∴ T_1 is not true.

In this case there is no uncertainty regarding the necessary numbers of premises or observations. A single observation can refute or falsify the theory. For example, in order to *verify* the claim that water boils at 100 °C at sea level, one would have to attempt to boil water at sea level and note that it boils at 100 °C. Then that experiment would have to be replicated at another sea level locale—then again and again . . . . But no matter how many observations confirm this claim, it can never be conclusively verified. There is always the possibility that a sea level locale exists where water would not boil at 100°C. However, to falsify this claim requires only one instance in which water did not boil at 100°C at sea level. The same point could be made at the level of scientific theories and systems.

Here, then, is where we find the difference between Einstein's theory and the other theories that Popper seemed to initially intuit. Since it is so difficult (if not impossible) to find disconfirming (refuting) observations for those three theories, they can be judged nonfalsifiable and hence nonscientific. Einstein's theory, however, can generate clear and specific predictive consequences, which, if they did not materialize, would refute the theory. An interesting consequence here, though, is that no scientific theory can be conclusively verified. Of course for Popper conclusive verification is not a criterion for science. So on that level that "shortcoming" is not a problem. But it does mean that no theory is "true" or a "fact" in the customary use of those words. Every scientific theory is forever open to new testing and forever vulnerable to a potential falsification. This aspect of science imbues the practice for Popper with a level of risk. In fact, he predicated risk itself as a quality of good science. The better, the stronger a theory is, the riskier it is. The problem with Marxism, psychoanalysis and individual psychology then is that they involve no risk. There is little, if any, chance of falsification, thus no risk. This criterion also suggests that a strong theory be specific. General, vague theories would be difficult to falsify. More specific theories take greater risks (of being falsified) but are bolder and move science and human knowledge forward more.

Popper also distinguished himself on this question from the logical positivists by a certain narrowing of the question. Unlike verifiability for the positivists, falsifiability for Popper does not operate as a general criterion for meaning, only as a demarcation criterion for science and nonscience or pseudoscience. Thus, for Popper, nonscientific claims can be meaningful. Indeed, he noted that many times science has arisen from nonscientific practices, such as chemistry from alchemy, and myths, metaphysics, or other cultural forms of knowledge may contain elements or the beginnings of science or a scientific theory without literally being science—according to the falsifiability principle (Popper, 1963/2000).

One possible weakness of the theory that Popper foresaw is that it might be possible for a theory to evade falsification "by introducing *ad hoc* an auxiliary hypothesis, or by changing *ad hoc* a definition" (2002, p. 20). The problem is that a theory could then become like psychoanalysis or Marxism in becoming nonfalsifiable through changes or interpretations engineered merely to "save" the theory. Thus, if all theories were susceptible to this form of reinterpretation through *ad hoc* changes, no theory would be nonfalsifiable and there would be no science. This would be an absurd conclusion. To avoid this absurdity, he argued that the point of empirical scientific method is not to evade falsification (note how he praised "risky" theories) but to expose a theory to falsification "in every conceivable way ... not to save the lives of untenable systems but ... to select the one which is by comparison the fittest, by exposing them all to the fiercest struggle for survival" (Popper, 2002, p. 20). This "fierce struggle for survival" brings a sense not only of risk but of rigor to science, establishing it as a practice with high epistemic standards and highly justified claims of knowledge.

KUHN: SCIENCE IS PUZZLE SOLVING

Much like the positivists, the problem of demarcation was not of primary importance to Thomas Kuhn, particularly in the context of his most famous work, *The Structure of Scientific Revolutions* (Hereafter, *Structure*). However, many found an implied statement regarding that problem in this work and Kuhn himself later commented on and expanded upon the implications of his theory on the problem of demarcation (1970). Early in *Structure* Kuhn writes,

> ... historians of science have begun to ask new sorts of questions and to trace different and often less than cumulative, developmental lines for the science ... Seen through the works that result ... science does not seem altogether the same enterprise as the one discussed by writers in the older historiographic tradition ... these historical studies suggest the possibility of a new image of science.
>
> —*Kuhn, 1962, p. 3*

These few introductory statements suggest challenges of long-held presumptions about science and new, "revolutionary" ways of looking at science. Merely appealing to historians of science represented a break from earlier philosophy of science, which largely ignored and discounted the lessons of history. This quote also implies that science may not be a simple unified phenomenon or practice but one that undergoes fundamental changes. A further, deeper implication here is that, in contrast to Popper and the positivists, the essence of science cannot be understood purely by an appeal to methodology, whether that methodology be verifiability or falsifiability. As revolutionary as Kuhn may seem from these statements and as revolutionary as he has come to be considered by reputation, he in fact discounted his disconnection with past philosophy of science and asserted a fundamental connection to past philosophy of science, particularly that of Popper. He believed that his agreements with Popper outnumbered his disagreements. Specifically, he asserted that he disagrees with Popper on the relation of the scientist to tradition and the sufficiency of the falsifiability principle as a criterion of demarcation (Kuhn, 1970, p. 2).

Kuhn's humility or admiration of Popper aside, these disagreements turn out to be quite profound. Kuhn identified two types of science: normal science and revolutionary or extraordinary science. Normal science, as Kuhn explains, "means research firmly based upon one or more past scientific achievements, achievements that some particular scientific community acknowledges for a time as supplying the foundation for its further practice" (Kuhn, 1962, p. 10). In other words, the practice of normal science presumes and employs a host of beliefs, practices, expectations, theories that are all part of the scientist's worldview, web of belief or mindset. Together, these beliefs, practices, expectations and theories compose a "paradigm." Kuhn has been criticized for employing this term in various ways throughout *Structure*, but a simple definition he provides early on is "an accepted model or pattern" (Kuhn, 1962, p. 23). Within the practice of normal science, a paradigm is accepted or presumed and not typically challenged or criticized. Prior to Kuhn, a scientist would not likely be conscious of working within a paradigm but merely employing the beliefs, techniques, and so forth that are simply proper for the field in question. Thus, the concept of paradigm begins to place into question the assumed ultimate rationality and objectivity of science, as one paradigm is simply one of many and it is questionable whether a scientist could observe her own paradigm from an external, objective viewpoint.

The simplest, most common example of two distinct paradigms covering the same area of science is the distinction between the geocentric theory and the heliocentric theory. The geocentric theory of course posited that the Earth was at the center of the solar system (or even the universe) while the heliocentric theory posited that the sun was at the center. The geocentric theory from a Kuhnian perspective cannot simply be dismissed as prescientific naïveté or religious-based belief. This theory was not only accepted as defining the structure of the universe but was developed, expanded upon, given support, and utilized by astronomers for centuries. The movements of planets were observed and measured. New concepts were introduced (epicycles and equants) in order to give the theory better explanatory and predictive power. It, for the centuries for which it was accepted, made sense. The adoption of the heliocentric theory about 500 years ago was a different, more complicated phenomenon, according to Kuhn, than has traditionally been believed. First, the idea of heliocentrism far pre-dated Copernicus, to whom of course is attributed the modern heliocentric theory. In the third century B.C.E., the Greek astronomer Aristarchus proposed a heliocentric theory. The theory would appear again, from time to time, in both Western and Eastern civilizations. Yet, it did not begin to "stick" until the age of Copernicus, Kepler, and Galileo. This change Kuhn calls a paradigm shift. A paradigm shift occurs when a number of observations are noted or results arise ("anomalies") that are not explainable within the presiding paradigm. Now the difficult part here is that there are always anomalies that occur within a paradigm. Most of the time, these anomalies are explained away, either as human or instrument error usually. However, at some point, a number of anomalies may culminate in a "crisis," which makes the paradigm unsustainable. At this time, another paradigm will be adopted. How many anomalies comprise a crisis is not a question that Kuhn addressed, which makes the change of paradigm seem not entirely rational. It also challenges the common view of scientific knowledge as growing cumulatively. The science that occurs at these paradigm shifts is called revolutionary or extraordinary science.

This extraordinary science, as the name suggests, is not the norm of science, though. Most science is normal science, research that occurs within an accepted, unquestioned paradigm. Within normal science, the paradigm provides a framework from within which to work and to provide standards and criteria for what can be accepted as justified knowledge, as answers to research questions. The paradigm is a "promise of success" and normal science is "the actualization of that promise" (Kuhn, 1962, pp. 23, 24). In actualizing that promise the scientist's function is one that Kuhn describes as puzzle solving. A research question represents a type of puzzle that the scientist sets out to solve within the parameters of the paradigm in which she works. Just as ordinary puzzles—be they Sudoku, crossword puzzles, or chess puzzles—test the ingenuity and skill of the puzzle solver, so do scientific puzzles test the ingenuity and skill of the scientist. Here arises an important distinction from Popper. For Popper, scientific research tests the presuppositions (theories, principles, etc.) of science. But for Kuhn, in normal science, it is the scientist (and her ingenuity and skills) that are tested. Kuhn describes this distinction as the difference between the scientist as "problem-solver" (Popper) and the scientist as "puzzle solver" (Kuhn, 1970, p. 5). In this formulation then problems test science and puzzles test the scientist. Also, like ordinary puzzles, rules are requisite. In order to solve a Sudoku, the puzzle solver must understand the rules restricting each digit, 1–9, appearing only once in each horizontal line, vertical line, and nine square box. In order to solve a chess puzzle, the puzzle solver must understand the rules defining and restricting the movements of the various pieces on the board, as well as the rules of castling, and so forth. The scientist too has rules to follow. These rules are provided by the paradigm and define what types of research questions can be asked, what is involved in experimentation, what standards justify a scientific conclusion, and so forth. Just like the Sudoku player, the scientist must stick to these rules. They are enforced by the community through peer review, replication, and other social oversight. Thus the normal scientist does not question these rules or the paradigm in general but instead maintains a deep commitment to the rules and the paradigm. This aspect points to a sharp distinction from Popper. For Popper, science was a constantly critical practice. The scientist must always question her beliefs, presuppositions, and even the rules guiding her research. This deep commitment noted by Kuhn once again points to a less than fully rational concept of the practice of science, as rationality is traditionally understood.

John Watkins cleverly describes Kuhn as up-valuing normal science and down-valuing extraordinary science (1970). Popper's motto would be *"Revolutions in permanence!"*—and Kuhn's motto would be *"Not nostrums but normalcy!"* (Watkins, 1970, p. 28). For Kuhn, science is the mundane, everyday practice of the scientist in the trenches. Extraordinary science exists, but it is not the norm. Normal science is also the "practice of science [for which] professionals are trained" (Kuhn, 1970, p. 6). Kuhn's focus then when he thinks about the nature of science is the nonsensational, mundane practice of science occurring in labs around the world every day. One can understand this focus. Comparing the occurrence of what he calls extraordinary science to what he calls normal science, the latter seems to be common; the former, rare. Thus, if we were to define "science" as extraordinary science, much of what we refer to as science today would in fact not qualify. "Science" would be restricted to the rare instances, its "occasional revolutionary parts," represented by Popper's examples of Lavoisier's experiment on calcination or the eclipse expedition of 1919

(Kuhn, 1970, p. 6). What happens in between, though, would be a state of limbo for Popper. Normal science is more accurately descriptive of "science" than extraordinary science, according to Kuhn, also because the critical attitude Popper identifies with science is not limited to what is typically accepted as science. One can find it in the study of philosophy as well. Thus, this critical attitude, according to Kuhn, is neither a necessary nor a sufficient property of science.

Kuhn was also critical of the focus of Popper's demarcation thesis, the principle of falsifiability. Kuhn took on this element of Popper's philosophy by addressing one of Popper's own examples of what turns out to be a pseudoscience according to his criterion of demarcation: astrology. According to Popper, astrology is not a science but is a pseudoscience because it makes no falsifiable claims (1963/2000). Any seemingly falsifiable or seemingly false claims could be explained away by the adherents uncritically *committed* to the belief system. Kuhn disputed this straightforward claim: "The history of astrology during the centuries when it was intellectually reputable record many predictions that categorically failed ..." (Kuhn, 1970, p. 7). The dispute here is less philosophical and more a claim of fact that history may answer. Although, arguably, there is room for some degree of interpretability in determining whether a claim is falsifiable or indeed has even been falsified (i.e., "categorically failed"). If Kuhn is correct in this factual dispute, then it would seem that astrology would qualify as a science according to Popper's criterion. He points this out not to argue that astrology is indeed a science but to identify a weakness of Popper's demarcation criterion. Essentially, the criticism here is that Popper's definition is too broad in allowing in practices not commonly or intuitively considered science. According to Kuhn's definition of normal science, the defining criterion is the practice of puzzle solving. It is true, he admitted, that astrology has rules, much like normal science. These rules, though, are not a function of its status as a science but as a "craft" (Kuhn, 1970, p. 8). A craft has pure utilitarian function, means-end engineering. Medicine prior to the introduction of biomedicine in the 19th century was also, according to Kuhn, a craft. Whereas crafts, such as astrology or premodern medicine, have rules, their practitioners do not, according to Kuhn, solve puzzles. In astrology, failed predictions do not "give rise to research puzzles, for no man, however skilled, could make use of them in a constructive attempt to revise the astrological tradition" (Kuhn, 1970, p. 9). So, according to Kuhn, astrology is not a science *not* because its claims are not falsifiable — for indeed, according to him, there have been instances of falsification. Rather, it is not a science because it presents its practitioners with no puzzles to solve.

Popper criticized Kuhn's theory as it applies to demarcation on at least two fronts. First, Popper noted, "few, if any, scientists who are recorded by the history of science were 'normal' scientists in Kuhn's sense" (Popper, 1970, pp. 53–54). This statement highlights how fundamental the distinction is between Popper's focus on what Kuhn would call extraordinary science and Kuhn's focus on normal science. Just as Kuhn did not deny the existence of extraordinary science — just that it exemplified the nature or essence of science — Popper did not deny the existence of normal science, or at least the existence of normal scientists. But, according to Popper's estimation, they are not real scientists. The normal scientist is someone who "has been taught badly ... taught in a dogmatic spirit ... a victim of indoctrination" (Popper,

1970, pp. 52–53). So the normal scientist does exist but only as one who does not live up to the expectations of real science, according to Popper. The normal scientist has not been properly taught the critical attitude of a scientist, that one should only provisionally accept any scientific claim or theory, that one should not maintain an irrational, dogmatic commitment to any position, theory, or claims. The normal scientist, in Popper's view, has not been taught science but been indoctrinated with a belief system. Kuhn's view is not only mistaken in taking the focus from the "real" scientists; it is also dangerous, claimed Popper. By normalizing the so-called "normal scientist," Kuhn discounted or "devalued" the critical aspect of science, leading to a normalization of dogmatism, which would be "a danger to science and, indeed, to our civilization" (Popper, 1970, p. 53).

Popper also referred to the normal scientist as an "applied scientist" as opposed to a "real scientist" whom he refers to as a "pure scientist" (Popper, 1970, p. 53). These designations may well point to a philosophical bias on Popper's part that discounts the workaday scientist who toils in her lab with no recognition. However, this person seems to be the focus for Kuhn. This person also seems to be more common and numerous than the scientific innovators "recorded by the history of science." Of course, no normal scientist has been recorded by history. That is part of what makes them normal scientists. Their existence, their work, and their accomplishments, however, should not be discounted or dismissed. Their accomplishments may not be as flashy or sensational as those of the extraordinary scientists, but they are often important in their own right. Many who study science or the philosophy of science may agree with John Watkins when he says, "Normal science seems to me to be rather boring and unheroic compared with Extraordinary Science" (1970, p. 31). The extraordinary, revolutionary parts of science may be what attract many to it. The normal scientist does seem dull in comparison to the Newtons, Galileos, and Einsteins of the world. Yet these geniuses, though geniuses they may be, do not operate in a vacuum.

Popper's second criticism of Kuhn's theory as it applies to demarcation was sounder. He questioned Kuhn's claim that at any one time in any one scientific domain there is but one dominant paradigm that rules. Part of the difficulty of assessing this claim is attempting to demarcate paradigms themselves. But at least in regard to theories of matter, Popper maintained that there has not typically been one dominant paradigm but "constant and fruitful discussion between the competing dominant theories..." (Popper, 1970, p. 55). And, depending on how one does demarcate paradigms from one another, it seems possible to raise other examples of not one but competing paradigms ruling within a scientific domain. This criticism reinforces Popper's view of science as essentially critical. It is this critical nature of science, for Popper, which guarantees the highest standards for knowledge, guarantees the rationality of science and guarantees progress in science that cannot be guaranteed in other fields of endeavor: "In science (and only in science) can we say that we have made genuine progress: that we know more than we did before" (Popper, 1970, p. 57). Of course, part of Kuhn's project seems to be to put this kind of belief (faith?) in the rational progress of science into question. Yet, even without this sense of progress, puzzles are still solved, progress made within paradigms and revolutions do occur from time to time.

IMRE LAKATOS: SCIENCE IS A RESEARCH PROGRAM(S)

At the risk of oversimplification, it might be said that Imre Lakatos carved a middle path between the Popper and Kuhn, attempting to retain a Popperian sense of falsifiability and critical rationality while integrating a Kuhnian sense of the traditionalism or conventionalism of normal science. Although the methodology he pursued in carving out this middle path was to criticize Kuhn while apologizing and (possibly) emending the work of Popper. According to Lakatos, Kuhn "fall[s] back on irrationalism" (Lakatos, 1970, p. 93), because the Kuhnian concepts of crisis, paradigm, and paradigm shift, which figure into his theory of scientific change (revolution), are not rationally determinable concepts. Leading science down a path of irrationality was beyond acceptable to Lakatos.

Largely, Kuhn arrives at this point of irrationality due to a misinterpretation of Popper on falsificationism, according to Lakatos. Two types of falsificationism can be gleaned from the work of Popper: naïve falsificationism and a more sophisticated version. Kuhn's error was to only see the naïve version in Popper's work, for only the naive version will fall to Kuhn's criticism of the falsifiability principle. Under naive falsificationism, "any theory which can be interpreted as experimentally falsifiable, is 'acceptable' or 'scientific'" (Lakatos, 1970, p. 116). This is the form of falsificationism discussed earlier in the sections on Popper and Kuhn, for this is the form that most patently comes out of his work. Lakatos, however, gleaned from Popper's work a more sophisticated version in which "a theory is 'acceptable' or 'scientific' only if it has corroborated excess empirical content over its predecessor (or rival), that is, only if it leads to the discovery of novel facts" (Lakatos, 1970, p. 116). Under the naïve version, a theory or claim is discarded once it is falsified or refuted. Yet, as Kuhn has pointed out, the history of science and the needs of scientific investigation dispute this version as a descriptive claim and likely also as a normative claim. Under sophisticated falsificationism, a claim or theory is not disposed of due simply to any disconfirming instance (refutation). Due to the complexity of theory design and the vagaries and variables of research in practice, the easy dismissal characteristic of naïve falsificationism would be imprudent and counterproductive. So, under sophisticated falsificationism, even though a theory may encounter disconfirming instances, it should be retained if it is corroborated, useful, and productive (of "novel facts")—particularly, more so than its rivals or predecessors. In more colloquial terms: Don't throw the baby out with the bath water.

Like Kuhn, however, Lakatos did not restrict his analysis to the level of "theory." Similar to Kuhn's "paradigms" he coined a broad concept referring to a large scientific view or grounding: the research program. Like a paradigm, a research program (or "programme" to use Lakatos's spelling) consists of the basic unquestioned beliefs and rules underlying the work of the scientist in any specific field. The rules he placed into two categories: negative heuristics which preclude certain paths of research (e.g., in modern biomedicine as a research program, hypotheses positing a demon etiology of disease) and positive heuristics which suggest or indicate proper research paths to follow (in modern biomedicine, the doctrine of specific etiology [Blaxter, 2004]). Science itself can be seen as one huge research program which is methodologically defined by "Popper's supreme heuristic rule: 'devise conjectures which have more empirical content than their predecessors'" (Lakatos, 1970, p. 132). Yet Lakatos's view, somewhat similar again to Kuhn's, is that science is composed of various research programs, such as Cartesian metaphysics (Lakatos, 1970, p. 132), Newton's gravitational theory (Lakatos, 1970, p. 133) or modern biomedicine. In addition to the two types of rules to be found within research programs, they are also structurally composed of two parts. First, there is a "hard core," from which the negative heuristics steer away criticism. Second, there is a "protective belt," composed of "auxiliary hypotheses," toward which criticism may be directed. The hard core remains intact while the protective belt is open to change. The negative heuristic of the programme forbids us to direct the *modus tollens* at this hard core. Instead, we must use our ingenuity to articulate or even invent "auxiliary hypotheses," which form a *protective belt* around this core, and we must redirect the *modus tollens* to *these*" (Lakatos, 1970, p. 133). In this way a research program maintains a sense of consistency without falling into dogmatism and irrationalism. Note also, the "ingenuity" he refers to as reminiscent of Kuhn's analogy of puzzle solving. While at the same time, the protective belt invites the kind of critical rationality of Popper's ideal. Regarding Newton's theory of gravitation, the hard core would be composed of Newton's three laws of motion and law of gravitation. The protective belt would be composed of "auxiliary, 'observational' hypothesis [sic] and initial conditions" (Lakatos, 1970, p. 133). This theory, though eventually widely accepted, was originally beset by anomalies. The adherents (as this designation suggests) of the theory stuck to it, or at least stuck to the hard core while adjusting the protective belt to preserve the theory as a whole.

So, according to Lakatos, contrary to Popper, not all scientific beliefs should be always questioned and criticized. Some hard core needs to be preserved in order to provide general, fundamental guidance for research. Yet, contrary to Kuhn, change in science is not simply a matter of "mob psychology." The protective belt changes for rational reasons. In this way, Lakatos claimed to rationalize conventionalism: "We may rationally decide not to allow 'refutations' to transmit falsity to the hard core as long as the corroborated empirical content of the protecting belt of auxiliary hypotheses increases" (Lakatos, 1970, p. 134). In other words, the commitment Kuhn proposed that scientists hold to the rules and beliefs of the paradigm in which they work is, in the context of a research program, not an irrational attachment. Within a research program, this commitment or conventionalism is rational, not religious, emotional, or irrational. Further, Lakatos allows for change not only within the protective belt but to the research program as a whole as well. Just as paradigms shift, so do research programs. But again, the shift will follow a rational process. However, the shift will not occur as simply or quickly as might be suggested by naïve falsificationism. As long as the program is still generating new data and a better program is not present, it will be retained. Not only does this standard allow for general, fundamental aims and purposes to scientific investigation, it allows for new theories (as in the example of Newton's gravitational theory above) to be given a chance to develop and take hold.

PAUL FEYERABEND: SCIENCE IS ANARCHISM

Austrian-born philosopher Paul Feyerabend carved out a theoretical position on this question different from the positivists, Popper, Kuhn, and Lakatos and one considered far more "radical" than any of theirs. Feyerabend studied with Popper early in his career and was influenced by him. He later developed theoretical views vastly different from and critical of those of Popper. Popper's view of science, according to Feyerabend's later work, is too reductionist. The logical positivists would be faulted in this regard as well. Feyerabend exhibited an influence of Kuhn in recognizing the historical and other "extra-scientific" influences on science itself. On this point, Feyerabend wrote that, "the actual development of institutions, ideas, practices, and so on, often *does not start from a problem* but rather from some extraneous activity, such as playing, which, as a side effect, leads to developments which later on can be interpreted as solutions to unrealized problems" (Feyerabend, 1975, p. 154). The institution of science, then, cannot be reduced to its supposed logical and empirical methodology. There will be many other influences outside of what is considered science (in a pre-Kuhnian mindset) that affect the development and essence of science itself.

Although showing influence of Kuhn, Feyerabend was highly critical of Kuhn's theory of science as well. Popper's form of critical rationality would exclude too much from scientific investigation due to the seeming ease with which any claim might seem to be falsified. But Kuhn's view of normal science might be too inclusive but also too exclusive of new ideas in its conventionalism. Feyerabend argued that Kuhn's puzzle-solving essence of normal science might allow more than we would want into the category of science, even allowing, possibly organized crime to be seen as a science (Feyerabend, 1970, p. 200). As conventionalist, normal science encourages too much loyalty to the status quo, inhibiting the new ideas necessary for science. However, strictly speaking, according to Feyerabend, there is no such thing as normal science as Kuhn described it. Normal science requires the existence and authority of one paradigm at a time within a discipline, yet, there are commonly, claims Feyerabe, "mutually incompatible paradigms" existing in a discipline at once (1970, p. 207).

Feyerabend referred to his view of science as epistemological anarchism. Science cannot be reduced to one logical/empirical methodology, nor can it be reduced to one methodology in general:

> The whole history of thought is absorbed into science and is used for improving every single theory. Nor is political interference rejected. It may be needed to overcome the chauvinism of science that resists alternative to the status quo.
> —*Feyerabend, 1975, p. 33*

Reduction to a methodology or to methodology itself would suffocate needed innovation. Since "the world which we want to explore is a largely unknown entity" (Feyerabend, 1975, p. 12), restricting our investigations to one methodology would needlessly, and possibly harmfully, narrow the scope of our perspective and limit our investigations. Even limiting science to what is considered "rational" (in terms of consistency, coherence, etc.) would be too limiting. To demand that new theories be consistent with old, that theories be wholly consistent with the facts, would again unduly restrict investigation and hypothesis creation. Not only that, such consistency cannot really be found in the history of science, especially regarding scientific progress (Feyerabend, 1975, p. 24). Feyerabend's primary principle of science is simply, "anything goes." Any rules are damagingly dogmatic. What scientists need more than methodological rules is creativity. Rules inhibit creativity. We see here also a political reflection of the freedom and democracy that characterize modern society. Though "anarchism," politically, implies more than the freedom promised by democracy. "Anarchism" implies a complete lack of structure and possibly chaos. But the practice of epistemological anarchism in science will not, according to Feyerabend, lead to chaos because "the human nervous system is too well organized for that" (1975, p. 13).

CONCLUSION

In 1981 the state of Arkansas passed a law that required public schools to provide "balanced treatment" in teaching both creation science and evolutionary theory. The state was quickly sued by a group including not only parents, biology teachers, and the National Association of Biology Teachers but various religious groups as well, representing Catholic, Protestant, and Jewish faiths. Put simply, the plaintiffs claim was that creation science, despite the name, was indeed not science but religion. Thus, for the state to require the teaching of creation science in public schools would be a violation of the First Amendment right to freedom of religion (the Establishment Clause) by imposing a specific religious view upon students. We have here a clearly important cultural issue regarding the problem of demarcation. In January of 1982, the U.S. District Court ruled in favor of the plaintiffs and the view that creation science is religion rather than science. The ruling of Judge Overton recognized the difficulty of the demarcation problem and provided reasoning that cannot be reduced to any one theoretical view. Elements of Popper, the logical positivists, and other theorists can be seen informing his argument. This decision did not of course put this issue to rest. It arose again in Dover, Pennsylvania when the Dover school board voted to include a statement on the limitations of evolutionary theory and the theory of intelligent design as an alternative as part of biology classes at Dover High School. This statement further guided students toward the intelligent design manual *Of Pandas and People*. A group of parents, with the help of the American Civil Liberties Union, sued the Dover school board. The plaintiffs contended that intelligent design was merely a thinly veiled version of creation science, and hence a violation of the Establishment Clause once again. Each side presented their arguments bringing in their own scientists and philosophers to support their respective views. In December 2005, Judge John E. Jones III agreed with the plaintiffs in his decision presenting much similar reasoning as employed by Judge Overton in 1982.

What is science? We may not have, as yet, answered that question. A simple response, given the multiplicity and uncertainty of theories presented here, is that there is no definition. Yet, given that we seem to be weighing these theories against what seems to be our intuitive or common sense notions of what is and is not science suggests that there is some definitional coherence to what we have in mind when we use this word. Each of these theories may contain some part of the truth.

So what we have here is a continuing debate but not merely an academic debate. This question can have important practical implications. Most simply, the determination of this question will affect what we fund as scientific research. And as indicated above, there are also deep cultural issues affected by this debate.

CRITICAL THINKING QUESTIONS

1. Is science primarily descriptive, predictive, or explanatory? Or can none of these be identified as primary?
2. Are certain specific sciences more primarily descriptive, predictive, or explanatory?
3. Is science prescriptive? Does it have its own values? Does it exist to tell us how to live? Or is that a function independent of science?
4. Which provides a more stable, justified criterion for science: verifiability or falsifiability?
5. Is it possible to have a meaningful statement that is not verifiable?
6. Based on the various definitions of science presented in this chapter, would creationism and intelligent design theory be considered sciences? Would biological evolution?
7. Based on the various definitions of science presented in this chapter, would nursing be considered a science?
8. Do nurses engage in puzzle solving in the manner that Kuhn describes?
9. Has there been a paradigm shift, a revolution as Kuhn describes in nursing?
10. Can science be anarchic, as Feyerabend advocates?

REFERENCES

Ayer, A. J. (1970). *Metaphysics and common sense.* San Francisco, CA: Freeman, Cooper and Company.

Ayer, A. J. (2000). The elimination of metaphysics. In J. McErlean (Ed.), *Philosophies of science: From foundations to contemporary issues* (pp. 28–34). Belmont, CA: Wadsworth Publishing. (Original work published in 1952.)

Blaxter, M. (2004). *Health.* Malden, MA: Polity Press.

Carnap, R. (1959). The elimination of metaphysics through logical analysis of language. In A. J. Ayer (Ed.), *Logical positivism* (pp. 60–81). Westport, CT: Greenwood Press. (Original work published in 1932.)

Carnap, R. (1967). *The logical structure of the world: Pseudoproblems in philosophy* (R. A. George, Trans.). Berkeley, CA: University of California Press. (Original work published in 1928.)

Feyerabend, P. (1975). *Against method.* London: Verso.

Feyerabend, P. K. (1970). Consolations for the specialist. In I. Lakatos, & A. Musgrave (Eds.), *Criticism and the growth of knowledge* (pp. 197–231). Cambridge, UK: Cambridge University Press.

Kuhn, T. S. (1962). *The structure of scientific revolutions.* Chicago, IL: University of Chicago Press.

Kuhn, T. S. (1970). Logic of discovery or psychology of research? In I. Lakatos, & A. Musgrave (Eds.), *Criticism and the growth of knowledge* (pp. 1–23). Cambridge, UK: Cambridge University Press.

Lakatos, I. (1970). Falsification and the methodology of scientific research programmes. In I. Lakatos, & A. Musgrave (Eds.), *Criticism and the growth of knowledge* (pp. 91–196). Cambridge, UK: Cambridge University Press.

Popper, K. (2002). *The logic of scientific discovery.* London: Routledge.

Popper, K. R. (1970). Normal Science and its dangers. In I. Lakatos, & A. Musgrave (Eds.), *Criticism and the growth of knowledge* (pp. 51–58). Cambridge, UK: Cambridge University Press.

Popper, K. R. (2000). Science: Conjectures and refutation. In T. Schick Jr. (Ed.), *Readings in the philosophy of science: From positivism to postmodernism* (pp. 9–13). Mountain View, CA: Mayfield Publishing. (Original work published in 1963.)

Reichenbach, H. (1951). *The rise of scientific philosophy.* Berkeley, CA: University of California Press.

Watkins, J. (1970). Against "normal science." In I. Lakatos, & A. Musgrave (Eds.), *Criticism and the growth of knowledge* (pp. 25–37). Cambridge, UK: Cambridge University Press.

Ziman, J. (1998). What is science? In E. D. Klemke, R. Hollinger, & D. W. Rudge (Eds.), *Introductory readings in the philosophy of science* (pp. 48–53). Amherst, NY: Prometheus Books.

8

Scientific Methodology

What is the foundation of all conclusions from experience? this implies a new question, which may be of more difficult solutions and explication.

DAVID HUME

INTRODUCTION

Many of us learned in grade school a rather simple and stilted process labeled the scientific method. A science education web site aimed at schoolchildren still proposes such a formulation in six steps:

1. Ask a question.
2. Do background research.
3. Construct a hypothesis.
4. Test your hypothesis by doing an experiment.
5. Analyze your data and draw a conclusion.
6. Communicate your results (Steps of the Scientific Method, 2009).

For schoolchildren this may be a good introduction, but it doesn't begin to hint at the controversies that the presumptions underlying this "method" have sparked. This method has been challenged both in theory and in practice. Philosophers of science have pointed to theoretical problems underlying this method; and historians of science (and some scientists themselves—see Bauer, 1992) have challenged the presumption that science is always, normally, ideally, or even ever performed according to this rubric. We begin with the most fundamental problem underlying this method and continue with various attempts to resolve this problem.

The Problem of Induction

An inductive generalization is the logical process of attributing a quality to a whole class of objects based upon our limited experience of some sample of that class. The interesting, and perhaps troublesome, aspect of this logical process is that it is common not just in scientific methodology but in daily life as well. We each make these types of inferences every day, often without even noting or realizing it. Merely

137

opening your front door requires what seems to be an implicit inductive inference that turning the knob has opened the door in the past and will do so today. Scientific claims, laws, and theories are largely based upon inductive inferences. Isaac Newton's law of inertia was inductively inferred from the observation of many individual objects that manifested this quality. From the continual confirmation of the hypothesis that all matter has the quality of inertia, the inference is made that the claim of inertia as a property of all matter is in fact a law about matter. In this example we see the direct correlation between induction and empiricism. Empiricism holds that knowledge is attained through empirical observation; perceptions from the eyes, ears, and so forth. Empirical observation is always observation of particulars. That is, we observe particular dogs, not the species dog or the concept of dog. We observe particular instances of matter manifesting inertia, not matter itself or inertia itself as general concepts or realities. Logical positivists/empiricists, being rather strict empiricists, noted this aspect of observation and saw at least part of the method of science to take these particular instances and generalize from them inductive inferences as a product of knowledge. The particular observations in themselves are not real or strong knowledge. The inferences based upon these observations are bolder, more useful forms of knowledge. The claim that a particular billiard ball has the property of inertia is a less bold and less useful claim than the claim that all matter has this property. The claim that a new antibiotic will kill a certain range of bacteria in one patient is a less bold and less useful claim than the claim that this antibiotic will kill such bacteria in all patients. However, the stronger claim in both instances is more difficult to establish and much riskier in terms of truth. As we learned in Chapter 4, inductive reasoning only leads to probabilistically supported conclusions. Thus, all inductively reached scientific claims, laws, and theories are true only to a degree of probability and always carry with them the logical possibility of being proven false. Yet there is an even deeper problem underlying this limitation. According to the classical empiricist David Hume (a person clearly admired by both logical positivists and logical empiricists), induction is not only limited by probability but is not even "founded on reasoning, or any form of understanding" (Hume, 1748/1974, p. 328).

Let's take a simple example of inductive reasoning. Most people accept, without giving it much thought, that the sun will rise tomorrow.[1] Why do they believe this? The simplest explanation is that the sun has risen every day in their lives and in recorded history in the past. So, the inference might be expressed in this simple argument:

The sun has risen every day in the past.
Therefore, the sun will rise tomorrow.

At first glance this may seem like a clear argument. Yet, there is an important premise missing:

The sun has risen every day in the past.
The future will continue to be like the past.
Therefore, the sun will rise tomorrow.

---

[1]Indeed, the fact that many will read this and accept this example as relevant and meaningful at indefinite points in the future reveals my implicit acceptance of this thesis, not only for tomorrow but for many tomorrows to come.

This new version provides a general principle that better connects the original premise with the conclusion, more clearly connecting the past to the future. But this new claim is clearly open to doubt and in need of evidentiary support. Being a general principle, it is not something known through direct experience, as explained above, but reached through some form of inference or as a self-evident, analytic claim. The denial of an analytic claim is a self-contradiction: for example, "All bachelors are unmarried." The denial of that claim would be "It is not the case that all bachelors are unmarried," or more clearly, "some bachelors are married." But to claim that any bachelor is married is a contradiction of the concept of "bachelor." However, the denial of the claim "The future will continue to be like the past" does not result in a self-contradictory claim. To say that the future will *not* continue to be like the past is an empirical and speculative claim. It can only be proven true by observing the future. One might attempt to provide support for this claim by adding the premise "In the past the future has been like the past." Yet to use this claim to support that "The future will continue to be like the past" claim would be to employ once again the type of reasoning we are trying to prove—to assume once again that the future will be like the past by again being like the past. This is a type of logical error philosophers refer to as begging the question: employing what is intended to be proven in order to prove it.

Another form of inductive reasoning is causality and is subject to the same type of criticism. Indeed, a causal inference may be understood as a type of inductive generalization. When one makes a causal claim, which is common in science, one asserts that some event A causes some second event B. This is an empirical, not an analytic, claim. For once again to deny it does not result in a contradiction. For example, one might assert that HIV causes AIDS. To deny this claim is only contradictory if we presume the definition of HIV as that which causes AIDS, but that again results in a question-begging argument. Indeed, if this *were* an analytic claim, it would not have been so difficult to reach. The early history of AIDS research shows the proposal of many possible causes of AIDS: amyl nitrate, a weakening of the immune system by a succession of (especially sexually transmitted) infectious diseases. And the fact that HIV as the cause of AIDS is so widely accepted and so strongly supported by research now that today those who will deny this claim are almost seen as maintaining a contradiction, they in fact are not. As small a possibility that this causal claim is false that there is, there still is that possibility. It is a claim that can only be justified through experience—in this case experience in terms of scientific observation and research—and inductive logic. This is because, to generalize again, to say that A causes B we are referring to two conceptually separable events. When we analytically say that all bachelors are unmarried, the two concepts (bachelors and being unmarried) are not conceptually separable because the concept of "being unmarried" is included in the concept of "bachelor." To say that HIV causes AIDS is again to synthetically connect these conceptually distinct events. For a simpler example, let us say the cue ball strikes the eight ball and causes the eight ball to move. Here again we have two conceptually distinct events: the cue ball striking the eight ball and the eight ball moving. As they can be held distinct in this manner, they are not necessarily or analytically connected. To connect them we must appeal to experience and something known as inductive inference.

The deeper problem, according to Hume, has to do with our concept of causality itself. This concept includes three primary elements. The first is temporality. That is, when we assert that A causes B it is presumed that A temporally precedes B. You never have an effect before a cause. The second element is spatial contiguity. The cause and the effect must come into physical contact. We say the cue ball causes the eight ball to move because it strikes the eight ball. We do not attribute the movement of the eight ball to the five ball which is resting still at the other end of the table. Even when we seem to attribute causality at a distance, we don't really. To say that pressing the power button on the remote control causes the TV to turn on leaves unsaid but implied that pressing the power button causes an infrared beam, which when operating on a sensor on the TV causes the TV to turn on. When we say the remote power button causes the TV to turn on, there is implied a causal chain. But beyond these two elements there is a third which is more conceptually troublesome. Saying that A causes B means more than that A precedes B and that A and B occur in the same place. Also part of our concept of causality is that there is some power in A to bring about B. Hume referred to this element as the necessary connection. The trouble with this element is that while the first two (temporality and spatial contiguity) are empirical, this necessary connection is not. A necessary connection implies that any causal claim is analytical, but as we have already seen, it is not. This necessary connection is something that we cannot see or perceive in any manner. "Causality" is, itself, beyond perception. Any causal inference we make can only be based upon the former two elements: repeated observations of A occurring before B, and A and B occurring at the same place. Thus, we inductively generalize from particular observations of these two elements to the claim that the two events are connected by this seemingly metaphysical concept of causality. Yet, Hume doubted that such an inference is rationally supported:

> The bread, which I formerly eat, nourished me; that is, a body of such sensible qualities was ... endued with such secret powers: but does it follow, that other bread must also nourish me at another time, and that like sensible qualities must always be attended with like secret powers?
>
> —*Hume, 1748/1974, p. 329*

As with the sun rising tomorrow there is no logical reason to accept that bread will continue to nourish me, that the cue ball striking the eight ball will in the future cause movement in the eight ball, or that HIV will continue to result in AIDS. He ultimately could find nothing more than custom or habit to attribute our inductive inferences to. That is, from viewing two events together again and again, we by habit or custom come to expect them to be conjoined in the future: a new day conjoined with a rising sun, HIV conjoined with AIDS, the striking of the eight ball conjoined with movement of that ball, the eating of bread conjoined with nourishment. But this expectation is merely psychological, not logical.

Now Hume did not completely reject causality or induction in general. As a human being he had to accept and work with those concepts on a daily basis, as we all do. His main problem was that as a philosopher, especially one interested in understanding and justifying scientific knowledge, he could find no logical justification for induction. And therein lay the problem: as a practical human being or as a scientist he has to employ and accept the practice of induction. But as a philosopher he can find no reasoning to back it up, leaving the status of inductively "inferred" claims as *knowledge* fundamentally uncertain.

Hypothetico-Deductivism

Empiricists in the 19th century (e.g., John Stuart Mill) and in the 20th century (logical positivists/empiricists) worked to find a better inductive methodology. In much of the logical positivist/empiricist work you can find many hopeful statements about the improvements on induction to come. A reliance on induction follows logically from the central logical positivist doctrine of verifiability. Many philosophers proposed strategies to solve the problem of induction. While none was successful in addressing the fundamental problem, a number of these strategies were valuable for highlighting problems attendant to the problem of induction and possibly making the problem of induction seem less intractable.

One simple strategy is the broadening of the role of the hypothesis. If we look back to the inductive method at the beginning of modern science, in the work of Francis Bacon (1561–1626), we see a very simple approach in his *Novum Organum*. He outlined his empirical investigation into the concept and phenomenon of heat. His method included merely listing everything that had the property of heat (fire, the sun, etc.) and those things which lack heat (ice, cold earth, etc.) then abstracting from all the hot things what they have in common, and which those things on the list of nonhot things lack, to determine what causes heat. There is a simple practical problem to this method which reflects the more general problem of induction. A list of hot things and a list of nonhot things would each be at least indefinite if not infinite in length.[2] Hypothetico-Deductivism, as employed by the logical positivists/empiricists, like Carl Hempel (1966/2000), was intended to address this problem. The basic structure of the method is to suggest a likely *hypothesis* to explain an event or predict the reoccurrence of an event, then logically deduce what would and would not follow logically (*deductively*) if that hypothesis were true—thus, "hypothetico-deductivism." Experiments then are structured to see if the logically deduced consequences follow. The introduction of a hypothesis provides some boundaries and guidelines, thereby limiting the observations that would be relevant to include in an investigation, for, in the words of Hempel, "a collection of *all* the facts would have to await the end of the world" (1966/2000, p. 45). But what exactly does "relevant" mean? What makes a fact or an observation relevant to an investigation? First, it means relevant to the hypothesis in question. A little more deeply it means that "either its occurrence or its nonoccurrence can be inferred from" the hypothesis in question. Hempel employs the example of physician Ignaz Semmelweis, who, while working in the 1840s at Vienna General Hospital, investigated the cause of childbed

---

[2]Of course this particular investigation into heat may suffer more fundamentally from some rather premodern misconceptions about the nature of the world as we understand it today. But this error would not necessarily be an error with the methodology itself.

fever, which took the lives of many new mothers in Vienna. What was particularly interesting and concerning was that there was much more childbed fever in the First Maternity Division than in the Second Maternity Division. One hypothesis he investigated was that the birthing position might be the cause. Women in the Second Division more commonly birthed laterally, and those in the First Division more commonly birthed on their backs. It seemed that those delivering on their sides had less incidence of childbed fever. Thus, the hypothesis was that birthing in a supine position causes childbed fever. The question of relevance then hinges upon what facts would be logically implied by this hypothesis. Most obviously a fact such as a rise or decrease in childbed fever upon changing the birthing position would be logically relevant. That is, if the hypothesis were true, we would expect a change in the First Division to lateral birthing to decrease the incidence of childbed fever. If the hypothesis were not true, we would expect no change in changing the birthing position in the First Division. In fact, he found that changing the birthing position had no effect on the incidence of childbed fever and concluded then that the hypothesis was false. The logical structure of such investigation would be as follows (where H is some hypothesis and E is a logically relevant event or fact):

If H is true, then E would follow (is true).
E does not follow (is not true).
Therefore, H is not true.

This is a logically valid argument. The form is known as *modus tollens*. Here is a simple example to illustrate the validity of the form in general:

If Bill is in Philadelphia, then Bill is in Pennsylvania.
Bill is not in Pennsylvania.
Therefore, Bill is not in Philadelphia.

Here it should be clear that the conclusion follows logically from the premises. If one is not in Pennsylvania, then one cannot be in Philadelphia—given that we are speaking of the specific Philadelphia that is in Pennsylvania, as the first premise asserts. The previous argument has the same *modus tollens* form and thus is deductively valid also. So it seems that childbed fever is not caused by birthing position. Another hypothesis he investigated was that "cadaveric matter" was the cause. Most of the women in the Second Division were attended by midwives, while most of the women in the First Division were attended by physicians and medical students who would often come directly from performing autopsies. To test this hypothesis he had physicians and medical students wash their hands before moving from autopsies to birthing. This may seem like a ridiculously obvious solution, but keep in mind that in the 1840s the germ theory of disease was still a contentious, not widely accepted theory. And, as we might expect, upon instituting a hand washing policy the occurrence of childbed fever decreased. Semmelweis thus concluded that childbed fever was caused by an infection delivered from cadavers by physicians and medical students to new mothers. The formal structure of the reasoning is a bit different in this case:

If H is true, then E would follow (is true).
E does follow (is true).
Therefore, H is true.

Logicians have a name for this argument structure also: Affirming the Consequent. For in a conditional (if–then) statement like the first premise, the smaller statement that appears between the "if" and the "then" is called the antecedent, and the smaller statement that follows the "then" is called the consequent. The second premise then affirms the truth of the consequent. The conclusion is the affirmation of the first premise's antecedent. The problem here though is that Affirming the Consequent is not a valid argument form. It is an invalid form—also called a formal fallacy. Compare this simpler example:

If Bill is in Philadelphia, then Bill is in Pennsylvania.
Bill is in Pennsylvania
Therefore, Bill is in Philadelphia.

It does not take much reflection to realize here that the conclusion does not follow with certainty from the premises. Given that Bill is in Pennsylvania and that Philadelphia is in Pennsylvania, it *might* be the case that Bill is in Philadelphia. But "might" is not good enough for deductive validity. There are hundreds of other cities and towns he might be in other than Philadelphia. A little reflection will demonstrate also how the argument above also does not guarantee its conclusion of the truth of the hypothesis. Thus, logically, Semmelweis has not established the truth of his hypothesis. Even replicating this test with the same results again and again will not logically verify the truth of the hypothesis. However, following the basic understanding of inductive reasoning—which as a matter of course sets aside Hume's actual conclusions and focuses on the hope that a better inductive mechanism will be found—"extensive testing with entirely favorable results ... provides ... more or less strong support for" the hypothesis (Hempel, 1966/2000, p. 48). This more or less strong support, something short of "proof" is commonly referred to by logical positivists and empiricists as "confirmation," leaving then scientific claims to be merely inductively confirmed through replicated tests, rather than deductively proven.

Probability Theory

Yet, how many positive results does a hypothesis need in order to be confirmed? No clear answer seems forthcoming. In order to provide such an answer, some philosophers of science turned, as did some early modern scientists like Isaac Newton, to mathematics. Particularly, they turned to probability theory. Most simply probability theory refers to the study of the likelihood that certain events will occur. This science/ mathematics began in the 17th century with the work of Blaise Pascal (1623–1662),

Christiaan Huygens (1629–1695), Jacob Bernoulli (1654–1705), and Pierre-Simon Laplace (1749–1827), as "classical probability." In classical probability any event we are sure will occur is given a value of 1, and any event which we are sure will not occur is given the value of 0. An example of the first case would be flipping a fair coin and having it land on either heads or tails. An example of the second case would be flipping a fair coin and having it land on both heads and tails. In between these extremes the probability of the occurrence of an event is expressed as a ratio of a number of possibilities of the occurrence in question over the total possible outcomes. So, in flipping a fair coin, the probability that it will land heads is $\frac{1}{2}$, as there is one heads side and two total possible outcomes. In rolling a fair die, there are six total possible outcomes. Any one of them on any one roll has a probability of $\frac{1}{6}$. The probability that an even number will be rolled is $\frac{3}{6}$, which can be reduced to $\frac{1}{2}$. In drawing a card from a randomly shuffled deck of 52 cards, the probability of drawing a spade is $\frac{13}{52}$ or $\frac{1}{4}$.

Classical probability is also called an *a priori* theory of probability, because everything can be known without any empirical foreknowledge. All that is needed are the initial conditions. In regard to coin flipping, what is needed to know is that the coin is "fair" and that the coin has two distinct sides. In regard to die rolling, all that is needed to know is that the die is "fair" and has six sides labeled 1–6. In regard to card drawing, all that is needed to know is that the deck is randomly shuffled, that there are 52 distinct cards and that there are four suits, each comprising 13 of the 52 cards. No experiments or trial runs are necessary in any of these cases. Probability can be calculated purely from these initial conditions.

Taken further, classical probability theory can calculate the probability of more complex events. Say we want to determine the probability of two independent events, two events each of whose occurrences have no influence on the occurrence of the other. For example, we might want to know what the probability of flipping a fair coin twice and landing heads twice. In this case we would multiply the independent probability of each event: P(a) x P(b), where "a" is the first toss and "b" is the second toss. Each toss of a fair coin has a $\frac{1}{2}$ probability of landing heads. So, to apply the formula: $\frac{1}{2} \times \frac{1}{2} = \frac{1}{4}$. Thus, the probability of two tosses landing heads is $\frac{1}{4}$. Alternatively, we might wish to calculate the probability of two events that do influence each other—are not independent. We might want to calculate the probability of drawing two kings from a randomly shuffled deck of cards with two draws. Here the formula is a little different: P(a) $\times$ P(b if a), meaning that we take the probability of drawing a king on the first draw and multiply that by the probability of drawing a king on the second draw. However, the probability of the second draw has been affected by the first draw because there is now one fewer king and one fewer card in total. So, on the first draw, the probability of drawing a king is $\frac{4}{52}$ or $\frac{1}{13}$. On the second draw, the probability is $\frac{3}{51}$. To apply our formula: $\frac{1}{13} \times \frac{3}{51} = \frac{3}{663}$ or $\frac{1}{221}$. We can also calculate the probability of getting two mutually exclusive alternative events. Mutually exclusive means that the two events cannot both happen, the occurrence of one excludes the occurrence of the other. For example, we might want to know the chances of getting either two heads or two tails. In this case, we would add the probabilities of the two events: P(a) + P(b). For the probability of two heads we return to our first formula: $\frac{1}{2} \times \frac{1}{2} = \frac{1}{4}$. The probability of two tails is the same. So then we apply our formula: $\frac{1}{4} + \frac{1}{4} = \frac{2}{4}$ or $\frac{1}{2}$. So the probability of getting either two heads or two tails is $\frac{1}{2}$. For the probability of alternative events that are not mutually exclusive, such as getting at least one head on two coin tosses, we amend this formula slightly. Let us call the coin landing heads at least once "a" and the coin landing other than heads on both tosses "not-a." Since we know we will end up with a result of either "a" or "not-a," the probability as a whole is 1, certainty. So the probability of the coin landing heads at least once will be 1 minus the probability of "not-a.' The probability of "not-a" will be the product of the probability of landing other than heads on each toss: $\frac{1}{2} \times \frac{1}{2} = \frac{1}{4}$. So, we apply our formula: $1 - \frac{1}{4} = \frac{3}{4}$. Thus, the probability of getting heads on at least one of two tosses is $\frac{3}{4}$. A little reflection or reapplication of the formula will demonstrate that this is also the probability of getting at least one tail on two coin flips.[3]

The ubiquitous examples of coin flips, die throws, and card draws are no accident. It is believed the study of classical probability began with a dispute between Blaise Pascal and Pierre de Fermat (1608–1665) over a game of chance (Copi & Cohen, 1994). This grounding in games of chance points to a limitation of classical probability, which lead to the development of more sophisticated theories of probability more applicable to scientific methodology. Classical probability contains a presumed principle known as equipossibility or the principle of indifference. Note the constant use of the word "fair" above to qualify die or coin. A fair coin is one that is not biased, not weighted or altered in some way to make landing heads or tails more than 50% likely. A fair die similarly is one that is not biased (or "loaded" in the vernacular) to land on any number more than the others. In other words, all possibilities are equally likely. The problem is that when we get beyond artificial games of chance to real-world questions of probability, equipossibility does not seem to hold. When it comes to games of chance, "the possible outcomes can be classified neatly into *n* mutually exclusive, completely exhaustive cases that fulfill the conditions of equipossibility" (Carnap, 1966, p. 25). But when it comes to more complex natural and human events (events studied by meteorology, physics, the social sciences, etc.), possible outcomes cannot be exhausted in an *a priori* manner. Of course, even games of chance are arguably not so simply determined, because the assumption of fair may not always be warranted and the number of variables may exceed those we can account for. Keep in mind that the purpose of probability theory, consistent with inductive logic and empirical science, is to utilize knowledge we do have to infer about knowledge that is beyond our direct perception. When flipping a fair coin we know that it will land either heads or tails. But we do not know which. However, if we could calculate not only the formal probabilities covered by classical probability but the infinitude of other variables, we could predict with certainty the outcome of each flip. Pierre-Simone Laplace proposed a thought experiment that has come to be known as Laplace's Demon. Imagine a being of immense knowledge and understanding who knows both the position of every particle of matter in the universe and every law of motion controlling that matter. Given some initial state of matter, this being would be able to predict the future with complete accuracy.

---

[3]Many of these examples borrowed from Copi and Cohen (1994, pp. 574–588).

It would be like us looking at the children's game Mousetrap. By following the Rube Goldbergian path that turning the crank will send the ball bearing, we can predict that the trap will fall upon the mouse. To Laplace's Demon the whole of the universe would be as simple to take in as the game Mousetrap is to us. Laplace's Demon would then be able to predict the flip of any coin by knowing not just the formal probabilities of a fair coin with two sides but the specific peculiarities of the hand flipping the coin, air currents that may affect the flip and even minor peculiarities of the coin itself that may make it slightly less than fair and any number of other seemingly incidental variables. One result of all this is that even with classical probability, the outcomes are "merely" theoretical, not absolutely conclusive. Thus, even though the chance of a coin landing heads is $\frac{1}{2}$, it is possible to have 10 heads flips in a row. It is possible to have 100 as well. Probability theory does not tell us that if you flip a coin 1,000 times that 500 will be heads and 500 will be tails. It does not even tell us that 1,000 heads in a row is not possible. The most it can tell us is that the ideal case will result, at least eventually, in a $\frac{50}{50}$ situation. It's worth noting that if a pair or one of a pair of gamblers suspected that a coin or die was not fair, they would test it empirically. Although in testing the coin or die, they would test it against the *a priori* expectations — perhaps not seeking perfect compliance, but not a very great deviation.

Yet experience has taught us that classical probability is good enough to provide us reliable knowledge in these limited situations with limited possible outcomes and limited "significant" variables. This is not the case in many real-world cases where the lack of equipossibility is a real problem. One development in probability theory to deal with this problem is probability based on relative frequency. Classical probability is based upon absolute frequency because we know, *a priori*, all the possible outcomes. With relative frequency we do not presume such knowledge. What makes this technique relative is that it is relative to the available evidence, not based on the absolute knowledge of only six sides to a die or two sides to a coin. Although, as noted above this absolute knowledge may not be as absolute as commonly presumed, but as also noted above it seems good enough to make classical probability a practical method for games of chance and other limited cases. This also means that probability of relative frequency is not *a priori* since the information needed cannot be attained merely from fully known initial conditions but requires empirical investigation. The probability of relative frequency is the type of probability associated with statistics. If we wish to understand how many Hispanic expectant women receive prenatal care, we would take a sample (e.g., 1,000 for simplicity's sake) of women who fit into the class of interest and determine how many of them received prenatal care. Let us say that number is 683, which would be 68.3% of our sample. For any pregnant Hispanic woman we could then attribute a 68.3% chance of receiving prenatal care. This is the type of probability deemed more appropriate for scientific investigation. Whether applied to physics, meteorology, or the social sciences, it takes into account the complexity of the world and provides not simply a vague sense of more or less strongly confirmed hypothesis but more quantifiable "degree of confirmation" (Carnap, 1966, p. 22). In addition, the formulae above, with appropriate consideration for a lack of the principle of indifference, function in statistical (relative frequency) probability as well.

Another theory of probability that many scientists and philosophers of science find more appropriate for scientific investigation is the subjectivist theory of probability. It is called subjectivist because instead of the objective information of the initial conditions utilized in classical probability (the number of sides of a coin, the number of sides of a die, and the number of cards in a deck) or the objective empirical information utilized in relative frequency probability, probability is based on the beliefs of individuals. Like classical probability, there is a gaming application to this technique. When betting on a football game, there are not the stable initial conditions found in flipping coins or throwing dice. The probability that one team will win is determined by what an individual is willing to risk in a bet. A football fan who is willing to take a 3 to 1 bet on her team believes that the team has a 75% chance of winning. This technique has the odd and seemingly counterintuitive consequence of assigning different, "valid" probabilities to any single event. The objective theories above worked to avoid this type of situation. But this variability is acceptable in part because it is recognized that probabilities do not inhere in events themselves. They are, rather, attributes of belief. This justification is acceptable, because both classical probability and relative frequency probability accept this principle, based on the recognition that probability is a function not of events themselves but of our limited knowledge of the world. There is an implicit appeal here to what social scientists call rational choice theory (see Chapter 14). In addition, for much scientific investigation and hypothesis testing, there are clearly not the *a priori* conditions assumed in classical probability but also not the empirical observations necessary for the theory of relative frequency. New hypotheses may have no history to draw from in order to assign a probability. The same may be true of new evidence. Absent these objective determinants, probability can subjectively be assigned to the initial conditions. Yet this theoretical approach is not wholly subjective, as these initial values will be plugged into the mathematical formulae of probability.

Philosophers of science who advocate subjective probability theory are often called Bayesians because of their application of a formula named for and designed by mathematician Reverend Thomas Bayes (1702–1761), known as Bayes' Theorem. Bayesians assert that scientists should or in fact implicitly *do* utilize Bayes' Theorem in testing and confirming hypotheses. Bayes' Theorem can be used to calculate the degree that evidence increases the probable truth of a hypothesis. Let us say a midwife hypothesizes that a particular birthing position reduces the pain and discomfort of childbirth. Call this hypotheses *H*. As a matter of subjective belief there is a probability that this hypothesis is true. If it were true, we would expect application of this technique to result in a decrease in pain and discomfort in childbirth. Call the occurrence of this outcome *E*. There is similarly a probability that *E* will occur. And there is a probability that *E* will occur assuming that *H* is true: $p(E/H)$. Once we (subjectively) assign probabilities to these basic elements, we can begin to plug them into Bayes' Theorem, which formally is structured thus:

$$p(H/E) = \frac{p(E/H) \times p(H)}{p(E)}$$

What we want to calculate, $p(H/E)$, is the probability that the hypothesis is true given this new evidence. So let us assign a probability of 0.7 to the midwife's hypothesis and a probability of 0.75 to the proposed evidence and a probability of 0.9 to the occurrence of the evidence assuming the truth of the hypothesis:

$$\frac{0.9 \times 0.7}{0.75} \frac{0.63}{0.75} = 0.84$$

Thus, the occurrence of a decrease in pain upon implementation of the proposed birthing position will increase the probability that the hypothesis is true from 70% to 84%. To some readers, this may all seem too arbitrary to be of any value, even given the justifications for the method provided in the previous paragraph. That is an understandable reaction. Yet Bayesians maintain that not only may the initial probability values be merely the subjective (though rational) beliefs of the scientists involved, but not even that minimal level of stability is necessary. Those initial values may be entirely arbitrary. This is because, according to Bayesians, as Bayes' Theorem is employed again and again and "more and more data come in ... the successive values of p(h/e) will converge on the correct value" (Rosenberg, 2005, p. 135). This is a remarkable claim, but one seemingly borne out by experience. It does not matter, then, what values one begins with. What matter are the logically derived results. And those appear to achieve the kind of universality and objectivity that we traditionally associate with knowledge.

Despite the seeming success of Bayes' Theorem, it remains a highly controversial concept. One odd problem is called the problem of old evidence. We would expect that a hypothesis which explains phenomena of the past or ongoing present to be provided more support by this fact. For example, our midwife's hypothesis might seem to be supported by the fact that women of a particular culture that traditionally employs the hypothesized birthing position are known to be unusually stoic during childbirth; whereas women from a culture that traditionally employs an alternative birthing position are known to be much more expressive about pain during childbirth. Let us for the moment set aside some obvious problems of interpretation that may taint this example. Any information that is known to be true already (old evidence) will be given a probability value of 1. It has already happened or is continuing to happen, so there is no question of its probable truth: $p(E) = 1$. Also, the truth or falsity of a hypothesis will not affect the probability of what we already know to be true. So, similarly, $p(E/H) = 1$. Now, let's plug these new numbers into Bayes' Theorem:

$$\frac{1 \times 0.7}{1} \frac{0.7}{1} = 0.7$$

So, contrary to expectations, old evidence, which is absolutely certain in truth, does not raise the probability that the hypothesis is true. Rather, it leaves that probability unchanged, according to Bayes' Theorem. One Bayesian response to this problem is to say that this unexpected, seemingly counterintuitive result is in fact consistent with an expression of a basic scientific value: hypotheses and theories should not be designed merely to fit preconceptions. Old evidence may instill in us certain preconceptions of how the world works and we may, consciously or unconsciously, shape our hypotheses according to these preconceptions. But we should describe and explain the world from an objective point of view, not from preconceived notions.

Although this answer may fail to properly distinguish from hypotheses improperly influenced by preconceived notions and those that simply (because they are right) are consistent with, and even descriptive or explanatory of, old evidence. One other Bayesian response might be to attempt to give old evidence not a value of 1 but a value that it would be given at a time before it occurred. The problem with this response is that it takes the most controversial aspect of Bayesianism to resolve this relatively simpler difficulty. Beyond the subjectivism of individually assigning probability values to events and hypotheses at question now, scientists now have to imagine themselves at another time before this old evidence is known to be true. And, as just mentioned, subjectivism in general is the most serious and fundamental problem critics of Bayesianism note. This fundamental use of subjectivity in this theoretical approach seems squarely at odds with the objective standards of knowledge traditional in scientific inquiry.

The Hypothetico-Deductive Method

Probability theory seems quite a strong method, and indeed it has proven so through much of modern science. It has proven quite fruitful and quite accurate in its abilities to predict and explain much of the natural and human world. However, all this empirical evidence aside, it still leaves untouched the basic problem outlined by Hume. No matter how much mathematics is added, the conclusions of inductive inferences are still not conclusive and there is no good logical reasoning to find belief in these conclusions. That is, we seem to be in the same place as Hume was 200 years ago. Induction, especially with probability added, seems empirically justified, but rationally, logically there is no clear justification. For this reason, some philosophers of science still resist reliance on induction as central to scientific investigation. Most important among these thinkers is the illustrious Karl Popper.

Popper proposed a variation on the hypothetico-deductivism of the logical positivists presented above. Popper's version remains truer to the deductive part of the method. Popper also proposes that a scientist must construct a hypothesis as a likely explanation for a phenomenon. That hypothesis must be tested with deducible results in mind. For the positivists, if those results are obtained, the theory is confirmed, not proven but confirmed. Taking the problem of induction more to heart, Popper is not ready to accept even this weakened standard of knowledge justification. So, according to Popper, positive results of an experiment do not "confirm" a hypothesis. However, following the employment of the *modus tollens* argument, Popper asserts that a hypothesis can only be refuted—never confirmed. In making a universal claim, as scientific claims typically do, merely one counterinstance can falsify such a bold claim. This then is an appeal to Popper's falsifiability thesis. It is Popper's position that scientists should not pretend to confirm hypotheses. The only real goal is to try to falsify or refute them. This strategy maintains a critical attitude toward scientific claims which would in theory lead to the strongest claims, as they are continually tested. Only the most likely to be true claims would be left, but no claim could ever be proclaimed true. To go along with this critical attitude only the riskiest, boldest hypotheses should be proposed and tested. Testing and failing to refute a weak hypothesis does not prove much. But to test and fail to refute a risky, bold hypothesis makes a stronger statement. And to test and refute a risky, bold hypothesis expresses the scientist's proper attitude and orientation as an objective knowledge seeker, not someone simply seeking to prove her hypothesis (and ultimately herself) right. Scientific investigation is not about any individual but about the method itself and about the cumulative effect of testing. The most that positive results can provide is what Popper called "corroboration." For Popper corroboration is a distinct concept from confirmation. Confirmation is meant to supply affirmative reasons to believe a claim, although, as noted earlier, confirmation is epistemically weaker than "proof" which provides irrefutable reasons for belief. Corroboration merely refers to a theory's track record of standing up to testing, its record of not being refuted in the face of good faith attempts to do so. An appropriate scientific attitude, according to Popper, will never put full faith and belief in any scientific claim, no matter how well corroborated. Scientific claims can only be accepted provisionally or tentatively, mainly for the purpose of testing further claims, building upon corroborated knowledge.

Popper's view of methodology may seem more logically coherent, yet there are both theoretical and real-world problems with it. Falsifiability falls to the same problem that W. V. O. Quine noted regarding verifiability. Recall from Chapter 6 that Quine's landmark paper, "Two Dogmas of Empiricism" (1951/2000) placed the logical positivist thesis of verifiability into question by noting that no statement can be tested in isolation. Every experiment tests not only the claim in question but a host of attendant claims or presumptions: the accuracy of measurement instruments, theoretical presuppositions, and so forth. This turns out to be a problem for Popper's falsifiability thesis as well—and by extension a problem for his form of hypothetico-deductive methodology. For, if a result appears to falsify a hypothesis, the hypothesis itself may in fact be true and the real problem may lie with one of the attendant claims being implicitly tested. This leaves us in a seemingly untenable logical position regarding scientific claims, succinctly described by Imre Lakatos: "Scientific theories are not only equally unprovable, and equally improbable, but they are also equally undisprovable" (Lakatos, 1970, p. 103).

Due to this problem, Popper replaced this simple form of falsificationism (sometimes called naïve or dogmatic) for a more sophisticated version. According to sophisticated falsificationism, merely producing a refuting instance to a hypothesis or theory is not enough to refute it. In addition, there must be another theory to replace the falsified theory. And this new theory must explain all that the falsified theory explains and more (excess content), and this new content must be corroborated. These new criteria make for a more stringent methodology and provide more stability to scientific knowledge. Under naïve falsificationism any scientific claim, hypothesis, law, or theory could be recklessly disposed of by some possibly sloppy scientific work or some untruthful attendant claims. With sophisticated falsificationism, claims are not so easily disposed of. The extra criteria noted above must be met, bringing about a more stable collection of knowledge claims of which science is comprised. However, these new criteria, while providing more stability, do not actually address the fundamental problem. The Quinean issue involving the inability to test a single claim in isolation still holds. In addition, there are claims that real science does not function as Popper described. First, scientists often do not reject a hypothesis following a single falsifying result, even with the more stable version of sophisticated falsificationism (Bauer, 1992; Kuhn, 1970; Rosenberg, 2005). More typically, with a cherished belief (theory, hypothesis) at stake, especially one upon which other important beliefs are connected (which following Quine's "web of belief" concept would be most), a scientist may be more likely to make ad hoc adjustments in order to "save the theory." These would be adjustments not necessarily implied by reason or empirical evidence but adjustments (in auxiliary hypotheses) that would keep the theory (for now) from being falsified. Similarly, a scientist may blame her equipment or other variables instead of the truth of the theory before accepting a conclusion of falsification. Second, it does not seem true from the history of science and actions of real scientists that science gives as little value to confirming instances as Popper does (Bauer, 1992; Rosenberg, 2005). Indeed, the piling on of confirming instances seems in real science to have far more epistemic value than Popper's concept of "corroboration" suggests.

CONCLUSION

We seem to be in a very similar position we started out with following Hume. That is, as for Hume, induction seems to work but he was unable to find a clear, philosophical justification for it. As for us, science seems to work. We see apparent successes throughout time, throughout the world. We have eliminated or nearly eliminated some devastating diseases, invented flying machines, and even traveled to the moon. Probability theory, even though it does not solve the fundamental question of the problem of induction, has proved invaluable to scientific progress. So, just as Hume had to accept the practicality of induction even though he could not justify it philosophically, we, it seems, must accept the practicality of a pluralistic scientific method, even though no complete philosophical justification seems forthcoming.

CRITICAL THINKING QUESTIONS

1. What do you remember being taught in grade school or high school about the scientific method?
2. What, simply stated, is the problem of induction?
3. You may have heard the moral dictum "Never generalize." Yet we constantly generalize, perhaps even necessarily generalize, often to our great benefit. So, why this apparent discrepancy between this moral dictum and our epistemic and even mundane needs?
4. Will the sun rise tomorrow?
5. Does HIV cause AIDS? Does smoking cause cancer? How do we answer these questions? How do we affirm causality in such cases?
6. What difficulties are there in establishing that HIV causes AIDS or that smoking causes cancer? In what way are these in fact different questions?
7. Construct your own, original argument in *modus tollens* form.
8. Construct your own, original invalid argument in Affirming the Consequent form.

9. If science is supposed to produce objective knowledge, why do many scientists affirm a subjectivist approach to probability?
10. Why, according to Popper, does "riskiness" mean better science?

REFERENCES

Bauer, H. H. (1992). *Scientific literacy and the myth of the scientific method.* Urbana, IL: University of Illinois Press.

Carnap, R. (1966). *Philosophical foundations of physics: An introduction to the philosophy of science.* In M. Gardner (Ed.), New York, NY: Basic Books.

Copi, I. M., & Cohen, C. (1994). *Introduction to logic.* New York, NY: MacMillan.

Hempel, C. G. (2000). The role of induction in scientific inquiry. In T. Schick (Ed.), *Readings in the philosophy of science: From positivism to postmodernism* (pp. 41–49). Mountain View, CA: Mayfield Publishing. (Original work published in 1966.)

Hume, D. (1974). An enquiry concerning human understanding. In Anchor Books (Ed.) *The empiricists* (pp. 307–430). Garden City, New York, NY: Anchor Books. (Original work published in 1748.)

Kuhn, T. S. (1970). Logic of discovery or psychology of research? In I. Lakatos, & A. Musgrave (Eds.), *Criticism and the growth of knowledge* (pp. 1–23). Cambridge: Cambridge University Press.

Lakatos, I. (1970). Falsification and the methodology of scientific research programmes. In I. Lakatos, & A. Musgrave (Eds.), *Criticism and the growth of knowledge* (pp. 91–196). Cambridge, UK: Cambridge University Press.

Quine, W. V. O. (2000). Two dogmas of empiricism. In J. McErlean (Ed.), *Philosophies of science: From foundations to contemporary issues* (pp. 115–128). Belmont, CA: Wadsworth. (Original work published in 1951.)

Rosenberg, A. (2005). *Philosophy of science: A contemporary introduction.* London: Routledge.

Steps of the Scientific Method. (2009). Retrieved November 28, 2009, from http://www.science-buddies.org/mentoring/project_scientific_method.shtml

9

Observation: The Scientific Gaze

There is more to seeing than meets the eyeball.
NORWOOD RUSSELL HANSON

INTRODUCTION

There is perhaps no more basic and fundamental element of modern science than observation. Premodern science certainly depended on observation as well but not as fundamentally. The study of nature that ruled from Aristotle till the scientific revolution depended more on presumed basic principles and the claims to be logically deduced from them. Part of the change that marks the scientific revolution and the cultural/intellectual movement of the Enlightenment in general was a suspicion of such inherited beliefs and the replacement of them with systematized empirical observation, to which would be applied inductive procedures rather than deductive inference. As basic and fundamental as the practice of observation would seem, the concept is not as simple or as unproblematic as one might expect. One merely looks (or possibly also, listens, smells, etc.) Nothing could seem simpler. Yet, throughout the development of the philosophy of science of the 20th century, close investigation revealed difficult problems with observation laying bare the presumptions of science and much philosophy of science.

SOME CONVENTIONAL NOTIONS

Merely the word "observation" and its basic uses raise complexities. The word brings to mind first the sense of sight. Observation has something to do with looking, watching, and seeing. This makes sense from an etymological point of view. The word derives from the Latin *observere*, which means to watch over. Additionally, we closely connect knowledge and seeing in our culture. Consider all the light and sight metaphors for knowledge: seeing the light, the light of reason, a light bulb turning on, "I see what you mean." Correlatively, consider the darkness and blindness metaphors for ignorance: being in the dark, blind leading the blind, blind spot, love is blind, the three blind men and the elephant. Yet, of course, observation refers to the empirical nature of scientific investigation and thus implies all the senses, not just sight. And of course there are cases in which a scientist will use senses other than sight in investigation. In medicine, for example, sounds and smells can be very important. "Perception" is the broader, more general concept here, of which observation, philosopher Dudley Shapere notes, is "a special case of 'the problem of perception'" (1982/2000, p. 150). The problems of perception then also affect observation. Philosophically, observation can be said to have two aspects: a perceptual aspect and an epistemic aspect (Shapere, 1982/2000). The perceptual aspect identifies observation as "a special kind of perception" including the "ingredient of focused attention" (Shapere, 1982/2000, p. 150). The epistemic aspect identifies "the *evidential* role that observation is supposed to play in leading to knowledge" (Shapere, 1982/2000, p. 150). Considering the perceptual aspect, etymologically, "observation" seems to be an appropriate word. "Watching over" seems to suggest a sort of "focused attention." So, perceptually, observation is not merely taking in sensory information but doing so in an intentional even formalized or systematized manner. Further, observation transcends even this intentional perception by its epistemic aspect as a means of evidence gathering. It is not merely perceiving and not merely intentional, focused perceiving but intentional, focused perceiving as part of a larger, formalized project of knowledge acquisition.

THE PRESUMPTIONS OF EMPIRICISM

Let us start not just with an idea but with the word "idea." Classical empiricism employed the term "idea" in a significantly technical, idiosyncratic way. Within the discourse of classical empiricism "idea" was not defined as a new or original thought springing from the mind of an individual person, as it typically is understood in colloquial English. Rather, "idea" referred to any content of the mind: "whatsoever is the *object* of the understanding when a man [sic] thinks" (Locke, 1690/1974, p. 9). With this use of the word an idea could be the color yellow, the sound of a bell, a Christmas tree, or even one's own mind. It was also generally held by classical empiricists that ideas have two origins: sensation and reflection. Sensation of course clearly refers to the powers of the body to take in information from the external world: sight, hearing, and so forth. Ideas from sensation would include such ideas as yellow, white, heat, cold, the sound of a bell, and a Christmas tree. Reflection refers to the mind turning its perception and understanding upon itself. Ideas from reflection would include perception, thinking, doubting, reasoning, and believing. It was also largely accepted that ideas "enter by the sense simple and unmixed" (Locke, 1690/1974, p. 15). For example, when sensing an ice cube, what enter our senses are discrete simple ideas: cold, hard, wet. Our mind then places these *simple ideas* into manifold wholes, creating *complex ideas*. An ice cube, then, and also a Christmas tree would be complex ideas, as they are composed of other simple ideas, whereas a simple idea is basic and irreducible to more fundamental elements (ideas). Another important type of complex idea is the general idea. Empirically, general ideas are problematic. They seem "simple" (in the colloquial sense of that term) but when considered from an empirical point of view become a problem. A general idea would be one such as "red" or "dog" as opposed to a particular experience of redness (seeing a red stop sign or a red fire truck or a vial of blood) or a particular dog (Lassie, Benji, or Rin Tin Tin). The problem from an empirical point of view is that whereas we have direct empirical experience of particular experiences of red or particular dogs, we do not have direct empirical experience of "red" or "dog" as general concepts. According to empiricists, our mind can abstract from simple ideas and particular observations to create general ideas like "red" and "dog" (Berkeley, 1710/1974, pp. 138–151; Locke, 1690/1974, pp. 37–38). For example, by repeatedly seeing red things (stop signs, fire trucks, blood) our minds abstract the similarity of color from these otherwise very different things to form the general idea of red.

Whereas the mind has the power to create complex ideas (as either manifold wholes or abstracted generalizations), classical empiricists held that the mind is passive in regard to simple ideas. Simple ideas are merely absorbed by the mind, perhaps much like how camera film absorbs light to reproduce the visual array of an external object as a picture. This passivity might seem like a weakness but it is important to the empiricist theory of knowledge. Since simple ideas are in themselves unmanipulable, they compose what can be called "brute data." Brute data simply exist as they are and are not in need of interpretation or analysis. From an epistemological point of view, this provides an independent stability to knowledge. By appealing to brute data, knowledge can be given a foundation beyond the subjective beliefs or the mental operations of any single person. Thus, for classical empiricists, simple ideas are the basis of all knowledge and any claims to knowledge should be reducible to a (or more than one) simple idea. Any philosophical or religious term or any claim to knowledge in general that cannot be traced back to at least one simple idea would be mere nonsense.

Two important presumptions can be drawn from this analysis. These are "presumptions" because they are not so much argued for as accepted as true without much question. And much subsequent philosophical study has placed these presumptions into question. First is the claim that ideas enter the senses simple and unmixed. This claim seems obvious and commonsensical given that, as Locke writes, "there is nothing can be plainer to a man than the clear and distinct perception he has of those simple ideas … one uniform appearance, or conception in the mind" (1690/ 1974, pp. 15–16). Yet, as obvious and commonsensical as this claim might seem, there are modern philosophical and psychological reasons to question and doubt it. Second is the claim that simple ideas are a type of brute data that merely enter the mind and endure no interpretation or any other subjectivizing mental processes. This presumption is particularly important, and not unrelated to the first, because it is this presumption which provides classical empiricism its ultimate epistemic authority, providing an objective, independent foundation for knowledge. Yet much philosophical and psychological study of the past 100 years has placed this claim into question as well.

While classical empiricism is not entirely coextensive with the empiricism accepted by later philosophers of science, the basic fundamentals of classical empiricism inform the epistemological views of 19th century empiricists like John Stuart Mill and 20th century empiricists like Bertrand Russell, G. E. Moore and of course Karl Popper, the logical positivists/empiricists and other important philosophers of science. In particular, the presumptions above—which relate back to questions of observation—seem intact. Yet by the mid-20th century these presumptions about observation began to be challenged, which by extension would challenge the objective, independent foundation of empirical epistemology itself.

PROBLEMS WITH EMPIRICISM

The classical empiricists recognized that empirical observation was not foolproof. They knew the error that optical, aural, and other sensory illusions could bring. The epistemological rationalists (e.g., Descartes, Spinoza, Leibniz) played upon the uncertainty brought about by the possibility of illusion to criticize empiricism as a philosophy of knowledge. Classical empiricists, however, did not presume—as the rationalists did—that knowledge must attain absolute certainty to qualify as true knowledge. The fact that we know we can be fooled by illusions, can recognize and fix that type of error, must mean that we can improve our perception and understanding. If we can look back and know we were fooled, whereas now we have clearer perception or understanding, then even with the possibility of sensory illusions empirical observation must be a strong enough standard for knowledge. However, as we will see, sensory illusions are only one type of challenge a fundamental reliance on empirical observation faces.

A Paradigm Case: Terri Schiavo

Let us begin with a story with which most of us are likely at least generally familiar. In 1990, 27-year-old Theresa Marie Schiavo suffered a cardiac arrest. She was eventually diagnosed as being in a persistent vegetative state due to anoxia secondary to the cardiac arrest. A persistent vegetative state is a type of cognitive pathology in which a person is awake but not aware. It is distinct from a coma in that the comatose patient is neither awake nor aware. The vegetative person may open their eyes and experience normal sleep cycles but lacks all cognitive function. The vegetative person has no consciousness as we understand consciousness in the human sense. She may respond to some external stimuli, such as tracking objects with the eyes, but has no experiential or cognitive understanding of those stimuli. Some patients recover from a vegetative state after a few weeks. However, the longer the patient is in a vegetative state, the less likely recovery is expected. After one year the state is referred to as a Permanent Vegetative State (PVS) (Jennett, 2002, p. 59). Hence in 1998, apparently accepting the irrevocable nature of his wife's condition, Michael Schiavo requested that Terri's feeding tube be removed to allow her to die on her own. Terri's parents, the Schindlers, disagreed with this decision, as they did not accept the vegetative diagnosis and the grim prognosis that accompanied it. In order to garner sympathy and support from the public, the Schindlers posted videos of Terri on the web. These videos showed Terri appearing to respond to the presence of her parents, watching the motion of a balloon, in general demonstrating the consciousness that a vegetative person would not have. Thousands, if not millions, viewed these videos on the web, including members of the U.S. Congress. As this case became a political issue, physician-Congressmen, Bill Frist (R-Tenn.), Dave Weldon

(R-Fla.), Joe Schwarz (R-Mich.), and Tom Price (R-Ga.), denied the vegetative diagnosis based on their viewing of these videos (Annas, 2006). Some viewed the videos of Terri Schiavo and saw a vegetative patient. Others viewed the videos and saw something different. This is the essential problem with observation in general: the possibility of two perceivers viewing the same visual stimulus yet seeming to see different things. This possibility further challenges the presumed objectivity of science itself. As we will see there may be several reasons why two people viewing the same thing may see different things.

Some Basic Problems

Before delving any more deeply into our paradigm case, let us take some simpler, classic cases of people seeing different things. One of these cases involves the Necker Cube (Figure 9.1).

As the two pictures below demonstrate more clearly, there are two distinct ways to perceive this drawing (Figure 9.2): as a cube in which the corner being pointed to is on the top right of the side facing the viewer and as a cube in which the corner being

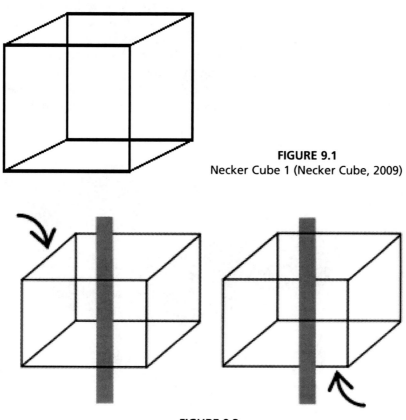

FIGURE 9.1
Necker Cube 1 (Necker Cube, 2009)

FIGURE 9.2
Necker Cube 2 (Necker Cube, 2009)

pointed to is on the top right of the side facing away from the viewer. Indeed, the same viewer can perceive the cube in both ways, but not simultaneously. With a little concentration, you can watch the cube switch back and forth—what is called flipping a gestalt switch (Kuhn, 1962, pp. 85, 111–114). But the mysterious thing is that when flipping this switch, the external visual stimulus you receive does not change. And when one person sees it as it appears on the left above and another as it appears on the right, again they are receiving the same visual stimulus. These facts point to the conclusion that an important part of seeing depends upon something that occurs inside of us and not simply what visual array of light rays reach our eyes. Another famous example like this is the duck–rabbit drawing (Figure 9.3).

At one moment it may appear to be a rabbit with its mouth to the right and its long ears pointing horizontally to the left. At another moment it might appear to be a duck with its bill on the left.

Now, one might protest that examples like these are quaint and even interesting, but they are artificial and intentionally designed optical illusions and not relevant to real-world perceptions. This may be so, but nonetheless they point to a variability in perception that does not depend on external sense data. Seeing these drawings in two different ways is called flipping a "gestalt switch" due to their development by Gestalt psychology. As we see a rabbit now and then a duck, a "gestalt switch" is flipped inside of us. Gestalt psychology (about which more will be said later) challenged the common sense view of seeing. The common sense view of seeing (and also the one seemingly held by classical empiricists and many other empiricists) is that the eye works simply like a camera: absorbing sensory information. Thus, just like a pair of cameras, "two people viewing the same object under the same circumstances . . . will 'see' the same thing" (French, 2007, p. 62). Yet what these two examples (and there are countless many others) begin to show is that there is something wrong

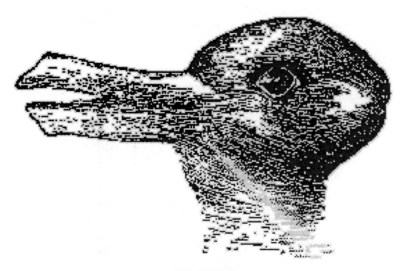

FIGURE 9.3
Duck–Rabbit (Rabbit–Duck Illusion, 2010)

with this commonsense view. And further, as Kuhn (1962) maintained, in real life also, gestalt switches are flipped.

For a real-world example, Norwood Hanson (1965) asks whether 17th century astronomer Johannes Kepler and 16th century astronomer Tycho Brahe "saw" the same thing when they looked up at the sun. The complicating factor is that Kepler held a heliocentric theory while Brahe a geocentric theory. Hanson's answer to this question is yes and no. When each of these men looked at the sun they had the same "retinal reaction" (Hanson, 1965, p. 6). Their eyes absorbed essentially the same sense data. On that level they saw the same thing. But, that is not all there is to seeing. For, "... seeing the sun is not seeing retinal pictures of the sun ... Seeing is an experience. A retinal reaction is only a physical state" (Hanson, 1965, p. 6). Hanson makes a quasi-phenomenological point here. Contrary to the classical empiricist presumptions, seeing (or indeed hearing, smelling, tasting, and tactilely feeling as well) is more than the accumulation and absorption of sense data. It is an experience of the person (using that word more expansively than did the classical empiricists) not merely a function of the senses. It is an experience that persons have as persons not merely as collections of sense organs. Because of differing theoretical presumptions, when Kepler and Brahe looked at the sun, there is a sense also in which they saw different things. For Brahe the sun was but one of many bodies that revolved around the central (and thus cosmically important) Earth. For Kepler the sun held a central and thus more important place in the universe. So, even though they took in the same sense data and had the same retinal reaction to these data, the objects that they, as persons (not merely as sensory input machines like a camera), saw were different.

For a related example, consider an X-ray as viewed by a medical student and that the same X-ray viewed years later when the student is an experienced physician. The student might see a representation of the inside of a particular person. This seems correct. And this is also what he will see as an experienced physician. Yet, as an experienced physician, there is much more that he will see. There are anomalies and pathologies that remain indistinct and essentially invisible to the student. The elements of their visual fields are the same, but they are not organized the same: "the same lines, colours, shapes are apprehended by both, but not in the same way. There are indefinitely many ways in which a constellation of lines, shapes, patches, may be seen" (Hanson, 1965, p. 17). There are some similarities and differences between the Brahe/Kepler example and the X-ray example and also between these two and the optical illusions raised earlier. Clearly with the X-ray example, there is a difference in knowledge that affects perception. Part of the reason the physician sees something different is that he has gained in knowledge over the years and come to recognize subtleties in an X-ray that the student did not see. One might say this of the difference between Kepler and Brahe as well, but the situation is a little different. In Brahe's time, geocentrism was the largely accepted theory. In Kepler's time, heliocentrism began to find greater acceptance. So each was working with what was considered knowledge and truth in their times. Yet, from our point of view, we might now be tempted to analogize Kepler with the physician and Brahe with the naïve, ignorant medical student. If we want to find a difference between these examples it might be that in the Brahe/Kepler example the difference is one of theoretical presuppositions, whereas in the X-ray example the difference is one of knowledge. This difference breaks down, however, if we come to understand that any claims to knowledge presuppose some theoretical commitments. Comparing these examples with the optical illusions of the Necker cube and the duck–rabbit, it does not seem that any particular knowledge or theory determines which cube or which animal is perceived. The drawings themselves are designed in an ambiguous fashion and sometimes called multistable projections (French, 2007). Yet, on another level, previous knowledge or theory does seem necessary. In order to view the Necker Cube and see a cube at all, one must first have Western conventions of perspective internalized as part of the way one sees the world. Because, literally speaking, the Necker Cube is not a cube. It is a pattern of intersecting and overlapping straight lines on a two-dimensional surface. A cube is a three-dimensional shape. One not culturally assimilated with Western conventions of perspective may see nothing more than intersecting and overlapping straight lines. No one who has not seen ducks or rabbits or both, or animals similar to ducks and rabbits will see what most of us see when looking at the duck–rabbit picture. It may just be an odd, indefinite shape. Another difference between the later examples and the multistable projections is that with the multistable projections there is a third perspective to be had over and above the two possible and ambiguous perspectives. With the Brahe/Kepler and the X-ray examples, that third, outsider perspective does not really exist, which may lead us down the dangerous road of relativism.

When presented with these ambiguities, a common response is to draw a line between "seeing" and "interpreting," so that everyone sees the same cube but *interprets* it as one type of cube or another. Everyone sees the same duck–rabbit drawing but interprets it either as a duck or a rabbit. Brahe and Kepler see the same sun but interpret it differently. The medical student and the physician see the same X-ray, but the physician has the requisite experience and cognitive tools to interpret the content of the X-ray. This approach has the benefit of preserving some sense of brute facts. Lying beneath all these interpretations are the same perceptions, the same brute facts. This approach will help retain the universality and objectivity presumed by empiricists. Hanson, however, argues that this distinction does not apply to what we are discussing here. There are times of course in which we interpret what we see. On a foggy night, seeing an indistinct figure in the distance, one might have to interpret this blur of a perception to make sense of it. Once the object is nearer and clearer, one's interpretation will be confirmed or denied. This example brings out the point, the difference which demonstrates why this distinction does not help us here: "To interpret is to think, to do something; seeing is an experiential state" (Hanson, 1965, p. 11). When Brahe looked at the sun, he did not have a retinal reaction to a stimulus and then apply a theory to that reaction. Rather, his geocentric theory shaped the experience he had of that visual stimulus. When Kepler looked at the sun, he did not have a retinal reaction to a stimulus and then apply a theory to that reaction. Rather, his heliocentric theory shaped the experience he had of that visual stimulus. They both simply saw the sun—though what each understood as the sun differed and led to different visual experiences of the sun.

The X-ray example provides some interesting complexities. On the one hand, it's true here also that when the physician views an X-ray he sees something different than the medical student and that difference is not due to a difference in interpretation. On the other hand, oftentimes with X-rays some actual interpretation is necessary.

Sometimes viewing an X-ray is more like seeing an indistinct figure on a foggy night. And like the indistinct figure on a foggy night, the radiologist's interpretation might only be confirmable (or deniable) through a closer look (exploratory surgery perhaps). But separate and prior to these indistinct or ambiguous images, a seasoned radiologist will look at an X-ray and see something very different from what a medical student, or even a physician of a different specialty, will see. But still, the radiologist just sees the X-ray. She does not see and interpret the X-ray, unless an indistinct or ambiguous image is determined to be in need of interpretation. Analogously, a trained musician may be able to hear an out of tune oboe in the midst of an orchestra, where such a subtlety is lost on the average music-lover (Hanson, 1965, p. 17). The musician does not hear and interpret the intonation problem. He simply hears it; whereas many others, receiving the same auditory sense data, do not. Similarly, the wine aficionado can detect subtle differences in high-quality wines that are lost on most wine drinkers. The better paradigm case of "seeing," according to Hanson, would not be the reception of sense data, such as patches of color, as the classical empiricists maintained, but seeing what time it is (1965, p. 16). Once a theory and practice of time-keeping is internalized one does not see the clock and interpret the time. One simply looks at the clock and sees the time. Similarly, for anyone fluent in speaking and reading English it is impossible to look at the marks on this page as mere marks. Seeing the marks is seeing the words. We challenge any reader right now to separate the visual experience of these marks from the apprehension of words.[1]

Philosophers of science refer to this quality of observation being affected by background knowledge and theory as the theory-laden quality of observation. That is, whenever we observe anything, or more generally perceive anything, there is inseparable theory and background knowledge that will shape that observation. Even when we try to separate observation from theory we run up against an infinite regress (Popper, 1935/2002, p. 75). We take a particular observation, identify the theory(ies) that underlies it, then identify the observations that support that theory(ies), then identify the theory(ies) that underlies those observations .... We never reach bedrock, brute facts. This lack of brute facts is a challenge to the presumed universality and objectivity of science. How do we address this lack of bedrock and possible relativism? We will address that question later. First, there are some further problems of observation we must look at.

Further Problems

There is a similar problem to this theory-laden problem that was raised in the Chapter 8 on method. Under most contemporary conceptions of the scientific method, a scientist brings to any experiment, any attempt at observation, a specific hypothesis—a provisional answer to the question at hand. The presumptions that in part comprise this

---

[1]Or consider the Stroop test in which subjects are shown words denoting simple colors (red, blue, green) but in type colored differently from the color that the word denotes. Most people are found to have a problem naming the color they see. When asked to name the color of the type, they more commonly name the color the word denotes.

hypothesis may well skew the scientist's perception. She is more likely to see what she expects, given the presumptions of the hypothesis. This does not mean that she will only see results or data that will confirm her hypothesis. What it means is that what counts as either confirming or refuting data will itself be based on certain presumptions and may limit what the scientist sees. This may be even truer today with the aforementioned reliance on technology. A particular instrument may truly only be capable of revealing certain types of data—the type of data that of course the experimenter presumes will be present. Other types may escape detection by the instrument. Advocates for creationism and intelligent design will point to these types of presumptions to attack the presumed objectivity of science in general and evolutionary theory in particular. The claim of course is that modern biologists are so imbued with evolutionary theory (and the hypotheses with which they design their experiments so constrained by) that they are constitutionally unable to detect any data that would be inconsistent with the presumptions of evolutionary theory, thereby calling into question the presumed objectivity of science, especially evolutionary theory (Intelligentdesignnetwork, 2005). But as noted in Chapter 8 there is a practical purpose to the use of hypotheses and even the limitations on perception that they impose. Without such limitations defining relevant data, data collection would be endless and without form. Hypotheses direct observations. This problem is really a more patent manifestation of the theory-ladenness of perception. For, when we say that a hypothesis brings with it certain presumptions, what we are talking about is a certain theory (or set of theories) about the way the world works informing and giving meaning to observations and observation statements. By extension then, theory-ladenness is not really an obstacle to observation but is in fact necessary to observation. Background theory and knowledge provide context and form for observation. Without this background, according to Thomas Kuhn, our experience would be as William James described that of a newborn baby: "a bloomin' buzzin' confusion" (Kuhn, 1962, p. 113).

Movements in 20th century psychology also note, develop, and explain some of these problems of perception. Gestalt psychology was developed as a response to psychological structuralism which understood perception in a manner quite similar to most philosophical empiricists: we perceive the world analytically as an aggregated collection of sense data. Gestalt psychologists like Max Wertheimer (1880–1943) endeavored to show that perception did not work that way. According to Gestalt psychology, we do not perceive discrete quanta of sense data that we then place into larger contexts—like Locke's theory of simple and complex ideas. Rather, what we perceive are complex wholes that have a meaning transcending their discrete parts. Contrary to Locke's theory we do not perceive coldness, hardness, and wetness and place these into a whole we call an ice cube. Rather, what we perceive is an ice cube. We might then, as a matter of analytical thought, reduce the ice cube to its constituent parts. We see wholes in a context of theory, not "piecemeal or item by item" (Kuhn, 1962, p. 128).

There is a famous story about Galileo often raised as an illustration of close-mindedness and a lack of critical reasoning (see, e.g., Copi & Cohen, 2002, pp. 139–140). From Ancient Greece until the beginning of modern science the heavenly bodies (planets, stars, the moon, etc.) were thought to be just that—heavenly, divine bodies, part of a perfect realm beyond and separate from this imperfect world we live in. Because the heavens are perfect, heavenly bodies must be in the most perfect shape. According to Ancient Greeks, that would be a perfectly round sphere. Many of Galileo's colleagues still thought in this manner. Thus, when Galileo looked through his telescope and reported observations at odds with traditional beliefs about the heavens (e.g., a moon pitted with craters and valleys, rather than being perfectly spherical) many of his colleagues refused to accept his findings. At first glance it might seem ludicrous to deny such facts—especially given our position now in which these claims about the heavens are undisputed givens—that these Schoolmen were simply being dogmatic, arrogant, ignorant, and refused to believe what was plainly before their eyes. Yet, to be fair, we can try to look at the situation more from their perspective. The telescope was a new and mysterious instrument at the time. An adequate theory of optics did not even exist to explain how the instrument worked or justify the authority and authenticity of the images seen through it. With this in mind some degree of skepticism seems reasonable. Such skepticism can be given further support when we compare Galileo's drawings of the moon as seen through his telescope to later drawings and contemporary photographs of the moon (French, 2007, pp. 65–66; Images of Scientific Breakthroughs, 2008; Pope & Mosher, 2009). To dismiss Galileo's detractors may mistakenly assume that there is some privileged perspective, as there is with the multistable projections, from which to judge differing observations.

This story raises the further problem that in modern science much observation is done not by the naked eye but through various forms of technology: microscopes, telescopes, X-ray machines, magnetic resonance imagers (MRI), neutrino detectors, and so forth. Some of these devices seem like pretty straightforward visual prosthetic devices (microscopes and telescopes), while others seem like more abstract forms of observing (neutrino detectors). Yet the straightforwardness of microscopes and telescopes can be misleading. For, even with those relatively simple devices, some distortion of what is being seen (e.g., refraction) is inevitable. All these instruments seem to place something between us and the thing to be observed that may justify a certain degree of skepticism toward what is observed. For those with experience with microscopes, think of your first time looking through a microscope. You likely saw nothing recognizable. You had to "learn" how to see through a microscope. This common experience suggests that microscopes (and other such devices) are not simple, straightforward visual prosthetic devices. They are tools that affect and change the world. Yet in modern science such tools are indispensable.

This necessity of observational instruments and the problem above that it raises point to an even deeper problem of observation in modern science. Much of what modern science studies is not directly observable. The most obvious example is subatomic particles. The problem with some such particles is more than a technological one. Even if adequate magnification were possible, some particles, such as electrons, would still not be visible, as light rays could not reflect off of them. We can observe what might be called the *effects* of electrons, such as a vapor trail in a cloud chamber. Here, though, many would say we are not observing the electrons but *inferring* them from their effects, or at best *indirectly* observing them. Electrons and other subatomic particles are often then put into a class of what are called "theoretical entities." These are contrasted with "observable entities" which are directly observable, at least in principle if not in practice. This problem became especially troublesome for the logical positivists because they endeavored to maintain a strict empirical outlook, yet they were especially inspired by modern physics which focuses on many nonobservables. So the problem they faced was how to maintain a strict empiricist approach while allowing for the positing of unobservable entities.

To understand the logical positivist response to this problem the first thing to remember is the school's emphasis on language. All claims to knowledge are expressed as statements. Thus, when we say we *know* something, what we know immediately is a statement or sentence. How do we know if any statement or sentence is true? Sentences are justified by other sentences. But ultimately we must reach some basic sentence (sometimes called a protocol sentence or atomic statement) which is directly related to a particular sense experience—a line of thinking obviously adapted from the classical empiricist (especially Humean) thesis that all meaningful concepts must be traceable to a sense impression. This sense experience was, for logical positivists, what gave claims to knowledge ultimate justification and ultimate authority. This seemingly simple process is made more complicated once a distinction between an observation language and a theoretical language is introduced: the recognition that there seems something different in principle between the way we talk about observable entities and the way we talk about theoretical entities; that is, a difference between observation statements and theoretical statements. Theoretical statements refer to theoretical entities, which are not directly observable. To make theoretical statements meaningful, they must be derivable from protocol sentences and ultimately the brute facts of basic sense experiences. However, as we have seen, due to the theory-ladenness of observation, such brute facts are not forthcoming. The logical positivists did not of course recognize this theory-ladenness and assumed that perception was unaffected by theoretical beliefs and then assumed "a source of neutral data that could be used to adjudicate among competing theories" (Schick, 2000, p. 164). Thus, to make theoretical statements (and ultimately theoretical entities) meaningful, the philosopher must "connect the observational components of a theory . . . with the theoretical components in order to insure . . . testability" (Matheson & Kline, 1998, p. 376). Yet, without appeal to the stability of brute facts the authority of protocol sentences has no basis and the very distinction between observation statements and theoretical statements begins to break down. Every observation statement implies a variety of other observation statements and theoretical presuppositions in support of it. What this means is that "No predicates, not even those of the observation language, can function by means of direct empirical associations alone" (Hesse, 1970/2000, p. 169). Like theoretical statements, observation statements are given support and meaning by a constellation of other statements and theoretical beliefs.

One can even take the erosion of the observation-theoretic distinction even further, as Dudley Shapere does, in arguing the counterintuitive primacy of theoretic language over observation (Shapere, 1982/2000). Because of the use of observational instruments noted before and the centrality of theoretical entities, "science has come more and more to exclude sense-perception as much as possible from playing a role in the acquisition of observational evidence" (Shapere, 1982/2000, p. 150). Ironically, what seems to have become more basic than direct perception through the senses is supposedly indirect perception through instrumentation. The authority of these instruments is dependent on (much the same but maybe more so) physical and other scientific laws. As new laws are discovered and old laws possibly revised or disposed of, the background knowledge that determines the authority of observation through instrumentation may change: "what counts as an observation, is a function of the current state of physical knowledge, and can change with changes in that knowledge" (Shapere, 1982/2000, p. 143). This realization leads us right back to the problem of relativism.

Observing PVS

In the Terri Schiavo case, particularly in reference to those videos on the web, we seem to be in a similar state as many of the examples above. Some viewing those videos saw a woman in a persistent (or permanent) vegetative state. Others saw something different. Perhaps like Congressman Tom DeLay (R-Tex.) they saw someone merely "handicapped, like many millions of people walking around today" (Annas, 2006, p. 106). One basic problem that might be pointed out here is the mix of expert and lay observations. Because of the public nature of this case, many with no experience with patients with neurological deficits (such as Tom DeLay) felt license to make a diagnostic judgment based on their observations of the videos. Physicians are advised to pay attention to the observations of those caring for a patient over several weeks time, including nurses and family members, when considering a diagnosis of vegetative state—while keeping in mind the possibility of such observations being skewed by wishful thinking (Jennett, 2002, p. 23). So, lay observations are not wholly irrelevant. Although, the kind of sustained observations suggested are not the kind to be had through watching these videos. If it is true, as noted above, that background knowledge has an effect on observation; it would not be surprising that experts and nonexperts viewing the same videos might see different things. Yet, of course, as noted earlier, a number of physicians in Congress denied the vegetative diagnosis based on these videos. One response might be that, though physicians, none of these were in fact neurologists. They had some level of expertise as physicians but not that of one who specializes in neurological disorders. One might also impute some amount of political skewing and prejudice to these observations. Given that these were all Republican congressmen and that it was mostly Republicans who allied themselves with the parents of Terri Schiavo, there seems some substance behind this claim. These diagnoses by physician/Congressmen raise another problem with observation in this case. Making a diagnosis purely on the basis of such videos is both epistemically and ethically suspect. There is no direct observation of the patient, only observation through the media of video and the internet. Thus, as above, the inclusion of instrumentation between the observer and the observed allows for dubiety. Further, there is the possibility of editing and the selective use of cuts to be placed on the web that could skew perception. Not only the fact of instrumentation being inserted between the observer and the observed can cause doubt, but the nature of that instrumentation to allow for manipulation can raise further doubt about what one is seeing.

Ultimately, the problem with observing the vegetative state is that this state relates to consciousness. As such, it raises the issue known to philosophers as the "other minds" problem. We are intimately familiar with our own consciousness (our own mind, not to be confused with our own brain, of which most of us know little) but have no direct contact with the consciousness of any other person. This raises the specter of solipsism. That is, for all we know the rest of humanity surrounding us may be a horde of mindless robots and may not have the type of feelings, experiences, and inner life—in general self-consciousness or self-awareness—that we do. One response to the other minds problem is that we can know others have minds by analogy. When we see others acting and reacting in manners similar to how we (as mind-having entities) act and react, we can infer that they do so also because they have minds. Leaving aside the problems philosophers have raised regarding this approach to the problem, we can note that neurologists will employ a similar standard in diagnosing vegetative state: "Much of the debate about diagnosis turns on what behaviours reflect cortical activity, and whether fragments of activity in the cortex necessarily indicates awareness—lack of which is the crux of the diagnosis of the vegetative state" (Jennett, 2002, p. 11). In simpler terms, people who have consciousness behave like *people who have consciousness*. Behavior is something we can see, consciousness is not. Yet certain problems arise here. Can we assume we know all the behaviors in which consciousness is manifested? Does this means of diagnosis reduce consciousness merely to its behavioral components? This is part of what makes a problem of the distinction of vegetative state from locked-in syndrome: a condition in which the "descending motor pathways from the brain are out of action" leaving the patient with little or no motor function but with sensation and consciousness fully preserved (Jennett, 2002, p. 20). If consciousness is to be inferred from behavior, yet a locked-in patient has no motor function, there will be no behavior to infer from, and such absence could lead to an inference of vegetative state. Behind the diagnosis of vegetative state lies a particular theory of consciousness, that consciousness includes certain subjective, mental states, that consciousness is somehow (in manners we do not fully understand) connected to brain states, that consciousness somehow transcends mere biological function, and so forth. Consciousness and, by extension, pathologies of consciousness like PVS become theoretical entities, not directly, empirically observable ones.

One might think that a simple solution would be to find pathological states of the brain to which PVS could be correlated. The first problem with that, however, is that such states have not been discovered. This is why PVS is a clinical diagnosis. The condition does not refer to any specific underlying pathological state of the brain. EEG (electroencephalography), CT computerized tomography), MRI, and PET (positron emission tomography) can all be used to observe states of the brain consistent with PVS but none of these results (or any combination of them) is diagnostically conclusive (Jennett, 2002, pp. 25–28). Also, as noted earlier, these are tools of observation (like microscopes and telescopes) that place technology between the perceiver and the thing perceived, thereby inserting room for doubt considering what is being observed (recall Galileo's inaccurate drawings of the moon seen through his telescope). Again, when we employ any of the diagnostic instruments above (EEG, CT, etc.), there is a plethora of theory lying behind our trust in these instruments and our perception of the information they give us—indeed our perception that what they provide us *is* indeed information. It seems that certain pathological states of the brain can be identified upon autopsy as indicative of PVS, but that is of no help in diagnosing a still living patient (Jennett, 2002, pp. 51–56).

But the deeper problem here is that we must remember what is under consideration here is consciousness, and none of these tools or tests "directly reflects consciousness" (Jennett, 2002, p. 28). Consciousness is a function of the mind that seems connected to but not defined by states of the brain. Minds are not (strictly speaking) observable (brains are, minds aren't) and neither is consciousness. Just as a diagnosis based on behavior has its limitations, one based on these diagnostic tools has even further ones—even though on the surface they might seem more "scientific," more objective, more sophisticated. None of the results we can attain from such tests is backed up by our long-held views (theories) of what consciousness is, whereas a behavioral diagnosis can be. This is due in part to the newness of these tools. In the future, our theory of consciousness may change such that these tools are a more direct reflection than our observation of behavior.

CONCLUSIONS: CAN OBJECTIVITY BE SAVED?

Perhaps the most fundamental problem we have come across is the theory-ladenness of observation. This seems to underlie many of the other problems raised: particularly the distinction between observation statements and theoretical statements, and the problem of observing through the medium of observational instruments. There is perhaps no greater defender of the objectivity of science than Karl Popper, yet he has to admit limitations to the objectivity of science. Science's objectivity is not, he wrote, "absolute" (Popper, 1935/2002, p. 93). Rather, due to the theory-ladenness of observation, the claims of science do not have the "bedrock" support once believed. Rather, science is like a building built in a swamp (Popper, 1935/2002). In order to attain any stability it must be built upon piles. Metaphorically, these piles would be long tested and widely accepted theories that shape our observations, justificatory strategies, and so forth. Yet these piles are driven into nothing more stable than the swamp itself. They need to be driven down in order to attain stability. That is, the theories must be embedded in our consciousnesses to help shape our belief system and worldviews in order to provide a framework for study. But, "if we stop driving the piles deeper, it is not because we have reached firm ground"—because we have realized, due to the problem of theory-ladenness, there is no firm ground to be had—"We simply stop when we are satisfied that the piles are firm enough to carry the structure, at least for the time being" (Popper, 1935/2002, p. 94). This last statement reflects Popper's falsifiability thesis and the fallibility built into science according to his view. No statement or theory is ever conclusively proven. It is only ever provisionally accepted "for the time being" as long as it is "firm enough to carry the structure."

Dudley Shapere (1982/2000) develops this type of answer further. When we note that observation is "laden" it is important that we consider that with which it is laden. To assume that the theory-ladenness of observation leads to epistemological relativism seems to assume that what it is laden with is itself arbitrary or at least uncertain. But what observation is laden with is "the best information [science] has available" (Shapere, 1982/2000, p. 153). Thus, "the fact that what counts as 'observational' in science is 'laden' with background information does not imply that observation is 'loaded' in favor of arbitrary, relative or even, in any useful sense, 'uncertain' views" (Shapere, 1982/2000, p. 153). Shapere's qualification of 'uncertainty' needing to be in a "useful sense" in order to be meaningful in this context is a restatement of the classical empiricist admission that empirical knowledge does not attain the level of absolute certainty that epistemological rationalists like Descartes strived for, but that that lack of absolute certainty did not disqualify it as knowledge. Uncertain in a useless sense is this broad recognition that absolute certainty is never achieved with any empirical claim. Uncertain in a "useful sense" would mean that there is a specific reason to doubt some specific claim—not simply the broad thesis that all empirical claims lack absolute certainty. This description develops Popper's claim that the piles must be driven down for stability but never reach firm ground, bedrock. Without any "useful uncertainty," however, they are "firm enough to carry the structure, at least for the time being."

This argument reaffirms the earlier claim that background knowledge and theory are in fact necessary to guide and limit observation and scientific investigation in general. They are "the means by which such further information comes to be attained" (Shapere, 1982/2000, p. 154). This recognition also begins to break down the observation/theory distinction even further. As observation (in general) depends upon background knowledge and theory, theoretical statements become just another form of observation statement—perhaps distinct only in the degree of reliance on background theory and knowledge, not distinct in kind from observation statements. Thus, both observation statements and theoretical statements (as much as we can continue that distinction) are only as strong as the theory and background knowledge that provide their foundation. Similarly, the authority of the results from any observation instrument depends upon background knowledge and a theoretical understanding of how the instrument works. This information is not merely indirect perception or inferred knowledge once the use of the instrument, just like the conventions of perspective or telling of time, has become an integrated, internalized to the way we see the world. Shapere (1982/2000) asks us to imagine a photograph from a powerful telescope. On that photograph is a mark, a tiny reaction of photosensitive paper and chemicals. The image is no bigger than a period on this page. Shapere suggests a sequence of descriptors for the mark: speck, dot, image, image of a star (1982/2000, p. 155), and so forth. As we progress through these descriptors, more background information is required. A "speck" seems very basic and formal, very "atomic" the logical positivists would have said. A "dot" seems a bit more meaningful, seems to rely on and appeal to more background knowledge. To call the mark an "image" clearly requires more background knowledge: at the very least knowledge of the function and purpose of telescopes and photographs, if not necessarily knowledge of all the theory and technological advancements lying behind them. To call it an "image of a star" requires even further background knowledge to distinguish the mark from other heavenly bodies or even artifact. The point is, an astronomer viewing this photograph does not first see a speck or a dot and then builds up from there adding theory and background knowledge. Because much theory is already internalized— because, according to Gestalt psychology, we do not see analytical parts first but theoretical wholes—when the astronomer views the photograph she starts more toward the right than toward the left.

Have Popper and Shapere saved objectivity? Perhaps, but only to an extent: As Popper explicitly notes and Shapere at least implicitly notes, we are not going to achieve absolute objectivity. But lacking absolute objectivity does not necessarily equate to or logically imply relativism. The continued, independent testing of knowledge and theory provides for a limited objectivity. Observation statements and claims to knowledge may not be reducible to subjective belief and relativism because the background theory and knowledge upon which they are based are not merely the personal commitments of any one scientist. They are part of the community knowledge-base and theoretically open to testing by anyone.

Yet we still run into the problem that our deepest commitments may be so deeply held that they cannot be tested. Placing them into question could destroy any basis we have for questioning and investigating in the first place. Ironically, an appeal to a philosopher often labeled a relativist may help us. In his *The Structure of Scientific Revolutions* Thomas Kuhn referred to and reaffirmed many of the same claims about the theory-ladenness of observation. Kuhn, of course reinterpreted the ideas in the context of his concept of paradigms. For Kuhn then what affects, informs, and directs observation is not merely theory but the broader concept of paradigm which may encompass a world of theory and may in fact be more accurate than simplistically referring to theory-ladenness. In Kuhn's concept of normal science, the student scientist doesn't simply study a history of discoveries and learn objective methodologies. She enters into the culture of science: in a sense, a world unto itself "determined jointly by the environment and the particular normal-scientific tradition that the student has been trained to pursue" (Kuhn, 1962, p. 112). Claims like these led many (critics and supporters) to label Kuhn a relativist, a label he denied, but an understandable charge given statements like these. He seemed to be saying here that the scientist's worldview, understanding of the world, and observations are determined by the culture in which she finds herself, not by clear perception and an objective mindset. Although many of Kuhn's investigations seemed leading toward a relativistic conclusion, it seems also in passages from *Structure* like the following that he was not ready to accept relativism as the proper and logical end of his studies:

> But is sensory experience fixed and neutral? Are theories simply man-made interpretations of given data? ... I find it impossible to relinquish entirely that viewpoint. Yet it no longer functions effectively, and the many attempts to make it do so through the introduction of a neutral language of observations now seem to me hopeless.
> — *Kuhn, 1962, p. 126*

Of course Kuhn's inability to deny the "Yes!" answer may reflect no more than a constitutional weakness, an inability to accept an unwanted but logically inferred conclusion. He also notes the lack of (or even possibility of) a neutral observation language. Thus, his affirmation of the answer from three centuries of philosophy may not be warranted.

Remember that Kuhn understood two types of science. Normal science was the focus of the previous paragraph. He also wrote of revolutionary science which occurs at periods of paradigm shifts, periods during which fundamental views and beliefs about the world change. One thing we might say that paradigm shifts indicate is that although our observations are theory-laden (or paradigm-laden), such influences on our perception are not immutable. The piles are driven deep but can be extracted. Kuhn referred to a psychological experiment by Bruner and Postman in which subjects are shown individual playing cards (Kuhn, 1962, pp. 62–63, 112–113). However, some of the cards are anomalous, that is, they are red spades or black hearts. At first subjects do not note anything unusual about the anomalous cards. They see the red spades as hearts or the black hearts as spades. As the experiment continues, the subjects are shown the cards for greater periods of time. Eventually most of the subjects begin to recognize the anomalous cards as anomalous. What this study seems to indicate on a small scale is that even though our perception is influenced by theory and back-ground knowledge, such influence can be overcome to bring out a new way of perceiv-ing the world. For a larger scale, science-oriented example, Kuhn noted that after Sir William Herschel discovered the planet Uranus where others had only seen stars, astronomers were "prepared to find additional planets" (1962, p. 116). Beliefs about that part of the sky kept many astronomers from seeing planets. Herschel was able to see past those prejudices, to see in a different way. Once he did, others were able to follow him. Yet we cannot privilege this new way of seeing the world, of seeing planets where previously others had seen only stars, as "fixed and neutral" as merely the world as it is without prejudice or theory-ladenness. No such way of seeing the world has been established. No observation language has been established as such. No paradigm presents a world to us in as brute and unproblematic a manner. In Kuhn's words, "It is hard to make nature fit a paradigm" (1962, p. 135). To think that it would fit a paradigm seems perhaps presumptuous; to assume that what is in one's head clearly and without distortion reflects what exists in the world. "That is why," according to Kuhn, "the puzzles of normal science are so challenging and also why measurements undertaken without a paradigm so seldom lead to any conclusions at all" (1962, p. 135). This ability to paradigm shift, to change one's long held, deeply cher-ished views of the world allows for some measure of objectivity. As wedded as we are to the way the world appears to us, when it no longer works, we have the ability to find another perspective. Yet, ultimately, we never reach a single, privileged perspective, one that nature will fit and reflect with no distortion or refraction. We never achieve that absolute objectivity Popper wrote about. But again, does this "failure" mean all we're left with is relativism? Let us keep such questions open as we extend some of these investigations into the next chapter on scientific theory.

CRITICAL THINKING QUESTIONS

1. What is the difference between observation and perception?
2. When Tycho Brahe looked at the sun and when Joahnnes Kepler looked at the sun, were they seeing the same thing?
3. When Michael Schiavo looked at Terri Schiavo and when the Schindlers looked at Terri Schiavo, were they seeing the same condition?
4. For students who have worked with microscopes—discuss your first experiences looking through the microscope and the "learning curve" needed before you could in fact "see" through the microscope. What does this learning curve tell us about observation?

5. What is the difference between seeing and interpreting what you see?
6. In what ways do you think your perception is "theory-laden"?
7. Assuming the theory-ladenness of observation, can we ever say we take an objective viewpoint? Can we ever attain objective knowledge in science?
8. What does Thomas Kuhn mean when he says, "It's hard to make nature fit a paradigm"? What does this tell us about observation and the pursuit of objective knowledge in science?
9. In 1967, Switzerland controlled 90% of the world watch market. It was at that time that the research arm of the Swiss watchmaking industry introduced the quartz watch. Traditional Swiss watchmakers upon seeing this new type of watch rejected it. Companies in the United States and Japan, however, adopted the new technology. Within a few years Switzerland had only 10% of the market (Barker, 1989). Does this appear to be a problem involving paradigms?
10. Can you think of any experience of seeing something at two different points in times and the presumed "same" thing appearing quite different to you? Think of a school or workplace on your first day and compare your perception after months there.

REFERENCES

Annas, G. J. (2006). "Culture of life" politics at the bedside—The case of Terri Schiavo. In P. Illingworth, & E. W. Parmet (Eds.), *Ethical health care* (pp. 103–109). Upper Saddle River, NJ: Prentice-Hall.

Barker, J. A. (1989). *Discovering the future: The business of paradigms.* St. Paul, MN: ILI Press.

Berkeley, G. (1974). *A treatise concerning the principles of human knowledge.* In *The empiricists* (pp. 135–215). Garden City, NY: Anchor Books. (Original work published in 1710)

Copi, I. M., & Cohen, C. (2002). *Introduction to logic.* Upper Saddle River, NJ: Prentice-Hall.

French, S. (2007). *Science: Key concepts in philosophy.* London: Continuum Books.

Hanson, N. R. (1965). *Patterns of discovery: An inquiry into the conceptual foundations of science.* Cambridge: Cambridge University Press.

Hesse, M. (2000). Is there an independent observation language? In T. Schick (Ed.), *Readings in the philosophy of science: From positivism to postmodernism* (pp. 167–174). Mountain View, CA: Mayfield. (Original work published in 1970)

Images of scientific breakthroughs: Astronomy—Galluci, Galileo, Kepler. (2008). Retrieved December 30, 2009, from http://longstreet.typepad.com/thesciencebookstore/2008/09/putting-a-grid.html

Intelligentdesignnetwork. (2005). Retrieved January 5, 2010, from http://www.intelligentdesign network.org/

Jennett, B. (2002). *Vegetative state: Medical facts, ethical and legal dilemmas.* Cambridge, UK: Cambridge University Press.

Kuhn, T. S. (1962). *The structure of scientific revolutions.* Chicago, IL: University of Chicago Press.

Locke, J. (1690/1974). *An essay concerning human development.* In *The empiricists* (pp. 7–133). Garden City, NY: Anchor Books. (Original work published 1690)

Matheson, C. A., & Kline, D. A. (1998). Is there a significant observational–theoretical distinction? In E. D. Klemke, R. Hollinger, & D. W. Rudge (Eds.), *Introductory readings in the philosophy of science* (pp. 374–390). Amherst, NY: Prometheus Books.

Necker Cube. (2009). Retrieved December 28, 2009, from http://en.wikipedia.org/wiki/Necker_Cube

Pope, T., & Mosher, J. (2009). *Galileo's observations of the Moon*. Retrieved December 30, 2009 from http://www.pacifier.com/~tpope/Moon_Page.htm

Popper, K. (2002). *The logic of scientific discovery*. London, UK: Routledge. (Original work published in 1935)

Rabbit-Duck Illusion. (2010). Retrieved January 3, 2010, from http://mathworld.wolfram.com/Rabbit-DuckIllusion.html

T. Schick (Ed.). (2000). *Readings in the philosophy of science: From positivism to postmodernism*. Mountain View, CA: Mayfield.

Shapere, D. (2000). The concept of observation in science and philosophy. In J. McErlean (Ed.), *Philosophies of science: From foundations to contemporary issues* (pp. 138–158). Belmont, CA: Wadsworth Publishing. (Original work published in 1982)

10

Theory and Reality

Evolution is only a theory. It is not a fact.
STATE OF OKLAHOMA, 2003,
HOUSE BILL HB 1504

JUST A THEORY

"But isn't evolution just a theory?" It is not unusual to hear such a question when the subject of evolution arises. It is an interesting question, as there is much implied behind it. First of course it is largely intended as a rhetorical question and hence not a real question but an implicit statement: "Evolution *is* just a theory." If we remove the word "just," it becomes a relatively trivial statement, as it is common knowledge that evolution is a biological theory. "Just" is clearly an important word in this statement then. It implies a lack of something, a "mere-ness," being less than in some way. Less than what? When prodded, the answer provided is that it is merely a theory rather than a "fact." The word "fact" carries a lot of weight, holds an elevated sense of epistemic significance, whereas the word "theory" for many people seems to hold little epistemic significance. Part of the problem is the equivocal nature of the term "theory" in colloquial English. It is used in various fields and studies and likely can be given a unique definition for its use within each. For some reason the epistemically weaker senses of these seem to stick with many in the nonscientific world, leaving them to conceive of scientific theory as nothing more than speculation, a guess, an unsupported "just-so" story.

On the other hand, "facts" are seen by many as epistemically superior, as true in an absolute sense. Of course, many don't recognize that "fact" is a highly equivocal term in our language. One interesting difference in meaning is that at times it is understood, as alluded above, as referring to that which is true and as referring to that which actually exists. At other times, it can be understood to refer to what is merely *alleged* to be true and to exist, but in actuality may or may not. Even if we univocally accept the former sense as the meaning of "fact," other problems arise. To say that a fact is true or refers to what actually exists is merely an analytic truth; it is true by definition. What such a claim elides is what the appropriate or adequate means of determining what does and what does not qualify as a fact. Without such an understanding, the accusation that a theory is just a theory and not a fact is vacuous.

But not only vacuous, such an accusation is also misguided, as it appears to misconceive or misinterpret the meaning of terms like "fact" and "theory" within the contexts of scientific investigation and scientific knowledge. Within the context of science, those things usually referred to as "facts," are actually not very interesting. "Facts" are typically observations. They are particular and limited: On such and such a date at such and such a time water boiled at 100°C at sea level. A fact such as this tells us nothing about water in general, how it will behave at other times in other places. Nor does it tell us about nature in general, the process of evaporation, the relation of heat and air pressure, and so forth. These more general subjects are the fruitful and interesting aspects of scientific knowledge and investigation. Merely recording a particular fact is far less interesting and fruitful. A fact is at best, then, a building block. It has value within the context of other facts, reasoning processes **and** theory. Yet by itself it has little significance.

A theory, on the other hand, is the boldest, most powerful statement made in science. Theories take us beyond the particular to the general, beyond empirical phenomena to underlying processes, from a plurality of experiences to a unified understanding. They make sense of so-called "facts." They are the expressions of what most people think of when they think of science. They provide access to that supposed arcane, almost mystical world that is science to many lay people. Some might say theories are what science is. Yet, the difficulties some students might have with "theory" are not wholly unfounded. Within science and the philosophy of science theory is not a completely univocal or unproblematic concept. It both carries certain inherent problems and raises further problems within the study and practice of science. What follows then is a close look at the concept of theory as it is used in science and the problems and questions it raises.

THE EPISTEMOLOGY OF SCIENTIFIC THEORIZING

Another misconception that leads many to underestimate the epistemic value of scientific theories is the confusion and conflation of the concepts of theory and hypothesis. Typically, a hypothesis is put forward by a scientist as a likely answer to a question about the nature of the world. According to Peirce (1955), hypotheses are inferred through the employment of abductive reasoning. Once posited as a likely answer, then, a hypothesis is tested: phenomena that would occur given the truth of the hypothesis are deductively inferred. Whether those phenomena occur, is empirically observed and recorded. From these observations further inferences can be made. One occurrence of an expected phenomenon does not transform a hypothesis to a theory. There is a problem of precision here, because one cannot specify how many affirmative experimental results move a hypothesis to the realm of theory—due to the problems and limitations of inductive reasoning as outlined in Chapter 8. Yet, at this point it is enough to say that repeated affirmative results eventually transform a hypothesis to a theory. Once at that point the theory takes on a more powerful epistemic authority. Yet, again due to the limits of inductive reasoning, it never has absolute epistemic authority. This limited epistemology leads to further problems and questions, problems and questions that extend some of the questions regarding unobservable entities from the last chapter and lead from problems of epistemology to problems of metaphysics.

As the boldest statements of science, theories can be seen to do the hard work of science. It is with theories that we find the purposes of description, prediction, and explanation (noted in Chapter 7) enacted and fulfilled. Prediction was more broadly covered in Chapter 8 in the context of induction. Explanation will be covered in Chapter 11. So, for the rest of this chapter, we will focus on theoretical description.

THE METAPHYSICS OF SCIENCE

One of the commonly accepted purposes of science is to describe the world, to tell us what is really there. On the one hand, this function seems rather simplistic. By simple empirical observation the world can be described. Yet, descriptions of the unobservable world have been central to scientific knowledge since the beginning of modern science and have progressively taken a larger role ever since—from Newtonian gravity to viruses, electrons, and bosons (the so-called "god particle"). The unobservable entities referred to in the previous chapter are also often referred to as theoretical entities, as their existence is predicated upon the acceptance of a certain theory or theory structure. Deny the theory, deny the entity. But of course, as noted again and again here, modern science is based upon an empirical outlook. To posit the existence of that which is not empirically verifiable seems at odds with a strict empiricism. This tension has led to a number of metaphysical views on this supposed descriptive function of science. These views can largely be placed into one of two general camps: scientific realism and scientific antirealism. We will look at these views in general, the reasons for and against them, and a few more specific views within these two general camps.

Scientific Realism

The term "scientific realism" seems straightforward enough, but even on its surface it is more complicated than it might at first seem. What it means first is that scientific theories are true. This is an epistemic claim and thus one about statements: the statement of an accepted scientific theory is "true." Those scare quotes suggest that we need a closer look at this concept of truth. Philosophers have proposed various concepts of "truth." The one typically implied in scientific realism is "correspondence," which means that truth is defined as a correspondence between the meaning of a statement and a state of the world. If a statement accurately reflects (corresponds to) a state of the world, then it is a true statement. Thus, if the statement of a theory corresponds to a state of the world, it too is true. If the germ theory of disease, which states that certain illnesses are caused by microscopic organisms, is true, then the world must be such that certain illnesses indeed are caused by microscopic organisms. This correspondence then leads to two other assertions as part of the thesis of scientific realism: scientific theories correctly describe what observable and unobservable things there are, and scientific theories correctly describe how those things are related. In other words, if genetic theory is correct, there are indeed structures called "genes" which determine physical and behavioral traits of living things and are responsible for the inheritance of these traits from previous generations. Further, if genetic theory is correct, it also accurately describes the relations between genes, DNA, and other biochemical structures. If atomic theory is correct, then matter is in fact composed of tiny entities called molecules, which are composed of more basic entities called atoms, which are composed of other, more basic entities, including protons, neutrons, and electrons. If gravitational theory is correct, then there truly is a force between material objects which explains why unsupported objects fall to the earth and that the fall of these objects can be predicted by the inverse square law of gravity.

But the complications do not end there. Since there are so many theories and so many have fallen by the wayside throughout history, the scientific realist cannot accept every theory as fulfilling all these metaphysical functions. Only the strongest or most mature theories can be accepted as fulfilling these metaphysical commitments. Of course, as noted earlier, the division between hypothesis and theory is unclear as it is; to try to divide immature and mature theories simply furthers such obscurity. Further, the claims of scientific realism may not be consistent with those of what might be called "common-sense realism." Common-sense realism (or naïve realism) might be described as the way in which most people (especially those who happen to be nonphilosophers and nonscientists) understand the world to be. According to common-sense realism, there is a world existing "out there" independently of any person's mind, perceptions, or beliefs that is at least roughly equivalent to our understanding of how the world is. Some individuals might misperceive or misunderstand the world from time to time, but generally we have direct access to the world through our senses and our minds. So we can know that the world is as we understand it to be. The problem is that many of modern science's claims have turned out to be inconsistent with "common sense." Prior to Copernicus and Galileo common sense told people that the sun revolved around the earth. Even as the scientific world began to accept the heliocentric view, much of the nonscientific world still accepted geocentrism, because it seems like the sun revolves around the earth. To assert the other way around seems counterintuitive. Yet, by this point in history, heliocentrism (at least as far as our solar system goes) has been absorbed into what we accept as common sense. But scientific realism would still affirm claims that would appear counterintuitive to common-sense realism. Common sense tells me, for example, that the desk upon which my laptop presently rests is a solid object. Modern physics, however, tells me that it is mostly empty space and the apparent solidity of the desk is due to forces between atoms and subatomic particles. These counterintuitive claims may also contribute to many people's distrust of science and low estimation of "scientific theory." It is still possible, however, that counterintuitive claims of science might be absorbed into common-sense realism, resolving the tension with but a short cultural lag.

No-Miracles Argument and Continua

The most common argument for the thesis of scientific realism is what is called the "no-miracles argument" (Hacking, 1983; Smart, 2008). This argument points to the obvious and prodigious successes of science: from technological achievements (flight, space exploration, the eradication of smallpox, and near eradication of many other diseases, etc.) to the predictive powers of science to the basic ability to manipulate nature. According to this argument the best explanation for why science has been so successful is that it is, in addition to being predictively and manipulatively powerful, descriptively accurate about both the observable and the unobservable world. The implication of the name of this argument is that if science did not accurately describe the world, its successes would seem to be a miracle. If science were wrong about the way the world is, it wouldn't be as successful as it clearly is. This argument is a form of abductive reasoning referred to as an "inference to the best explanation." That is, of the possible explanations for the success of science, the claim that it accurately describes the world (scientific realism) seems the most plausible, that is, the best explanation. Advocates for this argument attempt to strengthen it by claiming that scientists themselves use this form of argument to justify the truth and accuracy of their own individual theories. Thus, the use of this argument regarding science in general reflects this more piecemeal use by scientists themselves. However, that reasoning may be its own undoing. It becomes a question-begging or circular argument. One cannot support a reasoning process with the same reasoning process, merely at a different level of analysis. Of course this question-begging aspect of the argument is merely extra support provided to the argument. The no-miracles argument can still be addressed on its own. On its own, its status as an abductive argument must be taken into account. Abductive reasoning is presumptive. It infers to the best or most plausible explanation and just as its use in hypothesis creation, such presumption requires further support and investigation. In other words, to further establish the abductive conclusion of scientific realism, such reasoning must occur again and again. That is, the success of science must continue and continue as well to imply scientific realism, leaving us with a thesis supported by abductive reasoning itself supported through inductive reasoning—leaving the critic of scientific realism with much room for doubt.

Another argument in favor of scientific realism raises the question of the distinction between observables and unobservables explored in the previous chapter (Maxwell, 1962). This argument challenges this supposed distinction and affirms rather a continuum between that which can and that which cannot be observed. As we move from small, difficult to see items, such as a grain of salt, to microscopic entities such as bacteria, to smaller and smaller entities, there is no principled point at which one can assert a clear distinction between that which is observable and that which is unobservable (i.e., theoretical). Any line one draws would be arbitrary, not based on a principled difference. The limitation is not an ontological one in which the supposed unobservable is of questionable existence, but a problem of human perception. If we had evolved with different sensory organs, we might see the world differently, see things we do not now, such as viruses, electrons, and so forth. We may have evolved to see X-rays or hear the infrasonic calls of elephants. In such cases, the world would appear quite different to us (and the "infrasonic" range would be defined differently), but the world there is would be the same. It does not make sense to limit reality by the limitations of human sense organs.

This line of reasoning leads also to questioning the skepticism of observation prosthetics such as microscopes, telescopes, and electron microscopes. A continuum can be noted in such cases also: from the simple magnifying glass (the images seen through which are not typically doubted), to the microscope, to the electron microscope, and to the cloud chamber. Again, asserting no clear line between detecting what is observable and really there, and detecting what is merely theoretically and possibly not there, if we accept the reality of the magnifying glass image, we must accept these technologically produced images all the way down the line. The problem of basing these arguments on the imputation of continua rather than a clear, principled distinction is that our world is rife with such continua, yet we apply practical, meaningful distinctions nonetheless. The growth from childhood to adulthood is a continuum, yet the distinction between child and adult is a useful and meaningful one. Even the journey from life to death may be seen as a continuum, yet that distinction clearly is meaningful. Although in these examples there may be some marginal cases (adolescents, brain-dead, and vegetative patients), these marginal cases do not destroy the distinction that is so useful and meaningful in the great majority of cases.

Structural Realism and Entity Realism

One form of scientific realism that has received much attention over the last couple of decades is structural realism (Worrall, 1989). This form focuses less on the existence of things or entities and more on the existence of the relations between things, especially as expressed in equations like the inverse law of gravitation. According to the view of structural realism, often in science theoretical entities do not "survive" changes in theory due to new data and new experimentation, but the structural relations between them do. Thus, it is epistemically more justified to assert the existence of these structural relations rather than the supposed entities between which they are at any point in time said to exist. There is some practical support for this view, as such relations (especially in the form of mathematical equations) have become central to many sciences, have become the primary tools of further investigation. However, this support might also be a weakness, as this view might seem better suited for sciences expressed in terms of mathematics (such as physics or chemistry) than for less mathematically oriented sciences (such as biology). Further, this view might be weakened by examples of scientific progress leading to changes not just in theoretical entities but in theoretical structure as well. In many cases, theoretical structure may endure through changes in theoretical entities, but if theoretical structure changes also due to new evidence and new theories, the reality of structure may become just as uncertain as that of entities.

Whereas structural realism posits the existence of theoretical structures rather than theoretical entities, the theory of entity realism takes the reverse position. This theory is most identified with the work of philosopher Ian Hacking (1983, 1982/ 2000). Hacking does not appeal to the no-miracles argument but takes a more pragmatist position—in the philosophical sense of that word. Our belief in the existence of theoretical entities should be based not on logical inference but on scientists' use of these entities as instruments and tools: "engineering, not theory, is the proof of scientific realism about entities" (Hacking, 1982/2000, p. 199). Hacking uses the example of an electron gun named PEGGY II. This instrument of physics uses *"various well understood causal properties of electrons to interfere in other more hypothetical parts of nature"* (Hacking, 1982/2000, p. 193). It sprays electrons as a part of larger experiments in which the spray of electrons uncovers new phenomena. Hacking argues that this standard of belief in the reality of things is employed in the realm of observable entities also. We believe in the existence of observable entities not simply because we see them (directly) but "because of what we do with them, what we do to them, and what they do to us" (Hacking, 1982/2000, p. 193). They have practical effects on our lives and projects. Analogously, with the utilization of such devices as PEGGY II, since electrons have such effects also, we can similarly believe in their existence. One limitation is that though we might be able to say we can believe in the existence of unobservables like electrons, we cannot say what they are like. We can note their "*well-understood causal properties*" but nothing about the nature of the electrons (or other unobservables) themselves. But isn't this part of what we usually mean when we note the existence of an entity, some understanding of the essence of the thing? Also, are there entities we can't manipulate or use as tools and instruments toward the acquisition of further knowledge? It seems this understanding of realism would leave those out, though they may well exist, as a matter of principle.

Antirealism

The no-miracles argument and the specific theories of realism still leave room for doubt, for positions that might be called antirealism. First, there are a couple of general arguments raised against scientific realism, particularly in response to the no-miracles argument. The no-miracles argument points to the success of science as evidence that scientific theory accurately describes the world. The problem is that so many theories and so many theoretical entities have fallen into the dustbin of scientific history that it seems quite possible that those theories and theoretical entities accepted today may as well. This argument is called pessimistic meta-induction. It is an induction in that it infers from the past "mistakes" of science to the claims of today. It is a *meta*-induction, because it is an inference about the specific inductive inferences of science itself regarding theories and theoretical entities, and it is pessimistic because it raises doubt about the truth of theories and existence of theoretical entities largely held to true or existing at the present time. Another general argument against scientific realism is based on the underdetermination thesis, which says that due to the inductive methods of science the evidence for any theory does not fully determine (prove) the truth of that theory. This leaves open the possibility of the same phenomenon being explained by more than one theory, in which both (or all) theories are supported by equal empirical evidence. This may sound odd, but consider an analogy from criminal law. A person is murdered. Shot once. The prosecutor has two suspects. There is not enough evidence to demonstrate that one rather than the other committed the crime. It is at least theoretically possible that the prosecutor could choose to simultaneously but separately prosecute both suspects and in fact convict both suspects. Given the epistemic standards of criminal law, the prosecutor need only prove guilt "beyond a reasonable doubt." It is possible that such a level of evidence could be brought against both suspects. The contention here is not one of conspiracy: that one actually shot the gun but that the other was involved in some way. The contention is, a rather impossible one, that in the first suspect's trial *this person* pulled the trigger and killed the victim, and in the second suspect's trial, that *this person* pulled the trigger and killed the victim. Now, certainly it is not *true* that both suspects performed the same act, but truth in that sense is not what criminal trials are about. They are about "truth" as defined by the epistemic standard of "beyond a reasonable doubt," and it is possible that there is enough evidence to prove the guilt of each of these suspects to that standard. Similarly, in science it is possible that there may be more than one theory related to a specific phenomenon, and that each theory can be proven to the epistemic standards of science to an equal degree, leaving us with possibly inconsistent claims to what reality is.

Attempts to get past the underdetermination thesis typically appeal to other standards than evidence for choosing between theories to find the "correct" one, factors which may make one theory appear to be more plausible. One of these standards might be the coherence of the theories themselves. One of the theories may appear more coherent than the other. A less coherent theory may have aspects of it that are not as yet fully explained or understood. It may not all quite fit together yet and may seem less plausible. A similar standard is that the better theory will be more coherent with existing theories. If we presume that accepted knowledge and theory comprise a solid knowledge base, the competing theory that fits better with this knowledge base will seem more plausible. A third standard is the employment of Occam's razor, the principle that the simplest explanation is usually the best, or (more accurately) that we should not needlessly multiply entities. The theory that explains the phenomenon with the fewest theoretical processes, steps, or entities would seem more plausible. As commonly invoked as many of these plausibility standards are, the general problem with them is that plausibility is a weak claim to knowledge and truth. Also, each has been contravened at some point in the history of science. Regarding the coherence of a theory, it is entirely possible that a seemingly incoherent theory can become more coherent following future study and discovery. Regarding the coherence of a theory with accepted theories, since we have to assume that our present theoretical knowledge base is correct, we ignore the possibility of a future revolution (paradigm shift) that might overturn this knowledge-base. With Occam's razor, the simpler theory may in fact neglect important aspects of explanation that the more complex theory takes into account, which could then be the more accurate, truer theory. Ultimately, none of these are the kinds of rational, empirical standards that are typical of scientific justification. They appear to be much weaker standards, possibly on the level of mere preference.

The Problems of Empiricism

Locke, Berkeley, and Hume

It might seem common sense that an empirical position on epistemology would automatically produce a realist position on metaphysics. Yet, things are not that simple and common sense may once again lead us astray. Consider again the problems raised in the previous chapter regarding the observation of unobservable entities and empiricism. Those problems extend to these questions of metaphysics. If we look back to the classical empiricists and the more general question of metaphysical realism (as opposed to the narrower question of scientific realism), we see an interesting variety of views. John Locke held a form of naïve realism. Epistemologically, his empiricism led him to a representational theory of knowledge. This means that what we know directly are "ideas" in the mind. The sensual world impresses itself upon our minds through the senses, and it is these impressions and ideas that we "know." These ideas, since they were impressed upon our minds by the external world, represent this external world. Thus, we know the ideas that are the contents of our mind; these ideas represent the real world; transitively we have knowledge of the real world. The problem is, as you should be able to predict from reading the previous chapter on observation, that this position presumes that our ideas are accurate representations of some real, existing objects external to our minds.

George Berkeley, on the other hand, refused this assumption. We know, directly, the ideas in our minds, but we cannot know that these ideas are representations of some other things outside our minds. All we have, according to Berkeley, are our ideas. There is nothing outside our minds. According to him, then, there is no such thing as matter. Everything that exists is mental: either an idea or an entity that has ideas. Yet, how is it that we seem to have similar ideas. If we all look at a tree, we all see a tree. If there is no material tree causing this idea in each of us, how is it we all have the same idea of a tree? These ideas, says Berkeley, must come from God. Although, according to Berkeley, the tree is not real as a material object, it is still real. It is real as an idea provided to us by God. The interesting thing here is that he argues away the material world, leaving us with a form of metaphysical idealism: all that exist are mental entities like ideas and minds. Like many philosophers of his era, Berkeley was reacting largely to new developments in science. His religious orientation (along with this theistic thesis here, he was also an Anglican Bishop) did not sway him from seeing and accepting the importance of the new sciences. By arguing away matter and replacing it with divinely produced ideas, he was able to keep the theories and laws discovered by science (relations between entities) without the existence of matter (material entities). In addition, he made room for God. As science progressed through the Enlightenment, it may have appeared to some as replacing God. Much of what was once explained by God was now explained by physics and other modern sciences. Mechanistic physics and qualities that inhere in matter like inertia seemed to push God out of the picture. By removing matter and replacing it with God-produced ideas, God can be brought back to the center of the modern worldview. So, Berkeley does describe a scientific realism of a sort, but it is not a realism that includes a concept of matter as most positions of scientific realism would.

David Hume was far more equivocal on this question than either Locke or Berkeley. He did not uncritically accept the existence of matter, as Locke, nor did he flatly deny such existence, as Berkeley. The skepticism Hume demonstrated regarding the use of induction, as outlined in Chapter 8, also led him to be philosophically skeptical of the material world but recognize the practical necessity of belief in it. Ultimately, Hume did not address these questions of metaphysics much. One must extrapolate from his writings to reach any such conclusions. His skepticism about induction and causality can imply certain skepticism about what exists—particularly as one might understand causality as a real force in the universe existent between actual entities. So, although an empiricist, and arguably the most consistent empiricist of the British Empiricist school, Hume was most likely agnostic regarding the question of material realism. Metaphysical questions, in general, were not questions he had much respect for. Empirically, we can assert and verify claims regarding our sensations, but to posit a world beyond and independent of our sensations begins to extend one's knowledge claims past the empirical and into the speculative, metaphysical realm.

Logical Positivism, Phenomenalism, and Instrumentalism

The logical positivists, reflecting an influence of the classical empiricists and Hume especially, similarly had little regard for metaphysical questions, even those regarding scientific realism. Many logical positivists espoused a view known as phenomenalism, which is an extreme empiricist view that denies that claims about external objects are really about external objects but about our perceptions (the phenomena which exist within our minds). Phenomenalism does not actively deny the existence of an independent, external world but, much like Hume, asserts that all we can make claims about are those sensations we directly perceive: To go beyond that is to go beyond what is empirically verifiable.

Another view, similar to that of the logical positivists on this issue, that questions scientific realism is instrumentalism. According to instrumentalism, theories are not to be evaluated on the basis of their description of reality but on their usefulness as tools (instruments), especially as tools for predicting phenomena in the natural world. Whether theories accurately describe the world as it is, according to instrumentalism, is not relevant, is beside the point. If a theory accurately predicts phenomena regarding some aspect of the world, then that is justification for accepting the theory—as useful and validated, if not as "true." The logical positivists accept much of this but do not qualify as instrumentalists as they recognize more than a predictive function of theories, a function that will be covered in the next chapter. Both positivists and instrumentalists interpreted claims in a somewhat metaphorical sense. Since the existence of theoretical entities like electrons can be neither verified nor completely refuted, statements about electrons are really shorthand, metaphorical statements about the observable effects we theoretically attribute to electrons.

Constructive Empiricism

One of the more interesting antirealist positions is the view developed by Bas van Fraassen (1941-) which he calls Constructive Empiricism (1980). Note again, we have a form of empiricism which does not lead directly to a form of realism. This demonstrates the important distinction between epistemology and metaphysics, and the presumptions many lay people make about their sense impressions. This view is empiricist generally in the usual sense of the word that knowledge is gained through sensory experience. It is constructive in the sense that the world that we can know of through science is that world that we "construct" through empirical study. But what does it mean to "construct" our world?

Constructing in this sense is an oblique reference to epistemological and metaphysical views influenced by Immanuel Kant (1724–1804). Kant attempted to reconcile the epistemological views of the Continental Rationalist and the British Empiricists by inferring a collection of innate structures of the mind (what he called concepts or categories) through which sense impressions are "filtered" to construct knowledge. He borrowed but amended the rationalist thesis that the mind contains innate ideas from birth. Rather than ideas (e.g., God, the noncontradiction principle), though, the mind is comprised of these innate structures, such as causality, unity, and plurality, which allow us to make sense of the sense impressions we experience. But these structures do not have content like ideas; they are formal in nature. From the empiricists he took the idea that without sense experience there is no knowledge—or more specifically, no content to knowledge. That content comes from sense experience. This constructed knowledge corresponds to what Kant calls the phenomenal world. This is the world that we can know through our phenomenal experience. The complication is that there is also another world. This is the world beyond our sensations, the world as it is "in itself." If you hold a pencil in your hand, you can list a host of sensations by which you would say you know the pencil: the yellow color, the smoothness of the paint, the sponginess of the eraser, and so forth. As the empiricists pointed out, these are all phenomena that we experience directly within us and this is so under Kant's analysis also, as we structure these phenomena into coherent knowledge through the innate concepts of the mind. This other world is called the noumenal world. It is the world as it exists in itself beyond and independent of our perceptions of it. We cannot know this world, particularly as Kant understands what it means to "know." However, when it comes to the phenomenal world, because the innate structures of the mind are *a priori* and universal (they do not vary from person to person), we can achieve certainty (especially through the rigor of empirical science) about our knowledge of this (phenomenal) world. This is the sense, then, for Kant, that we "construct" the world we experience and our knowledge of it.

Van Fraassen does not attempt to deduce innate structures of the mind or concern himself with a proposed world beyond our sensations. He does, however, accept only a world we can construct through our perceptions of it. He rejects the views of logical positivism and instrumentalism which accept theories as metaphorical or symbolic of observation statements, in their denial or agnosticism regarding the correspondence of these theories to unobservable entities. He accepts theoretical statements as they stand but does not hold them as "truth-claims." Put simply (perhaps too simply), when it comes to theories he replaces "truth" with the concept of "empirical adequacy." To assert the truth of a theory would imply adequate knowledge of a correspondence between the statements of the theory (both observation and theoretical) and a world beyond and independent of our senses. As knowledge is limited by sense experience, such assertion of truth is either fruitless or meaningless. Empirical adequacy, on the other hand, is not asserted as a truth claim but "displayed" (van Fraassen, 1980). It is displayed through empirical investigation. A theory is empirically adequate if "what it says about the observable things and events in this world are true—exactly if it 'saves the phenomena'" (van Fraassen, 1980, p. 12). As an empiricist he allows truth to be predicated of observable things and events, if our sense experience corresponds to our observations statements of such things. A theory must correspond to what we can observe—in the past, the present, and the future. This is what is meant by "saving the phenomena." Unexpected empirical results or other empirical data that do not fit into the theory raise problems, prevent empirical adequacy. If the theory "saves the phenomena," then what it says about the unobservable world could be true. Epistemically, that is as much as can be hoped for.

Van Fraassen's view depends upon a distinction between observable and unobservable entities. Because theories refer to unobservable entities, they are not susceptible to determinations of truth, but merely empirical adequacy. Theories also refer to observable entities, of which truth claims can be made and the empirical adequacy of the theory as a whole depends upon. But, as noted earlier, some philosophers have challenged this distinction, arguing in favor of a continuum between the observable and unobservable that makes any distinctive line drawn between them arbitrarily placed and thus not a rational, justifiable distinction (Maxwell, 1962). Van Fraassen responds that "observable" is a "vague predicate." Our world and our language are rife with vague predicates: attributed qualities which are in many cases clearly and easily predicated but in some marginal cases, not so easily. "Bald" is commonly raised as an example of a vague predicate. The term is often applied to men who are not completely devoid of head hair. Yet how much lack of head hair, how much exposed scalp must there be to appropriately apply the term? There are some men who are clearly and unequivocally bald and some clearly not bald. There are also marginal cases, but these marginal cases do not invalidate the general application of the concept. Even asserting a continuum between the observable and the unobservable, there is a clear difference between observing the moon through a telescope and "observing" subatomic particles in a cloud chamber. Somewhere between those extremes, van Fraassen argues, there is a distinction even if we cannot nonarbitrarily indicate where. The fact that human sense organs limit our capacities to sense the world around us *is* ontologically relevant, argues van Fraassen contradicting Maxwell. For, the only world we can assert as "there" is the world we construct out of our sense experiences. He makes a much closer connection (as Kant did) between epistemology and metaphysics than Maxwell (1962) seemed to.

Postmodernism and Reality

Perhaps the most radical and controversial metaphysical position on science and scientific theory is social constructionism (sometimes social constructivism). This idea grew out of the broader movement of postmodernism in philosophy and sociology. Postmodernism is a contemporary skeptical movement that challenges modern claims to knowledge, especially knowledge as part of a unified system like science. Postmodernism was given a strong voice in the sociology of science with the advent of the Strong Program in social science, initiated by sociologists David Bloor (1976) and Barry Barnes (1974) at the University of Edinburgh. In the philosophy of science, Thomas Kuhn was a major influence on postmodern thought—whether he would admit to such an influence or not. His paradigm-oriented analysis of science and scientific change downplayed if not totally dismissed the role of rational deliberation and calculation in the acceptance of scientific theory, including the replacement of old theories by new. This analysis suggested the type of epistemic relativism indicative also of postmodern thought. Postmodern thought has spread through the fields of humanities and social sciences since the 1970s. It has much less effect and influence in the natural sciences. Because one if its central tenets tends to be relativism (epistemic and sometimes moral), it has met with much resistance from more traditional and more conservative researchers and theorists, who often found postmodern thought sloppy and vacuous, compared to the precision and rigor of analytic philosophy and empirical science.

Social constructionism refers similarly to the notion of constructed knowledge and a constructed world initiated by Kant. Like van Fraassen, social constructionists separate from Kant in refusing to make any claims regarding innate, universal categories of the mind and in disregarding any ideas of a noumenal world beyond the senses. Unlike van Fraassen, social constructionists do not elevate sense experience as the ultimate standard of knowledge. There is among postmodernists and social constructionists a recognition of the problems of observation noted by the likes of Hanson (1958/2000) and recognition of the influence of nonrational (social, cultural, and psychological) factors as illustrated by the likes of Kuhn (1962). The claim of social constructionists is that many entities which have been uncritically accepted in their essence may not really have that essence traditionally associated to them. These supposed essences are influenced strongly by social forces which skew the way we see and understand the world. Oftentimes, these reputed essences reflect the function of retaining *status quo* power relations in society. For example, philosopher Michel Foucault famously analyzed such concepts as madness (1961/1988), illness (1963/1994), homosexuality (1976/1990), and even the basic structure of knowledge (1966/1990). According to Foucault, these are concepts constructed through discourse, writing, power, and other social and cultural practices, rather than "natural kinds." Interestingly, just as more conservative commentators resisted relativistic thinking for moral and political reasons; social constructionists often also had moral and political motivations. By demonstrating that previously believed natural entities and concepts are in fact constructed, and often constructed by those in power to retain power, by revealing this constructedness (deconstructing supposed essences), new paths of being are opened up. People are not restricted by false essences meant to define them in a narrow sense. This allows us to question our presuppositions about who is and is not insane or ill and how we treat such people, about what homosexuality means and what it means to apply labels of sexuality.

Many, especially critics of postmodernism and social constructionism, assume that to affirm an entity or concept as a "social construction" is to deny its reality. This idea of social constructionism spread through academic disciplines in the decades of the 1970s through the 1990s such that it took on the appearance of a fad. And certainly critics like Alan Sokal and Jean Bricmont made such charges (1998). Nearly everything imaginable was described as a social construction, from gender to nature to quarks to postmodernism itself (Hacking, 1999). Although, through this plethora of concept application was much equivocation. Social construction did not always go "all the way down." That is, some concepts of social constuctionism allowed for the possibility of some independent existence upon which we apply social interpretation. If we change this interpretation of a particular concept we essentially change *our* concept of it, though leaving possibly existent some reality beyond. Or, as Hacking (1999) demonstrates, a concept like child abuse may be based upon real, independently existing behaviors. These are behaviors that we aggregate and collect within a human constructed concept like child abuse. The particular acts of child abuse are independently, objectively real, but the manner in which these acts are coalesced into the singular concept "child abuse" is a matter of social construction. Indeed, even when social construction goes "all the way down," simply because something is constructed does not mean that it does not exist. The fact that it is constructed implies that it exists. The difference between more traditional views about naturally occurring, independently existing entities, and social constructionism is that under social constructionism, entities are conceived as far more plastic and malleable. Even though homosexuality may be a social construction that does not mean that there may not be homosexuals as that term is understood. There is an echo of Berkeley in this. Just because our perceptions are not based on sensations of physical matter does not make them unreal. But since homosexuality is a construction of our culture and society, not God or nature, we can change our ideas surrounding it, our treatment of homosexuals, and our presumptions about what kinds of people homosexuals are.

In a famous or infamous example of social constructionist analysis, sociologists of science Bruno Latour and Steve Woolgar (1986) observed the laboratory at the Salk Institute. Taking jobs as lab technicians, they acted as anthropologists observing a foreign culture. They noted the negotiations, power relations, rhetoric, and other nonrational factors that went into knowledge construction. The knowledge produced in this lab (and by extension, in labs in general), they attempted to illustrate, is not a result of simple empirical investigation and logical inference. Rather, it is also the result of many psychological, cultural, and social factors that earlier philosophers of science (e.g., the logical positivists and Karl Popper) defined as distinct from science as a concept and science as a practice. Yet, what they intended to show is that these nonrational factors are and have been integral to the creation of what we call scientific knowledge. Further, as social constructionists, they held that such laboratories do not take a reality which is simply sitting there, passive (a collection of brute facts) and draw knowledge out of it. They described, rather, such laboratories as factories in which raw data go in at one end and an artifact called scientific knowledge comes out at the other end. In Latour and Woolgar's terms, reality is the *consequence* of this process, not the *cause* of it (1979/2000, p. 204). Perhaps the most interesting aspect of this view of knowledge construction (called Actor-Network Theory) is the diminished role of intentional human action. Humans (scientist-humans, lab-tech-humans, etc.) are reduced to their function within the lab. Even when Latour and Woolgar write of the negotiation and resolution of disputes among scientists which are inevitable parts of the knowledge construction process, this seemingly human behavior is described more in terms of robotic action. All the humans fill their roles like the parts of a machine and out comes knowledge. This diminishment of the human, rational contribution has certainly been met with much resistance and criticism (e.g., Amsterdamska, 1990).

CONCLUSION

Lay conceptions of science and its theories run the gamut from naïve acceptance of its authority and what it says about the world to simplistic, ideological dismissal of all science has to say about reality—whether that be global warming, evolution, or far more modest claims about the health effects of foods. Philosophical conceptions run a similar gamut, though hopefully excluding those extremes. Yet even the most realist of realists must admit of some skepticism as part of a general scientific outlook. And even the most relativist social constructionist must accept some authority to the claims of science. This chapter has focused on the function of theory to describe the world that is there. Also mentioned in relation to logical positivism and instrumentalism was theory's predictive function. The next chapter will focus on another central function of science and scientific theories.

CRITICAL THINKING QUESTIONS

1. Is saying that evolution is "only a theory" a way of demonstrating its lack of epistemic authority?
2. Identify a scientific theory in nursing or medicine. Lay out specifically what the theory claims, in terms of entities, explanations, and predictions. What evidence is there supporting this theory? Are there competing theories or an obsolete theory that this theory replaced?
3. Identify a disproven scientific theory in medicine or nursing. What specifically did that theory claim? What led to its being disproven?
4. What theoretical entities are commonly referred to in medicine and health care?
5. How does the "no-miracles" argument support the thesis of scientific realism?
6. What is the difference between structural realism and entity realism?
7. If one were a structural realist regarding nursing science, what specific structures might be referred to?
8. Consider the application of pessimistic meta-induction and the underdetermination thesis in the history of medicine.
9. In what ways might disease be said to be a social construct?
10. Apply Actor-Network Theory to the running of a hospital.

REFERENCES

Amsterdamska, O. (1990). Review: Surely you are joking Monsieur Latour! *Science, Technology and Human Values, 15*(4), 495–504.

Barnes, B. (1974). *Scientific knowledge and sociological theory.* London: Routledge.

Bloor, D. (1976). *Knowledge and social imagery.* Chicago, IL: University of Chicago Press.

Foucault, M. (1994). *The birth of the clinic: An archaeology of medical perception* (A. M. Sheridan Smith, Trans.) New York, NY: Vintage Books. (Original work published in 1963)

Foucault, M. (1990). *The history of sexuality: An introduction*, Volume I (R. Hurley). New York, NY: Vintage Books. (Original work published in 1976)

Foucault, M. (1988). *Madness and civilization: A history of insanity in the age of reason* (R. Howard). New York, NY: Vintage Books. (Original work published in 1961)

Foucault, M. (1994). *The order of things: An archaeology of the human sciences.* New York, NY: Vintage Books. (Original work published in 1966)

Hacking, I. (2000). Experimentation and scientific realism. In J. McErlean (Ed.), *Philosophies of science: From foundations to contemporary issues* (pp. 189–199). Belmont, CA: Wadsworth. (Original work published in 1982)

Hacking, I. (1983). *Representing and intervening: Introductory topics in the philosophy of natural science.* Cambridge, UK: Cambridge University Press.

Hacking, I. (1999). *The social construction of what?* London, UK: Harvard University Press.

Hanson, N. R. (2000). Observation. In J. McErlean (Ed.), *Philosophies of science: From foundations to contemporary issues* (pp. 129–138). Belmont, CA: Wadsworth. (Original work published in 1958)

M. Isaak (Ed.). (2005). *Index to creationist claims.* Retrieved May 11, 2010, from http://www.talkorigins.org/indexcc/CA/CA201.html

Kuhn, T. S. (1962). *The structure of scientific revolutions.* Chicago, IL: University of Chicago Press.

Latour, B., & Woolgar, S. (1986). *Laboratory life: The construction of scientific facts.* Princeton, NJ: Princeton University Press.

Latour, B., & Woolgar, S. (2000). The social construction of scientific facts. In T. Schick, Jr. (Ed.), *Readings in the philosophy of science: From positivism to postmodernism* (pp. 201–207). Mountain View, CA: Mayfield.

Maxwell, G. (1962). The ontological status of theoretical entities. In H. Feigl, & G. Maxwell (Eds.), *Scientific explanation, space, and time: Minnesota studies in philosophy of science* (Vol. III, pp. 3–27). Minneapolis: University of Minnesota Press.

Peirce, C. S. (1955). Abduction and induction. In J. Buchler (Ed.), *Philosophical writings of Peirce* (pp. 150–156). New York, NY: Dover.

Smart, J. C. C. (2008). *Philosophy and scientific realism.* London, UK: Routledge.

Sokal, A., & Jean, B. (1998). *Fashionable nonsense: Postmodern intellectuals' abuse of science.* New York, NY: Picador.

van Fraassen, B. C. (1980). *The scientific image.* Oxford, UK: Oxford University Press.

Worrall, J. (1989). Structural realism: The best of both worlds? In D. Papineau (Ed.), *The philosophy of science: Oxford readings in philosophy* (pp. 139–165). Oxford, UK: Oxford University Press.

11

Explanation and Laws

To explain the phenomena in the world of our experience, to answer the question "why?" . . . is one of the foremost objectives of empirical science. While there is rather general agreement on this point there exists considerable difference of opinion as to the function of the essential characteristics of scientific explanation.

Carl G. Hempel

INTRODUCTION

The previous chapter on theory focused on the descriptive function of scientific theories. As indicated, this function has been highly contentious. Debates between different forms of realists and antirealists persist. The previous chapter also noted the predictive function of theories, which is less contentious and the function that is most relevant to the practical application of science. However, the predictive function is susceptible to the same criticisms and limitations that we have noted regarding inductive reasoning. There is another generally recognized function of scientific theory. Scientific theories also explain. To claim that scientific theories *describe* the world is to say they answer the question "What?" To claim that scientific theories *predict* phenomena might be to answer the questions "When?" and "Where?" To claim that scientific theories *explain* phenomena is to say they answer the question "Why?" For many it is just this question which represents the deepest knowledge possible of science. It is, in the words of Hempel, "one of the foremost objectives of empirical science" (1965, p. 245). Simply describing what is there can seem superficial. Most anyone can describe what a computer is and what it can do. Far fewer can explain why or how it works. Of course when we are discussing description in theoretical sciences (in which entities such as genes, atoms, electrons, etc. are referred to), things are not exactly that simple. But there is still this sense that description only takes us so far. Predicting what will occur is highly practical. However, to reduce science to this function may seem to reduce science to technology. Even with a perfectly predictable science, it is arguably an element of human nature to want to know more: to know not just *what* will happen but *why* it will happen. Salmon (1978/2000) points to Laplace's demon in describing the distinction. Pierre-Simon Laplace (1749–1827) was a French physicist who composed a famous thought experiment in which he asks that we consider the possibility of a super-intelligent being who knows (a) the

189

location of every bit of matter in the universe and (b) all the laws that govern physical matter (Laplace, 2007). Given such knowledge, this "demon" should be able to predict the future with complete accuracy. Salmon's point is that even with such incredible knowledge and ability, it seems like something would still be missing. A deeper understanding would still be lacking. Unlike description, an explanatory function of scientific theories is not in itself that contentious. Rather, *how* this explanatory function is fulfilled is largely where the contention lies. Accordingly, we will look at several views regarding how science explains phenomena.

THE DEDUCTIVE–NOMOLOGICAL MODEL

The Deductive–Nomological model (D–N model for short) of explanation, also called the Covering Law Model, was a product of logical positivism. This fact points to one reason, as noted in the last chapter, that logical positivists are not instrumentalists. Both positivists and instrumentalists recognize the predictive function of theories. But positivists also recognize an explanatory function, largely in terms of the D–N model. This model is called "deductive" as explanation in this model is conceived as a form of deductive argumentation. It is called "nomological" because of the central position that laws play in the model.[1] Before we begin in detail on the model, then, let us take a look at the narrower concept of scientific law.

Laws

The term "law" brings a sense of universality, indubitability, of the absolute. To call a claim a scientific law seems to settle the question. There is nothing further to ask. Yet such rhetorical power holds little weight among most philosophers. A deeper look at "law" in a scientific context is in order. Let us take as paradigmatic (not in the Kuhnian sense) Isaac Newton's first law of motion, the law of inertia: an object in motion remains in motion until acted on by an external force; an object at rest remains at rest until acted upon by an external force. This is a law that is well known among scientists, nonscientists, philosophers, and nonphilosophers. Also, among nonphilosophers and nonscientists, it seems to be conceived in the absolutist sense alluded to above: it is a principle of reality to be found everywhere without exception—but also, at least anymore, without critical reflection.

The statement of a law, then, is most clearly expressed in the form of what logicians call a universal affirmative statement (All A's are B's) or a conditional statement (If. . .then. . .). For example, the law of inertia can be expressed thus: "All objects at rest/in motion are objects that will remain at rest/in motion until acted upon by an external force"; or "If an object is at rest/in motion, then it will remain at rest/in motion until acted upon by an external force." In either form it predicates a common quality upon some subject in question. Here, that subject would be material objects. The universal affirmative form clearly indicates the generalized aspect of a law: that the predicate applies to all material objects, which points to generalization as a necessary condition

---

[1]"Nomological" derives from the Greek "*nomos*," which means law, custom, or tradition.

for a law. Although a necessary condition, generalization is not a sufficient condition for a law. There are many generalizations that are clearly not laws. Hempel (1966) presents this instructive example: "All solid spherical masses of pure gold weigh less than 100,000 kilograms." This is a true generalization as far as we can tell. That is, anywhere you look you are not going to find a mass of gold weighing more than 100,000 kilograms. Although true and a generalization, this is not a law. It is what is called an accidental generalization. Here, "accidental" is used in the philosophical sense to mean not an unintended error or mistake but merely contingent. A contingent truth is true due to specific circumstances which may have been different themselves, thereby not leading to the situation held to be contingently true. In this case, the fact that it is true that there are no 100,000+ kilogram boulders of gold *could* be true—given different contingencies. It may even be possible to construct such a boulder if we could collect enough gold. Compare this accidental generalization to this second example: "All solid spherical masses of pure plutonium weigh less than 100,000 kilograms." Although similar in form, this is a different type of statement. It is different because of why it is true versus why the "gold" statement is true. As noted, the "gold" statement is an accidental generalization, which is only contingently true, true because of the way in which gold has been distributed around the universe. The "plutonium" statement is true because any mass of plutonium (due to the nature of plutonium) would become unstable and explode before reaching 100,000 kilograms. So there *could not* be a 100,000+ kilogram of plutonium. This indicates that laws are something more than contingent truths. The same seems to be so with our inertia example. It seems like more than an accident or contingency to say that all material objects at rest remain so. To call it a "law" suggests something deeper.

Here is where the conditional statement of law may be helpful. Let us restate the "plutonium" claim as a conditional statement: "If x is a mass of plutonium, then x will weigh less than 100,000 kilograms." The conditional expression of a law brings out the logical connection involved. For analysis' sake, let's introduce some terminology. Any conditional statement can be broken down into two simpler statements. The first is the statement that is placed between the "if" and the "then." In this case, that would be "x is a mass of plutonium." That statement in the context of the conditional statement is called the "antecedent." The second is the statement following the "then." In this case that would be "x will weigh less than 100,000 kilograms." In the context of the conditional statement that is called the "consequent." To assert the truth of a conditional statement is not to assert the truth of either the antecedent or the consequent. Rather, it is to assert a logical relationship between the two. Take for example the conditional statement, "If I am in Philadelphia, then I am in Pennsylvania." This is true (assuming that we are referring to the Philadelphia that indeed *is* in Pennsylvania. Not to allow that assumption would be sophistry), regardless of whether you happen to be in Philadelphia or not. This statement is true if you are in Pittsburgh or Paris or Philadelphia. Consider in addition the statement, "If it's night time, then the sun is down." Again, this statement is true, whether it happens to be day or night. For what a conditional statement asserts is a logical connection between the antecedent and the consequent. The connection asserted is that any time the antecedent is true, the consequent will be true also. Conditional statements are also called hypothetical statements: given the hypothesis that it is night time, then the sun must be down. Given the hypothesis that I am in Philadelphia, then I must be in Pennsylvania. So, regarding the "pluto-nium" claim, what is asserted is a logical connection between the statement that some given thing "x" is a mass of plutonium and the statement that that "x" is no more than 100,000 kilograms. Any time it is true that some "x" is a mass of plutonium, it will also be true that the said mass will weigh no more than 100,000 kilograms. That is a true assertion, given what was noted earlier about the instability of plutonium. Compare this amended claim though: "If the Moon had been composed of pure plu-tonium, it would weigh less than 100,000 kilos." This too is a true conditional state-ment. Even though the moon that we know (the large orb in the sky that is 3,474 kilometers in diameter) would certainly weigh much more were it composed of pure plutonium, it could not have reached that size and mass if it were composed of pure plutonium. Thus, it would have to be under the given mass limit. But if we make the same type of claim about gold, we get a different result: "If the Moon had been composed of pure gold, it would weigh less than 100,000 kilos." This statement is false. There is nothing about gold to prevent the moon (hypothetically) from being composed purely of it and retain the size we identify with the moon in actuality. Thus, the assertion of the logical connection between antecedent and consequent for this statement is false. There is then some necessity in the logical connection between the antecedent and the consequent in the conditional expression of a scientific law.

And here is where things become difficult. What is the nature of this necessity? When discussing necessary truths in contrast to contingent truths, the most common meaning is *logically* necessary truth (or statement). But as we have learned earlier, logi-cally necessary truths (analytic truths) tell us nothing new about the world. They merely assert relations between concepts. And certainly we expect scientific laws to tell us something about the world. Secondly, logically necessary truths are typically obvious and knowable through rational contemplation, whereas we typically recog-nize scientific laws as in need of empirical study and support to be asserted. Thirdly, a sure test of any proposed logical truth is that its denial should be a contra-diction. For example, refuting the logically necessary truth "All bachelors are unmar-ried" would result in a contradiction because denying that each and every bachelor is unmarried is inconsistent with the definition of "bachelor." Or even more simply, negating "The red truck is red" would also result in a contradiction. Denying a scien-tific or natural law does not result in a logical contradiction. Denying that a pure plu-tonium moon would have a mass less than 100,000 kilograms is not in itself a contradiction. Denying that a particle of matter will exhibit the properties of inertia is also not a logical contradiction. It is perfectly conceivable that some piece of matter would not exhibit the properties of inertia or that a hunk of plutonium might have a mass over 100,000 kilograms, while it is not conceivable that a bachelor could be married and still be a bachelor or that a red truck could not be red.

These questions of necessity fall within the branch of logic known as modal logic. Modal logicians refer to different forms of necessity. We might say that a natural law may not be *logically* necessary but may instead be *physically* necessary. To be logically necessary is to be necessitated by the laws and structure of logic. To be physically necessary is to be necessitated by the laws and structure of the physical world. The per-spicuous reader should see the problem with this answer. Such physical necessity is precisely what we are trying to establish with scientific laws. Thus, to base the necessity of natural laws on the concept of physical necessity is to beg the question. What seems to be part of the concept of a scientific law is that it is grounded in reality in some metaphysical sense. In descrying the laws of nature, scientists are plumbing the deep structure of the universe. Once these studies turn metaphysical, empirical science—its methods, its justifications, its authority—begins to fall away.

So let us return to the empirical method. Scientific laws are established largely through empirical observation and inductive inference—they usually make reference to other laws also. Our studies have already established the limitations inherent in observation and inductive inference. The only way to tell that matter has the property of inertia is to test it. The only way to know with absolute certainty that *all* matter does is to test every piece of matter. Not only that, we would have to test every piece of matter for all time, since it is at least conceivable that some bit of matter might gain and lose the property of inertia. We are epistemically left then with the limitations of induction, as well as the limitations of perception we studied in Chapter 9. "Law" in that deep sense of scientific law that is often suggested in the use of that word can never be established. This leaves many scientists and philosophers of science more modestly conceiving of scientific laws as mere observable patterns. Recognizing them as established patterns allows us to use them as elements of theories without making unfounded metaphysical presumptions. But that still seems to strip away what seems to be a cherished sense of what scientific *law* means.

Another problem with scientific laws is that even if we could establish them with certainty, they are often in an important sense not really true. Yet they are still accepted as true. This is because scientific laws are often conceived and structured in terms of ideal conditions. Take our law of inertia exemplar again. Has anyone ever observed an object truly (cosmically?) at rest? Certainly, we can observe objects at rest relative to the earth. That is, practically, how Newton established and tested his laws. Yet, conceptually, they refer as well to rest relative to the universe. It's not even clear whether there is such a thing. They are also conceived as in a friction-free environment. Take the third law of motion (for every action there is an equal and opposite reaction) for a clearer example here. Because friction operates on matter (friction of surfaces or friction of air), most experiments testing this law will be slightly imperfect. The reaction will usually *not* be precisely equal and opposite. The more general point here is that laws (again conceived ideally) leave out many small, difficult to control for variables. Largely, these variables are of little significance. As a practical matter the laws turn out to be "close enough." They work. They allow us to predict and explain phenomena. Yet in a technical sense, they are not "true." They do not reflect the world we have, the phenomena we observe, but only approximations of those phenomena. The problem is that to precisely describe such phenomena (taking into account all variables big and small) would be impractically complex and not generalizable. And it is the generalizing feature of laws that makes them useful and helps theoretically bring together disparate phenomena into a comprehensible statement about the world we know.

One way to conceive these "approximate" laws of nature is as elliptical generalizations in which variables are elided but if included would accurately reflect the real structure of the world. These are sometimes called *ceteris paribus* generalizations. "*Ceteris paribus*" means "all things being equal" in Latin. All things being equal, an object at rest will remain at rest until acted upon by an outside force. All things being equal, there will be an equal and opposite reaction for every action. The point here is to attempt to retain the force of the law (as an absolute, true statement), while recognizing that it is not really true. Yet some critics still find this too speculative, too metaphysical (Cartwright, 1980/2000). But here we get to the underlying problem of this analysis for the last few paragraphs. Remember the focus here is supposed to be on explanation. However, we have been conflating this discussion of explanation and a discussion of description. In order to accept laws as successful in constructing explanations, we need not accept them as true descriptions about reality (Cartwright, 1980/2000). The two goals are distinct and should not be confused. This way of thinking leads toward a more pragmatic conception of laws and explanation.

Back to the D–N Model

First some basics: It is customary in philosophical discussions of explanation to employ a little Latin because English does not provide the same simple and accurate terminology. We will use the term "explanandum" to refer to the phenomenon to be explained. "Explanandum statement" will be the sentence that refers to that phenomenon. The term "explanans statements" will refer to the specific explanatory sentences, those sentences that do the explaining. And the term "explanans" will refer to the collection of explanans statements within a given explanation.

The D–N model, as described by Hempel (1966), includes two basic requirements for a good explanation. First, "the explanatory information adduced affords good grounds for believing that the phenomenon to be explained did, or does, indeed occur" (Hempel, 1966, p. 48). This is called explanatory relevance and refers both to some basic intuitions about what an explanation is and to the deductive form by which the D–N model is understood. The second requirement is that the explanans must be empirically testable, which of course conforms to the empirical standard held by logical empiricists like Hempel as well as most scientists and philosophers of science.

According to the D–N model, the explanans of an explanation composes a set of premises that deductively imply the explanandum statement, which of course refers to the explanandum itself. Let us attempt an explanation of the operation of a mercury thermometer.

1. Mercury expands as heat is introduced to it.
2. A mercury thermometer is composed of an airless glass tube with an amount of mercury.
3. Normal body temperature is higher than that of normal room temperature.
4. At T_0, the thermometer is at normal room temperature.
5. Therefore, at T_1, when the thermometer is introduced into a person with normal or above normal body temperature, the mercury will expand and rise in the tube.

Statements 1–4 are the explanans statements and statement 5 is the explanandum statement. There are two types of explanans statements. Statements 1 and 3 are general laws. Statements 2 and 4 are empirical facts. These two types of statements work together as premises leading deductively to the conclusion that given these laws and these empirical conditions, the mercury will rise. Because these premises lead conclusively to the explanandum statement, this explanation form meets the requirement of explanatory relevance. In other words, deductively this explanation provides good reason to believe that, given the truth of the explanans statements, the explanandum statement will also be true and thus the explanandum itself will occur. Knowing what laws and conditions will bring about the explanandum is taken to be an understanding of why the explanandum occurs. Each of the laws is empirically testable. Also, each of the empirical conditions is directly empirically verifiable. Therefore, this explanation also meets the requirement of empirical testability.

THE INDUCTIVE–STATISTICAL (I–S) MODEL

According to Hempel (1966), though, not all scientific explanations can be made to fit this model. This is due to the fact that not all scientific laws operate on the universal standard as natural laws are typically conceived. Some laws hold in only a probabilistic sense, for which we develop a different model, the inductive–statistical model (I–S model). If a teacher unwisely comes to class with a bad cold, speaking in front of class, spraying germs with every word and breath, one cannot say with certainty that any one student will contract a cold from the teacher. Yet, one would not be surprised if a few students did come down with colds. Thus, it appears unjustified to compose a law such that "if a person is exposed to another person with an active rhinovirus infection, then that person will become infected also." That clearly is not true. Why it is not true may be no different in principle than why we noted earlier that other (presumably) universally true laws are not really true. Yet, the case seems clearer here. Rather, we might accept a law structured as such: "if a person is exposed to another person with an active rhinovirus infection, then the probability that that person will become infected is high." If we place this probabilistic law into an argumentative schema as we did before regarding the mercury thermometer, we get an argument of similar structure but one that is inductive rather than deductive:

1. If a person is exposed to another person with an active rhinovirus infection, then the probability that that person will become infected is high.
2. Student A was exposed to her teacher who had an active rhinovirus infection.
3. Therefore, it is highly probable that Student A will become infected also.

Note here that the inductive structure allows for the possibility that all the explanans statements are true but that the explanandum does not occur, that "on the information contained in the explanans, the explanandum was to be expected with high probability, and perhaps with 'practical certainty'" (Hempel, 1966, p. 59). This type of inductive explanation can be relatively rough and approximate like this, or it can take on a more rigorous probabilistic/statistical aspect. Take the medical claim that smoking causes cancer. It is not a simple fact that each person who smokes a single cigarette or more will develop cancer. It is not even a simple fact that a person who smokes x number of cigarettes a day for y number of years will develop cancer. There are no known numbers we can substitute for "x" and "y" that will make that statement true. Yet it is statistically undeniable that there is a link between smoking and cancer. This is a link that can be expressed mathematically as a statistical correlation, providing a more specified type of explanation than that given regarding rhinovirus infection. This type of explanation, some advocate, should supplant all attempts at the D–N model, given the difficulty of establishing laws as absolute invariance (Suppes, 1994).

THE CAUSAL MODEL

The more commonsensical model that the D–N model and the I–S model seem to be trying to avoid is what is called the causal model. The reason for this avoidance is the theoretical (and practical) difficulties of the concept of "cause" that we surveyed in Chapter 8. It is because of these difficulties that cigarette companies were able for so long to deny the link between cigarette smoking and cancer in the face of so much overwhelming evidence. It is not that they truly had the evidence on their side or good arguments but that they exploited the uncertainties of "causation" to construct arguments that were clear examples of sophistry but seemed good enough for those who wanted to be convinced by them. Indeed, the necessity that is considered part of natural laws referred to in the previous section is often conceived in terms of causality. A 100,000+ kilogram ball of plutonium will explode *because* of the nature of plutonium itself. The law of inertia *causes* an object at rest to remain in that state. The laws governing matter *cause* the mercury in a heated thermometer to rise. The laws governing biology and biological systems *cause* those exposed to the rhinovirus to become likely to be infected. There is no law that causes all quantities of gold to have a mass less than 100,000 kilograms. That just occurred by happenstance (contingently or accidentally). Of course all this talk of laws "causing" events begins to sound a little queer. People cause things to happen. Animals cause things to happen. Even inanimate objects and forces can cause things to happen: such as the storm causing a tree to fall on my house. However, to refer to something as abstract and ontologically vague as "laws" being an agent of causation sounds a little strange. This strangeness is compounded by the fact that 200+ years since David Hume we still do not have an adequate conception of what causality is. Empirically, we can refer to nothing more than regular patterns. But causality seems to be something more than that. So, employing the concept of causality does not solve the metaphysical problem we ran into in our earlier discussion of laws; it only reinforces it.

PROBLEMS OF INFERENTIAL EXPLANATION

Critics have identified problems with both the D–N model and the I–S model. We can refer to them collectively as inferential explanation, as they both present explanations as forms of argumentative inferences. With their attempt to avoid all hints of metaphysics, some critics complain that their development of inferential explanation does not amount to an explanation at all (Salmon, 1978/2000). The model appears too close to the example of Laplace's demon above. An explanation comprised of explanans statements that are merely premises leading deductively or inductively to a conclusion explanandum statement appears quite similar to mere prediction. An explanation is supposed to provide deeper knowledge and understanding than just a prediction. Laplace's demon also takes a set of covering laws and empirical conditions to *predict* what will occur. Yet, this prediction would not presume any deeper understanding of why things happen the way they do. In addition, just as we can predict events with the employment of covering laws and empirical conditions, there are cases in which we can take a phenomenon and covering laws to retrodict an earlier state or phenomenon (Salmon, 1978/2000). This would appear to have a similar if not the same form of an inferential explanation, but no one would call it an explanation. It is counterintuitive to suppose that later events can be used to explain earlier events. This reaction points again to the idea that there is something missing in the inferential model. The problem is that this something may be of a metaphysical nature, like causation.

A problem similar to that of retrodiction was suggested by philosopher Sylvan Bromberger (Losee, 2001). Utilizing laws of geometry and light as well as the height of a flagpole, one can explain why its shadow is a certain length. Yet this process can be reversed. Beginning with the length of the shadow, adding principles of light and geometry, one could appear to explain the height of the pole. But it would seem odd to say that a flagpole is x feet high because (implicit appeal to laws of geometry and light) its shadow is y feet long. Again, something seems missing from the inferential model.

THE PRAGMATIC MODEL OF EXPLANATION

Bas van Fraassen (1980) recognized these problems with the inferential model and developed what is called a pragmatic explanation instead. Being an empiricist he wanted to avoid appeals to metaphysics, just as the logical empiricists did. He argued that the inferential model did leave something out but not something metaphysical. The inferential model, as he described it, was based on a two-term relation. These two terms were "theory" and "facts." Laws as parts of theories and empirical or initial conditions as facts are all that the inferential model takes into account. According to van Fraassen, explanation is a three-term relation between theory, fact, and *context*. When we ask why some phenomenon occurred, we are asking that question in the midst of a particular context and a change in context can change what we accept as an appropriate answer. When we ask why a cancer patient experiences a remission, we might want to know what internal processes preceded the remission. We might want to know what therapies may have led to the remission. We might want to know what genetics may have influenced the remission. All questions occur within a context. All questions contain presuppositions. A proper response to a question must recognize those presuppositions.

Context also affects appropriate answers in another way. When a patient requests an explanation from a physician and the physician responds in highly technical language beyond the understanding of the patient, that may be a true or accurate explanation but it would not count as a good one. It is not good because it does not provide the understanding sought by an explanation—for the person requesting the information. So who is seeking the answer can also be part of the context. This explanation could be appropriate when requested by another physician. Also, just as an explanation might be bad but true, it can also be good but false. Explanations of the past in science that appealed to theories and theoretical entities that are no longer held to be true or exist (e.g., phlogiston, aether, vitalism) could be good explanations but not true. Here, good would be predicated largely upon the usefulness of these theories. Untrue theories have oftentimes in the past proven to achieve some degree of empirical adequacy and even been useful in application of science. In the 19th century, the germ theory of disease was in competition with the miasma theory of disease. The miasma theory held that diseases were caused by poor sanitation. Before the mid-19th century, many cities were filthy. Garbage littered the streets and the smell of decomposing matter wafted through the air. Under this theory it was the smell and the decomposing matter in the air that caused disease. Thus, to combat disease under this theory, urban areas began public sanitation projects. These projects led to a decrease in diseases like cholera and bubonic plague—and led to the practices of public sanitation we have today. These results seemed to justify the miasma theory. Yet the theory was wrong and the germ theory eventually won out. And of course, referring back to the section on laws, it may well be that no law is really true, but that does not preclude their usefulness in explanations.

One possible shortfall of this pragmatic model of explanation is that by denying a particular syntactic model like an inferential form distinction between scientific and nonscientific explanation becomes difficult. From a pragmatist perspective, though, van Fraassen would discount the importance of such a distinction. The adequacy of the explanation as an explanation is what is important. Less important is whether it is "scientific." The only criterion he alludes to for distinguishing scientific from nonscientific explanation is that a scientific explanation draws upon science for the information contained within. This response, however, appears too circular to satisfy most critics of the pragmatic model.

THE UNIFICATION MODEL OF EXPLANATION

A final proposed model for scientific explanation is the unification model (Friedman, 1974; Kitcher, 1976, 2000). This model also appeals to theoretical laws to construct an explanation. The focus of this model, as opposed to the D–N model and the I–S model, is less on structure to distinguish scientific from other types of explanation than on the nature of understanding. The unification model similarly attempts to avoid bald appeals to metaphysical concepts. What makes an explanation a scientific explanation is not merely an appeal to laws but a standard for how those laws work, what are criteria for better laws. All models of explanation aim for generality, which makes sense given the generality of laws themselves. That is, even when a particular event is explained, it is explained in such a way that that explanation can be generalized to distinct but relevantly similar cases. The unification model focuses on this aspect of explanations in elaborating the notion of understanding as it is to be drawn from scientific explanations. Understanding is increased by reducing the concepts we need to hold to explain the world. If one can only explain a particular event in terms equally particular, no real understanding is achieved. Indeed, that could hardly be called an explanation. Thus, according to the unification model, we should be seeking ever greater generality to "reduce the total number of independent phenomena" (Friedman, 1974, p. 15) and to replace "a large number of independent laws with a smaller number of laws from which the old laws follow" (Kitcher, 1976, p. 208). Unlike the D–N model or the causal model, the unification model does not purport to identify some necessity or inevitability of phenomena based on laws and other phenomena. Rather, it increases our "over-all understanding of the world," simplifying nature "via a reduction in the number of independent phenomena that we have to accept as ultimate" (Friedman, 1974, p. 18).

A good explanation under this model will encompass more than previous explanations, bringing together previously unconnected phenomena under "more general patterns" (Kitcher, 1981/2000, p. 95). As an illustration, Kitcher provides the example of a magician who purports to make salt dissolve in water by use of a hex (Kitcher, 1981/2000). Every time he waves his hand over the salt and water mixture, the salt disappears. From this information, what would appear to be an explanation could be composed according to the D–N model. The problem with the D–N model in this case, according to Kitcher, is that the "hex" explanation for the dissolving of salt in water will not explain cases in which salt dissolves in water when it is not hexed. Thus, two explanations (at least) will be needed. An explanation which appeals to the chemical properties of salt and of water can cover all these cases, thereby providing a more unified explanation and both broader and deeper understanding. Fewer explanations, broader, more encompassing theories are better under this model. On the one hand, this thinking follows the progress of much natural science of the last few centuries. As natural science has progressed, new theories have often encompassed old theories to provide deeper understanding. In fact, this tendency could be seen as an integral element of modern natural science. Premodern (Aristotelian) physics held that different rules applied to the earthly realm and to the celestial realm, the realm of the moon, the planets, and the stars. This is so in part because the objects of the celestial realm are made of a different substance than the objects of the earth. Whereas objects of the earth are made of the four elements earth, air, fire, and water, objects of the heaven are composed of a perfect fifth element called aether. Motion of the earthly realm and motion in the celestial realm are explained using different principles because the realms themselves are essentially different. One of the major advances of modern physics and astronomy was to reduce the principles governing motion such that the same principles apply here and beyond the earth. Another reduction involved here is in terms of elements. The four elements which compose everything of which the earth is made plus the fifth element of the heavens were reduced in the modern era to the one substance of matter.

Interestingly, however, the epistemic basis of this approach of reduction and unification is premodern. The underlying principle here is Occam's razor first introduced in Chapter 10. Also known as the principle of parsimony, Occam's razor is attributed to medieval philosopher William of Occam (1285–1349) and asserts that one should not unnecessarily multiply entities. That is, any hypothesis, theory, or explanation that asserts or assumes fewer or the fewest entities, laws, and so forth is preferable and more likely to be true. More simply put (following Occam's razor to explain Occam's razor?), the simplest answer is usually the best. Occam's razor is appealed to not just in science or philosophy of science but in many areas of study and research. It has great intuitive appeal. Yet, epistemically speaking, it can never be anything more than an axiom or an assumption. It is not subject to proof, and in that way may be outside of what we understand as empirical science. Despite the apparent historical evidence alluded to above, an evaluative appeal to reduction and unification does not have a strong epistemological basis. Indeed, the apparent historical evidence can be countered with historical evidence to the contrary. The five elements of premodern physics were supplanted by the one substance of early modern physics. Later, matter and energy were reduced to a single concept. But matter itself in modern chemistry has been complexified into 117 distinct elements.

Related to this final criticism are criticisms regarding possible metaphysical pre-suppositions. As explanations are functions of theories, reduction and unification can also be applied to theories and sciences. Such a view as applied to theories would hold that simpler, broader theories describe the world better. As applied to sciences, such a view would hold that there is something of a hierarchy of sciences, from the more specific to the most general. At the far end of specificity might be found the human sciences: psychology, sociology, anthropology, and so forth. A reductionist would hold that the claim made by these sciences could be reduced to (and thus explained and described better by) the biological sciences. The biological sciences could be reduced to chemistry, and chemistry could be reduced to the (presumably) most basic and the root of all sciences, physics. Metaphysically, views such as these presume that we do have a "simple" world, an apparently complex world that can be reduced to simpler, more general parts. Of course, an explanatory unificationist might attempt to avoid this problem by separating explanation and description and denying any metaphysical presuppositions in the unification model. Yet there is another problem raised by critics of unification. Recall that van Fraassen emphasized that when giving an explanation, a particular context and a particular request for infor-mation is implied. When requesting an explanation at the "level" of social science, an answer in terms of physics may not be adequate, and may not provide the information and the understanding needed. To ask why a certain sample of the population of preg-nant women tend not to seek prenatal treatment, receiving an answer relating to the motion of basic particles of matter will not help. Or, to stay within the natural sciences, to ask why a particular species has a specific trait, an answer in terms of the chemistry of DNA may not provide the information and understanding needed. These different sciences may not be completely reducible. They may be distinct enough that not all claims can be adequately translated into the more general language of the presumably more basic science.

CONCLUSION

Clearly, the concept of explanation is still a matter of debate and discussion. These various models highlight important aspects of explanation. Yet these models do not exhaust the formal study of explanation. We will revisit this question in Chapter 13 to survey models and questions about explanations from within the context of the social sciences. Yet, we may ask if these social science models might also shed light on problems of explanation in the natural sciences. Such a claim would reverse much conventional knowledge that the social sciences should reflect the natural sciences. But such a reversal may be well worth considering.

CRITICAL THINKING QUESTIONS

1. Identify at least three laws in nursing or medicine—not just true generalizations but laws.
2. Identify at least three merely true generalizations in nursing or medicine. What is the difference between these statements and the laws identified in Question 1?
3. Use one of the laws identified in Question 1 to compose an inferential explanation.
4. Is the explanation you formulated in Question 3 subject to the problem of retrodiction?
5. Consider the children's game Mousetrap™. Imagine you are Laplace's Demon and the game is the universe. What more is necessary in order to say that you *understand* what is happening in the game?
6. Compare the advantages and the disadvantages of the various forms of explanation outlined in this chapter.
7. Compose an explanation that is true but bad.
8. Compose an explanation that is good but false.
9. Are sciences like biology and physiology reducible to "more fundamental" sciences like chemistry and physics?
10. Are social sciences like psychology and sociology reducible to natural sciences like biology, physics, and chemistry?

REFERENCES

Cartwright, N. (2000). The truth doesn't explain much. In J. McErlean (Ed.), *Philosophies of science: From foundations to contemporary issues* (pp. 175–180). Belmont, CA: Wadsworth. (Original work in published 1980)

Friedman, M. (1974). Explanation and scientific understanding. *The Journal of Philosophy, 71*(1), 5–19.

Hempel, C. G. (1965). *Aspects of scientific explanation: And other essays in the philosophy of science.* New York, NY: The Free Press.

Hempel, C. G. (1966). *The philosophy of natural science.* Englewood Cliffs, NJ: Prentice-Hall.

Kitcher, P. (1976). Explanation, conjunction, and unification. *The Journal of Philosophy, 73*(8), 207–212.

Kitcher, P. (2000). Explanatory unification. In T. Schick, Jr. (Ed.), *Readings in the philosophy of science: From positivism to postmodernism* (pp. 89–98). Mountain View, CA: Mayfield. (Original work published in 1981)

Laplace, P. S. (2007). *A philosophical essay on probabilities.* In F. W. Truscott & F. L. Emery (Trans.), New York, NY: Cosimo.

Losee, J. (2001). *A historical introduction to the philosophy of science.* Oxford, UK: Oxford University Press.

Salmon, W. (2000) Why Ask, "Why?"? In T. Schick (Ed.), *Readings in the philosophy of science: From positivism to postmodernism* (pp. 79–86). Mountain View, CA: Mayfield. (Original work published in 1978)

Suppes, P. (1994). *Patrick Suppes: Scientific philosopher, Volume 1: Probability and probabilistic causality* (P. Humphreys Ed.). Dordrecht, The Netherlands: Kluwer Academic Publishers.

van Fraassen, B. C. (1980). *The scientific image.* Oxford, UK: Oxford University Press.

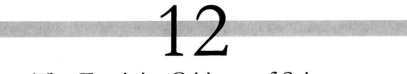

12

The Feminist Critique of Science

Why Can't a Woman Be More Like a Man?
ALAN J. LERNER

DIFFERENCE AND SUPERIORITY

This well-known question of Professor Henry Higgins from Lerner and Lowe's *My Fair Lady* brings with it many assumptions and crystallizes much that feminism in general and in relation to science in particular criticizes about the place of women in history and society and how women are conceptualized. First, such a question assumes that there is some significant difference between men and women. Such differences can be predicated upon biology, politics, or society. Of course there are differences, but the controversial aspect of the assumed distinction is about what makes a difference "significant." In what context is a difference significant? According to what other presumptions is a difference significant? What are the implications of holding a difference as significant? Is a presumed significant difference a real difference? Second, such a question also seems to assume that being "like a man" is superior to being "like a woman." What presumed qualities of men are superior to the qualities of women? Why are the presumed qualities of women inferior? Are the male qualities truly superior to female qualities? Are these qualities truly qualities of men and of women, and if so, how are they engendered?

As science is our focus here, any possible cognitive differences between men and women would be particularly relevant. A common feminist claim is that thought is structured around an indefinite set of dichotomies: reason/emotion, mind/body, universal/particular, culture/nature, production/reproduction, active/passive, singularity/plurality, individual/community, and reductionism/holism. In each of these dyads, the former has been held in higher esteem in our society and our intellectual history. The latter has been viewed as less valuable, as less geared toward truth and knowledge creation. At the same time, the former of each has generally been identified with men and the way men think. The latter of each has generally been identified with women and the way women think. So, just as these latter terms have been devalued, women, as associated with these terms and concepts have similarly been devalued. Let us take a closer look at some of these dyads. Traditionally, men have been identified with rational capacities and women with emotion. And it is reason that, throughout intellectual history in the West, has been identified as the locus of knowledge acquisition, ethical judgment, and successful functioning in the public and political realms. Thus, women have in the past often been excluded from fields that require this type of thinking: the sciences, academic philosophy, business, and political office. Put simply, women simply are not rational. They are, rather, emotional. They make decisions based on feelings and affective attitudes rather than cold, rational deliberation. It is this type of thinking that in the United States kept women from having the right to vote until 1920—132 years after ratification of the U.S. Constitution!

This presumed distinction between men and women can be connected to many of the other dyads. As men are identified with rationality, they are then also more identified with the mind. Mental and cognitive activities have been considered the proper realm of men. The association of women with emotion is consistent also with an association of women with their bodies, as emotions have been largely identified more with the body than the mind. Part of the function of mind and reason has traditionally been to set aside emotions as irrational obstructions to clear thinking. Women have been more associated with the body due largely to reproductive activities. Certainly men have a role in reproduction, but it is women who carry and give birth. In addition, the menstrual cycle is a monthly reminder of embodiment. Presumably, men would be more able to focus on their minds, work out problems, discover new truths, and create new technologies. Women would be blocked from these functions by this constant reminder of embodiment. The answers reason provides are also typically universal and singular. The goals of traditional ethics, science, and philosophy have been to reach conclusions that apply not to any particular situation but all similar situations—that is, universally. Additionally, reason operates within the individual, not communally. Women's connection to their bodies, taken more broadly, also points to a connection to nature. Take the menstrual cycle again. This cycle follows (roughly) the phases of the moon, suggesting a deep connection to nature. Men have no such recognized connection to nature. Men, rather, have been identified with culture: politics, science, philosophy, and the arts. Childbirth, again, points to women's connection to nature and raises another of the dyads. Childbirth is (merely) reproduction, whereas the creation of culture is production. Reproduction has been perceived as a natural function, not a real achievement. Production (of culture, science, knowledge, etc.), on the other hand, is seen as a real achievement, something new, rather than a mere biological copy. This production of culture, etc., achieved through the rational function of the mind, also reflects the active nature of men. Mere reproduction, a bodily function, is conceived as passive.

The traditional association of men and women across the various dyads has established and reinforced the presumed superiority of men over women and furthered the inequality between men and women in society. Feminist critiques have challenged many of the presumptions involved in this conceptualization of gender difference. These critiques have had the ultimate goal of emancipation and equality of women.

HOW MIGHT A FEMINIST ANSWER PROFESSOR HIGGINS?

One of the most important points about feminism to note initially is that there is no one thing that is feminism. There are many feminisms. What connects them is simply a recognition of past and present inequality, oppression, and marginalization of women. But feminisms differ widely on what the source of this inequality is, the degree to which it still exists, and what the appropriate strategies for addressing it are. Regarding the way the issue has been framed so far, a feminist might deny that the traditional attribution of qualities outlined above is in any way accurate. Rather, dividing up men and women across these dyads amounts to mere stereotyping rather than an accurate and justifiable analysis. Although there may be some superficial differences between men and women, essentially men and women are the same. Interestingly, this thinking has its roots in the usually masculine thinking of Ancient Greece. In Plato's *Republic*, Socrates maintained that women in the ideal state would hold any position that men could, based on the claim that the only difference between them is that women bear children and men beget children.

Alternatively, a feminist might argue for the need to transcend these dualities. The idea is that these dyads are mere constructs that constrain our thinking. If we can begin to think across them instead of constraining our thinking to one side of them, we could achieve a broader, more inclusive conceptualization of ourselves, reality, and thinking. Achieving an improved, more equitable, more inclusive science would require "transcending antitheses" (Sayers, 1986/2000, p. 233). Or, a feminist might instead embrace the traditional differences. She would then argue that though there are differences, those differences do not imply a hierarchy: that one type of thinking or one type of person is superior to another. Rather, there are identifiable differences between men and women, but these are differences among equals that may complement one another. Finally, there will be feminists who will argue that a female or feminist approach to knowledge and science is due to certain social circumstances superior to a male approach. The traditional, patriarchal hierarchy is reversed. So, there is no one feminist answer to Professor Higgins. All feminists would certainly say he is wrong, but for a variety of different reasons.

TRADITIONAL (MALE) SCIENCE AS EXCLUSIONARY SCIENCE

The 1960s and 1970s were a time of great change in this country and in Europe. A number of historical and cultural events gave birth to movements that challenged long-held beliefs, practices, institutions, and supposed verities. The practice and institution of "science" was no exception. Cultural critique of science at this time resisted the traditional philosophical analysis of science as purely logical and empirical by attempting to uncover the oppressive and discriminatory elements of science relating to race, class, culture, and gender. Modern science, as a product of the Enlightenment, is supposed to be coldly rational, progressive, and antiauthoritarian. Yet, by the late 20th century, due to much of scientific research being funded and co-opted by the government (especially in terms of defense) and big business, science had come to be seen, rather, as part of the *status quo* (Godfrey-Smith, 2003). No longer progressive and anti-authoritarian, science had come to be seen as part of the power structure—particularly, the white, middle and upper class, male power structure. Any single one of these critiques—from race, class, culture, or gender—would be worthy of study here. But we will focus on gender as, in the words of feminist philosopher of science Sandra Harding (1935–), "gender difference is the most ancient, most universal, and most powerful origin of many morally valued conceptualizations of everything in the world around us" (1986, p. 17). Since genders exist in all cultures, classes, and races, gender issues cut across all of these. In addition, many feminist philosophers of science integrate these other cultural concerns and differences into their analyses and arguments, since women *qua* women are affected also by differences in culture, race, and class. It is important to note that feminists do not simply wish to criticize science or merely to destroy its authority, which in essence would mean to destroy science itself. Rather, most feminists merely resist "science in so far as it reflects and contributes to the maintenance of existing social inequalities between the sexes" (Sayers, 1981/2000, p. 230). The goal then is to improve science by removing its prejudices and blind spots, by making it more inclusive in a variety of ways. Along these lines, many feminists were clearly influenced by the other mid to late 20th-century criticisms of science from Quine's criticism of empiricism's dogmas to Hanson's critique of observation to Kuhn's challenge to science's presumed objectivity, rationality, and progress. The most interesting feminist work, however, moves from mere criticism of presumptions and cherished beliefs to a restructuring of science and knowledge acquisition in a more holistic, inclusive, perhaps less presumptuous manner.

The most basic, although more historical than philosophical, feminist criticism of science is the neglect of the contributions of women to science. As science has traditionally been a pursuit of men, the great heroes of modern science have been men (Copernicus, Galileo, Newton, Boyle, Bohr, Einstein, Watson/Crick, etc.) and the history of science has been recorded largely by men, the focus has been on the contributions of men. The view of women as emotional and less rational has also contributed to this neglect. If women are seen as not having the intellectual capacity for contributing to science, it is unlikely that any real contributions would be acknowledged when they do occur. Feminist historians and philosophers of science then have taken it upon themselves to uncover and publicize the forgotten and ignored contributions of women, to what feminist and zoologist Sue Rosser (1989) calls "Compensatory history" (p. 5). They have taken a number of different approaches toward this goal. One approach is what Sandra Harding (1991) calls the "women worthies" approach. This approach focuses on great women who have made singular and important contributions to scientific progress and discovery: for example, Ann Sayre's *Rosalind Franklin and DNA* (1987), exposing the largely uncredited and unappreciated work of Franklin in discovering the structure of DNA. Some feminists, however, find this approach too close to the "great men" approach to history and thus too androcentric in style, too exclusionary in presuming (as male-oriented history has) that history is made solely or primarily by supposed great individuals and not by collectivities of people at all levels of culture and society. So, some advocate instead an approach that reveals the contributions that are "less public, less official, less visible, and less dramatic" (Harding, 1991, p. 26).[1] Often, women have contributed in relatively more modest, unsung ways as assistants, technicians or even through "domestic support" to famous (male) scientists (Hubbard, 1989; Schiebinger, 1987). Also included in this approach is sometimes a revisiting of the demarcation question, interpreting many traditional activities and duties of women as sciences, as *gynocentric* sciences. Such activities include midwifery, cooking, and homemaking, which, according to Ginzberg (1989), if they had been activities associated with men would have been called "obstetrical *science*, food *science*, and family *social science*" (p. 71). As doubtful as that might be, a more interesting part of this approach is the claim that these activities are more than simple, mundane chores but that real, effective, and consistent knowledge has been generated by these activities. A third approach broaches more philosophical questions. This approach is epitomized by biophysicist Evelyn Fox Keller in her work *A Feeling for the Organism: the Life and Times of Barbara McClintock*. On the surface, this book may appear to follow the "great men" approach labeled as androcentric by some feminists. But what Keller did that was different was to demonstrate McClintock's different, even feminine/feminist way of thinking and approaching scientific investigation. In studying genetics she challenged the (male) "Master Molecule" model and "focused on the interaction between the organism and its environment as the locus of control" (Rosser, 1989, p. 9). In other words, rather than an authoritarian, one-dimensional view of genetics as controlled by the DNA molecule, she worked from a more inclusive, holistic, interactive position, one which also reflected "a unity with and deep reverence for nature" rather than a more masculinist attempt to conquer nature (Schiebinger, 1987, p. 16). This approach, according to Keller, allowed McClintock to make discoveries that likely would not have been made with a more masculine approach to investigation.

Similar to the concern for the neglect of female contributions to science in the past is a concern for the ratio of women presently in science. According to Rosser (1991/2000) and the U.S. Congress's Office of Technology Assessment, women constituted only 9% of scientists and engineers in this country in 1976. By 1986 that number had increased to 15%. According to the National Science Foundation (National Science Foundation, 2008), in 2006, 39% of doctorate holders in science and engineering were women. However, "women were higher fractions of people employed in temporary positions than of those in top leadership positions" (National Science Foundation, 2008). The reasons for this underrepresentation are manifold. The most obvious of course is the traditional dearth of women in the sciences and the already noted neglect of the women that there have been. But feminists point to other problems. Some charge that the manner in which science is taught in primary and secondary schools is often exclusionary as being geared toward boys and young men (Rosser, 1991/2000). Some suggestions to ameliorate this situation include removing sexism from textbooks, increasing the number and length of observations, considering problems outside the traditional scope of science (especially from female dominated fields like nursing and home economics), and focusing on gender in hypothesis formulation (Rosser, 1991/2000, pp. 395–399). Some of these suggestions focus on a deeper

---

[1]See, for example, Gornick (2009) and Rossiter (1982).

question already alluded to in the reference to Keller's book above. The reason female students are less likely to enter scientific fields, some argue, is that science and scientific education reflect "male ways of thinking" which are not commensurate with "women's ways of knowing," which in fact was the title of a well-known book on this subject (Belenky, Clinchy, Goldberger, & Tarule, 1997). Echoing Kuhn, Ruth Hubbard argues that science is comprised of "accredited fact-makers" (1989, p. 120). That is, science is not merely the practice of great individuals but a "social enterprise" (Hubbard, 1989, p. 119). Science students are not merely guided to think in a purely rational manner but "socialized to think in particular ways" (Hubbard, 1989, p. 120). In addition, these students have traditionally been drawn from particular populations, particularly the male, upper-middle and upper class, while generally excluding women and the working and lower-middle class. Hubbard, thus overturns the Enlightenment view of science as antiauthoritarian, progressive and objectively unbiased and perceives it rather as "made, by and large, by a self-perpetuating, self-reflexive group: by the chosen for the chosen" (Hubbard, 1989, p. 120). What are sometimes called women's ways of knowing tend to reflect the right hand side of the dyads we started with. As with Keller's analysis of McClintock (1983), some feminists assert that women do not strive toward reduction, analyticity, and rational objectivity but instead think in more holistic manners that include the contribution of subjective, even value-oriented aspects. We'll take a closer look at some of these claims later.

Another criticism of exclusion involves the manner in which science has treated women as objects of study. These complaints are usually leveled at the biological, medical, and social sciences. In the past, the sciences of biology and medicine have claimed that women's brains were smaller than men's, thus implying the intellectual inferiority of women and asserted dubious medical problems based on women's unique biology (Hubbard, 1989; Schiebinger, 1987). The biological differences between men and women have also been used to perpetuate women's inferior social position by affirming the "anatomy is destiny" thesis, the notion that women's capacity for reproduction mandates their restriction to home and hearth and other less authoritative, more nurturing roles such as nurses, secretaries, and domestic help. Finally, a form of this complaint has been leveled against medical research that in various ways medical research underserves women and is geared more toward the interests of men. French existentialist philosopher Simone de Beauvoir wrote one of the most influential works in 20th-century feminism, *The Second Sex*. The meaning of that title is clearly reflected in this concern of feminist philosophers of science. What de Beauvior meant was that the male sex has been considered the norm, while "female" is always secondary, different, the other. This idea is reflected often in our language. Words such as "mail*man*," "police*man*," "chair*man*," and "busi-ness*man*," convey a male presumption. We expect and assume those in these positions will be male. When they happen to be female, this is seen as an exceptional case. Some might defend these roles as traditionally male, so it makes sense to use such words. Other words may be more difficult to defend. The term "coed" to refer to a female college student is still used and assumes that female college students are somehow unusual or out of the ordinary, when in fact women have overtaken the population of men in higher education. To refer to a female physician as a "female physician" rather than simply as a "physician" also reflects this attitude. Of course a similar corollary way of thinking can be manifested by terms such as "male nurse" or "male secretary." The difference is that these are traditionally less powerful positions than their presumed male counterparts of physician and businessman. The point is that this is about more than just words, or that words themselves are about more than just words. This language reflects and perpetuates certain disparities in social power.

In regard to medical research men have in many ways been taken as the norm, leading to what would appear to be an inconsistent practice in science. On the one hand, science has focused on, developed, and theorized on the inherent differences between men and women. On the other hand, medical research has often inferred from research performed solely on men and applied it to women, without taking into account how differences in female physiology might limit such application. One might point to a concern of utilizing women as research subjects that reproductive functions could be affected. Yet Longino and Doell (1987) note also the use of male *rodents* in hormonal research, the results of which are then inferred to claims about human females. Feminists have complained of the focus of research on cardiovascular disease on men when cardiovascular disease is a serious problem for women. Alternatively, research on contraception has focused on women. This focus is interpreted as reflecting the assumption that due to anatomy, women are presumed to have the primary responsibility in reproduction and family planning. Little research beyond the condom has been done regarding men's role in contraception, whereas the 20th century saw numerous technological advances in female-oriented contraceptives.

According to some feminists, the very nature and attitude of traditional science is not only biased toward men but even hostile toward women. Here, often many of the aforementioned dyads are appealed to. In particular, the association of men and culture and women and nature is often implied. Feminist historian of science Ludmilla Jordanova (1980), for example, points to a statue in Paris of a nude woman removing a veil inscribed, "Nature unveils herself before Science" (p. 54). With this aesthetic example the metaphor of woman as nature is as explicit as it could ever be. This metaphor then transcends gender and sex and appeals to sexuality as well. The implicit idea seems to be that laying nature bare (discovering the secrets of nature) is similar to a woman physically baring herself. The woman is a passive object upon which the male gaze operates and nature too is a passive object upon which the scientist's gaze acts. Evelyn Fox Keller (1985) and Sandra Harding (1986) take this line of argument further, both identifying Francis Bacon as particularly guilty in establishing this attitude in modern science. Bacon, an important and influential figure in early modern science, described the scientific mind as virile and masculine and nature as an object not only to be known but also to be penetrated, dominated, and mastered (Keller, 1985). This language reflects (and ultimately perpetuates) many traditional views of men toward women. Not only does this possibly perpetuate negative attitudes toward women, but it may even lead to a somewhat limiting perspective of science in which humanity is seen as ontologically and irretrievably separate from nature. This separation, though due in large part to the presumably objective attitude of traditional science which led to many discoveries and important advances, may also have prevented other insights and discoveries. This attitude is in direct opposition to that of Barbara McClintock as described by Keller (1983). Rather than separate from nature, McClintock saw humanity as one with nature, as having a subjective interest in nature, not an objective disinterest.

FEMINIST EPISTEMOLOGY: DO WOMEN REALLY THINK DIFFERENTLY FROM MEN?

To attribute differences, especially cognitive differences, between men and women can be quite controversial. Throughout the feminist movement of the 1960s and 1970s, most feminists downplayed and denied any difference between men and women (especially cognitive differences) in search of an androgynous political ideal in which women are equal in capacity to men and thus should have equal rights. By the 1980s, a new feminism arose that recognized potential problems with this andro-gynous political ideal. For one thing, women *qua* women may have needs distinct from those of men—particularly needs associated with childbirth and other health issues. An androgynous political ideal would be ill-suited to deal with such problems. Thus, in the 1980s, "difference feminism" rose. Difference feminists asserted that there are significant, politically and morally important differences between men and women. Often, these differences included cognitive differences. There is a risk in making such a claim that feminist critics of difference feminism pointed to. Such claims of differ-ence risk affirming the old sexist claims of difference and inferiority that feminists began fighting against. But of course difference feminists argue that though women may be different from men, that fact, in itself, does not imply that women are inferior. "Different" may mean just that: simply different, not better or worse. Although there are some feminists who go further and argue for the superiority of women.

To attribute differences between men and women raises another, important, difficult, and politically volatile question. What is the source of this difference? The classic, sexist assertions of difference were typically based upon some notion of the essences or natures of men and women. That is, in some deeply ontological sense men and women are different. Often, these claims of essential difference (and the claims of inferiority they implied) were dubiously supported and rationalized through appeal to biological and medical sciences. Difference feminists tend to eschew these types of explanations for difference. Either such explanations are left open, or more social, sociological, or anthropological explanations are appealed to. This seems to be the case with those feminist philosophers of science who assert cognitive differences between men and women.

Three Feminist Epistemologies

As with any other question feminism addresses there is no one homogeneous feminist response. Sandra Harding (1986, 1987, 1991) identifies three general strains in feminist epistemology. The first she calls feminist empiricism. This is the most conservative of the three. Essentially, feminist empiricists accept the traditional standards of scientific empiricism. The standards, methods, and methodologies of science need not be changed or reconceived themselves. The criticism of feminist empiricists is that science itself does not live up to its ideals, that it "has not adhered rigorously enough to its own norms" (Harding, 1991, p. 113), particularly in relation to its attitude toward women and the contributions of women. Thus, the remedy is relatively simple. Identify those areas where science does not meet its own norms and encourage it to do better. In particular, the ideal of objectivity has often not been met by science in its dealings with women and women's issues. The sexism and androcentrism found in science and scientific study are then adventitious elements that can be extricated merely by following the standards of logic and empiricism inherent to the true study of science.

Less conservative is the strain Harding calls standpoint theory. According to standpoint theory, knowledge acquired by investigation will to some degree depend upon or be influenced by one's social status, role, or position. To put it simply, men and women look at the world differently and will produce different knowledge. Different perception and thinking asserted by standpoint theorists is caused not by biological differences but historical and social differences—particularly "men's dominating position" as opposed to "women's subjugated position" (Harding, 1986, p. 26). Further, and more controversial, standpoint theorists argue that the women's point of view is not only different but superior, in relation to knowledge acquisition or construction, to men's.

The most progressive strain is feminist postmodernism. As the name suggests, feminist postmodernists borrow and apply to their own purposes from postmodern thinkers, including the Strong Program of the sociology of science and philosophers Michel Foucault, Jean-François Lyotard, and Richard Rorty. Like postmodernism, in general, feminist postmodernism emphasizes the fractured, fragmented nature of existence and identity in the contemporary world. We are no longer composed of seamless, cohesive selves and traditions but fragmented collections of traditions and a sense of self that likewise lacks coherence and cohesiveness due to the variety of roles we play and the plurality of cultures we draw from in constructing our being. Due to such radical fragmentation, feminist postmodernism adopts a skeptical attitude toward universalizing claims, the power of reason, the assumption of progress (political and scientific), and essences and essentialism (Harding, 1986). Thus, the critique of feminist postmodernism goes further than the other two epistemologies, challenging not only traditional modern science but also the very "assumptions upon which feminist empiricism and the feminist standpoint are based ... (Harding, 1986, p. 27).

Harding argues that the conservative view, feminist empiricism, is too conservative. Following traditional "norms of inquiry" is precisely what led us to developing sexist and androcentric sciences (Harding, 1986, p. 26). These parts of science are more than adventitious, more deeply embedded in scientific inquiry and scientific knowledge than feminist empiricists suppose. So a deeper, more radical approach is needed. Yet, feminist postmodernism, in Harding's estimation, goes too far. Feminist postmodernism would undercut the emancipatory goals of feminism and feminist philosophy of science. Postmodern analyses that attempt to show the world, selves, and knowledge as fractured and fragmented would preclude the identification or creation of "one, true, feminist story of reality," needed to provide coherence and direction to the movement. The relativistic views that seem integral to postmodernism would also, according to Harding, undercut the feminist epistemic goals of achieving "theories that accurately represent women's activities as fully social, and social relations between the genders as real ... components in human history" (Harding, 1986, p. 138).

Harding endorses standpoint theory. In a deep manner, the differences between men and women, she contends, are not merely differences among equals which give no advantage to one side. Male perceptions of the world lead to understandings that are "partial and perverse," whereas female perceptions result in "more complete and less perverse understandings" (Harding, 1986, p. 26). Ironically, this difference is due to men's culturally superior position and presumed superiority in general (Harding, 1991). In our patriarchal society where men are the "first sex" and women the "second sex," men and male views define the *status quo* and common wisdom. Women are positioned in something of an outsider position. Yet, women are not complete outsiders. They are equivocally part of and outside of culture and society, whereas men are more completely and integrally insiders. This equivocal position of women provides a unique perspective and perception. They can understand and partake in the male perspective, yet offer their own outsider perspective as well. As such, women can more readily perceive the prejudices and biases inherent to scientific study. They are less likely to being scientific thought by devaluing themselves, as feminists have claimed much male-oriented science has. As strangers to the social order of science, women are not as bound to the rules that have evolved around science as a social practice, which may provide unique creativity and insight. Further, as women have been oppressed, they would be less wont to maintain the *status quo*, again leading to further creativity and insight. Women, coming from positions of less power can also provide a less lofty, intellectually removed, more grounded perspective based on the experiences of everyday life. Women's standpoint as insiders/outsiders would be more prone to allow for the transcendence of the ideological dualisms we began with, whereas men would more likely be stuck on one side of those dualisms. All these advantages provide for, according to Harding, "a morally and scientifically preferable grounding for our interpretations and explanations of nature and social life" (Harding, 1986, p. 26). Harding emphasizes that the differences she identifies between men and women are not based on biology but socialization, so as to avoid the stereotyping and oppression that characterized androcentric views of the differences between men and women (Harding, 1991). Standpoint theory would ultimately lead to a redefinition of objectivity, in which an "objective" viewpoint is not presumed to be some ideal external position (a view from nowhere) outside of all interests and investment, but one that recognizes the greatest totality of perspectives, perceptions, and their attendant values, interests, and investments.

Subjectivity, Objectivity, and the Values of Science

A common point of feminist epistemological critique is the subjective/objective dyad noted at the beginning of this chapter. Scientific/male thinking is traditionally assumed to strive for objectivity and eschew subjectivity. Objectivity presumes an independent standard, possibly even an independent reality, and a lack of bias (subjective interest) which provides for value-free inquiry, ensuring the most rationally supportable answers. Objectivity and value-free inquiry is assumed to provide for "the integrity and autonomy of scientific inquiry" (Longino, 1990, p. 5). That is, subjective or value-laden science would lack integrity and autonomy by not being ground in the pure search for objective truth but guided by what would be considered extraneous (political, moral, etc.) goals. It would not have integrity by having at one and the same time the presumed goal of the search for (objective) truth and some other personal, political, partisan goal that may not be consistent with a search for truth. It would not be autonomous from the presumption that science is identified with the search for objective truth. If some extraneous values or interests are influencing the direction of research or even inference, then science (particularly science as merely a logical and empirical practice) is not in control of its own investigation and conclusions. Thus, the traditional (male) view is that "value-laden or ideologically informed science is always bad science" (Longino, 1990, p. 7). Feminist philosophers of science often claim, however, that objectivity is a specifically male standard, not one connected to some neutered sense of nongendered persons. Other feminist critiques include that objectivity does not provide all that seems promised by it. Finally, it is even claimed that in a real sense objectivity is not even a possible standard to strive for.

If it is the case that, for whatever reason, women's thinking tends more toward the subjective than the objective, or that the very dichotomy of subjective/objective is a species of male thinking, then orienting science around objectivity may in fact exclude women from science and scientific studies. This sense of "exclusion" works along several dimensions. If women are largely understood, stereotypically or not, as being less than capable of objective thought, then women may not be accepted by the male scientific establishment, girls and young women may not be encouraged as students to enter the sciences, actual contributions of women to the sciences may not be accepted as science, and women themselves may not see science as a pursuit for which they are suited. Of course the claim from feminists is rather typically framed not that women are less than capable of objective thought but that women's thinking (due to biological factors, social factors, or some combination of the two) is more broadly encompassing, transcends the simple dichotomy, and includes both objective and subjective elements, without dismissing or completely suppressing the subjective. Further, but more generally, objectivity, as indicative of the *status quo*, would tend to reinforce and perpetuate the traditional exclusivity and marginalization that feminists have identified in science, making a continued commitment to objectivity and value-free inquiry, in the words of Helen Longino (1944–), "not just empty, but pernicious" (1989, p. 54). And of course, if such exclusivity and marginalization is indeed part of science this fact begins to put into question the very claim that science and scientific investigation is truly (purely?) objective and value-free.

In actuality, it is a relatively uncontroversial claim to assert that science and scientific study is laden with *some* values. These values would include truth, accuracy, simplicity, predictability, and breadth. That is, what makes good science is that it is guided by the search for truth and/or produces true (or as true as possible) claims, that its claims and investigations are as precise and accurate as possible, that simpler explanations generally are preferred, that theories allow for prediction of future events and world-states, and that scientific claims and investigation be applied across a broad spectrum of reality and human experience. The reason that these values are not controversial and do not problematize science's presumption of value-free inquiry is that these values are what Longino calls "constitutive values," meaning that they are internal to science and essential to our very understanding of science, to its practice and progress (1990). As such, these values are more often assumed or taken as axiomatic than explicitly recognized as values. More controversial are feminist claims about "contextual values": values within the personal, social, and cultural realms, belonging to "the social and cultural context in which science is done" (Longino, 1989, p. 48). Traditionally, constitutive values and contextual values are seen as "distinct and separable" (Longino, 1989, p. 48). Feminist approaches to epistemology can challenge this presumption, asserting instead that these two types of values are inextricable and intertwined and perhaps less distinguishable than previously thought. Following this challenge might then come a challenge to the presumption that inclusion of contextual values in scientific practice results in bad science, that inclusion of contextual values necessarily compromises the integrity and autonomy of science might then come. In other words, contrary to traditional claims, science is not devoid of (contextual) values and is indeed value-laden rather than value-free. The problem is that science has largely failed to recognize this value-ladenness. Such failure can lead to unintended bias—or once again, bias that intentionally or unintentionally reinforces the *status quo*, the prevailing power structure. The surprising conclusion of this line of reasoning, however, is that science which does indeed include a masculine bias may not necessarily be bad science (Longino, 1989).

One area in which contextual values seem unavoidable is in what to choose to study. Sometimes it may seem that scientific questions and problems simply present themselves. As we, as a race, as a people, travel through this world, problems and puzzles arise. We merely address those that confront us. There may be some scientific problems that can be described like this. But without a doubt many paths of investigation are intentional choices. These choices are guided not by mere human curiosity but cultural or personal values. There are many avenues to follow in scientific investigation. We cannot follow all of them. Science cannot be ruled by an attitude of complete disinterestedness, as objectivity is often defined. Otherwise, we would have no motivation for choosing any particular research project. Thus, contextual values will inevitably play some role in choosing what questions and puzzles to pursue. If the prevailing values in science are those of men, then there will likely be a bias toward men and against women in the choice of what to investigate.

Further, feminists also emphasize that knowledge acquisition is not the individualist act it is often conceived as in modern science and modern philosophy. This individualist view of epistemology traces back at least as far as René Descartes, who in his *Meditations* developed the concept of the lone, contemplative thinker, working out the problems of the world from within his own mind. This view has been unofficially adopted by science and the philosophy of science, as reflected in the "great men" approach to the history and philosophy of science. Popper, for example, seems to imply this view by his falsificationist view of science that lauds the great individuals who are able to innovate through critical experimentation. This view is in stark contrast to Kuhn's view of "normal science" as exemplary of most science that is done.

Normal science is the majority of scientific work done by the great mass of scientists and engineers working anonymously in labs—as opposed to the supposed greats whose names we remember. These normal scientists run their experiments, publish papers that lay people will never read or likely ever hear about, but they still may make important steps within intraparadigm puzzle solving that contribute significantly to social knowledge. The feminist view is consistent with and likely influenced by this picture. Of course the individualist picture has been contested throughout the modern history of both science and philosophy, because it is so obviously incomplete at best. Both philosophers and scientists employ journals and conferences and salons and professional organizations to provide for and enhance interaction and discourse—all toward the goal of furthering knowledge acquisition and justification. But feminists have emphasized more strongly than critics of the individualist picture of the past, the idea that scientific inquiry is a "group endeavor" (Longino, 1990, p. 13). The practice of science is not an individual one and the results are not the results of individual effort or individual application of reason. The contribution of society will inevitably bring with it the values and norms of that society. This will include not simply constitutive values like truth and accuracy but the values inherent in the culture itself.

This line of thinking leads to the further claim that not only has science not been value-free as has been supposed, it cannot be. And if that is the case we would have to reconsider our criteria for good science. To achieve pure, disinterested objectivity would require stripping away all context, interest, bias, preconceptions, in short, subjectivity, from our perception, thinking, judgments, and inferences. The position of many feminist philosophers of science is that this stripping away is just not possible. We are, whether men or women, context-dependent, interested, tendentious beings with preconceptions that are not only an inevitable part of our thinking but even a necessary part. One fact that bolsters this feminist argument is that they were not the first to begin down this road. Many nonfeminist philosophers of science in the mid- to late 20th century had already begun this form of critique. Feminist philosophers took it further and in a specific emancipatory direction. The work of Quine, Kuhn, and Feyerabend was influential in this regard. From Quine, feminists took the insight that empirically we cannot test any claim alone. But the acceptance or testing of any claim presupposes a host of other claims (a web of beliefs), not all of which can be tested simultaneously. From Kuhn, they built upon his insights into normal science and the inescapable influence of paradigm. And from Feyerabend they were influenced by his radical openness to method. And later there was much influence and cross-influence between feminists and postmodern thinkers.

"Awareness of our subjectivity and context," writes Ruth Hubbard, "must be part of doing science because there is no way we can eliminate them" (1989, p. 127). Following the arguments of Quine and Kuhn, we cannot leave behind our subjectivity in any human activity, including science. It informs everything we do. Traditional philosophy and science has turned subjectivity into a bad word. And there may have been good reasons for this. But to believe that we can reduce ourselves to nothing more than objective perceivers who produce pure rational judgments is a patent denial of human nature. It also is another strategy for excluding women, as women have long been associated more with a subjective orientation than an objective one. Some feminists may also appeal to quantum physics to bolster this argument (Hubbard, 1989;

Keller, 1985). Unlike Newtonian physics, quantum physics denies a clear subject–object distinction which is the root of objective thinking. According to quantum physics, the very act of observation affects what is being observed. So, there can be no clear distinction between the two—no radical separation, no objective viewpoint, and no stripping away of all subjective influence.

Certainly those feminists who critique science's claims to objectivity do not typically advocate a complete abandonment of objective standards in favor of complete subjectivity. Such a position, most feminist philosophers of science realize, would be self-defeating. Validating mere subjectivity would mean exclusionary male views and practices are no better or worse than feminist views. That is, without some appeal to objective thinking and criteria, there would be no ground to stand on to criticize the traditional views and methods of science. Such subjectivism or relativism would undermine the feminist aim of identifying "the objective ways in which the sexism of our society affects its science both in its theory and in its practice" (Sayers, 1983/2000, p. 234). In addition, completely embracing subjectivity would destroy any attempts at demarcation or clear criteria for good science. In which case, any pursuit or belief system could be defined not only as science but good science. This might include vitalism, Lamarckism, creationism, or astrology. Instead, this critique usually leads to a blurring or transcendence of the subjective/objective distinction. True thinking and knowledge creation is neither purely subjective nor purely objective, but "an interplay between objectivity and subjectivity" (Hubbard, 1989, p. 119). Or, as Longino (1989) argues, objectivity itself should be "reconceived as a function of the communal structure of scientific inquiry rather than as a property of individual scientists" (p. 50). This communal reconception of objectivity brings in elements typical more of subjectivity, as well as a critique of the individualism that is part of the traditional male view of reasoning and science.

Recognizing the subjective elements of scientific thought has its own advantages. First, following Feyerabend, science would be more open, more pluralistic, and more tolerant of "multiple, competing, complementary and partial explanations" (Rosenberg, 2005, p. 182). This attitude of openness, pluralism, and tolerance has the potential for bringing in new ideas, leading to new and important insights into nature and humanity. Indeed, recalling modern science's Enlightenment orientation as antiauthoritarian and progressive, one might think that such a result of rethinking science would be welcome. Second, and along the same lines, Longino (1990) argues that a more inclusive approach would lead to better theories, theories which both flow from and serve "the cognitive needs of a genuinely democratic community" (p. 214). Finally, recognizing the "assumptions, values and interests" (Longino, 1989, p. 54), not just the logic and empirical data, that shapes our knowledge, rather than leaving them to lie under the surface, allows us to better guide scientific investigation to serve all people.

CONCLUSION

So, why can't a woman be more like a man? From within feminist philosophy of science we've seen various responses to this question. One might be that women should not be more like men if that means narrowing one's thinking in an ideological manner, maintaining a stifling *status quo,* and enacting oppressive and exclusionary practices. The feminist empiricists might argue that women should be more like men as far as committing to the traditional norms of scientific inquiry but certainly not in bypassing those as may have been done in relation to women's position on science. The standpoint theorist might argue that women are already enough like a man, having been raised within a patriarchal society, they have been socialized and enculturated into men's ways of thinking, while simultaneously developing a separate, outsider understanding of the world. The postmodernist would deny that "being a man" or "being a woman" really means anything coherent or corresponds to some natural state. Ultimately, whether women are or should be more like men, or whether men are or should be more like women; the goal should be the best science possible that serves the interests of all and makes emancipation in thought and in action ever more possible for all.

CRITICAL THINKING QUESTIONS

1. Beyond the obvious anatomical differences, are there substantive differences between men and women?
2. Consider the dyads listed at the beginning of the chapter. Does one side of these dyads accurately describe you, your personality, and your thinking?
3. Do men and women think differently?
4. Would a feminine science be different from a masculine science?
5. Would the science we know today be different if it hadn't been developed mostly by men for the last few hundred years?
6. Given that nursing has been and is still largely dominated by women, has that fact affected the nature and development of nursing as a science?
7. Is what Harding calls "feminist empiricism" too masculine? Does it concede the masculine authority in science and neglect the unique contributions that could be made by women?
8. Is what Harding calls feminist standpoint theory too women centered? Does it suggest too much of an animosity toward men?
9. Can good science be something less than objective—even subjective?
10. Can/should a woman be more like a man? Can/should a man be more like a woman?

REFERENCES

Belenky, M. F., Clinchy, B. M., Goldberger, N. R., & Tarule, J. M. (1997). *Women's ways of knowing: The development of self, voice and mind.* New York, NY: Basic Books.

Ginzberg, R. (1989). Uncovering gynocentric science. In N. Tuana (Ed.), *Feminism and science* (pp. 69–84). Bloomington, IN: Indiana University Press.

Godfrey-Smith, P. (2003). *Theory and reality: An introduction to the philosophy of science.* Chicago, IL: University of Chicago Press.

Gornick, V. (2009). *Women in science: Then and now.* New York, NY: The Feminist Press at CUNY.

Harding, S. (1987). The instability of the analytical categories of feminist theories. In S. Harding, & J. F. O'Barr (Eds.), *Sex and scientific inquiry* (pp. 283–302). Chicago, IL: University of Chicago Press.

Harding, S. (1986). *The science question in feminism*. Ithaca, NY: Cornell University Press.

Harding, S. (1991). *Whose science? Whose knowledge?: Thinking from women's lives*. Ithaca, NY: Cornell University Press.

Hubbard, R. (1989). Science, facts, and feminism. In N. Tuana (Ed.), *Feminism and science* (pp. 119–131). Bloomington, IN: Indiana University Press.

Jordanova, L. J. (1980). Natural facts: A historical perspective on science and sexuality. In C. MacCormack, & M. Strathern (Eds.), *Nature, culture, and gender* (pp. 42–69). Cambridge, UK: Cambridge University Press.

Katz, J. C., & Warner, J. L. (Producers), & Cukor, G. (Director). (1964). *My fair lady* [Motion Picture]. United States: Warner Bros. Pictures.

Keller, E. F. (1983). *A feeling for the organism: The life and times of Barbara McClintock*. New York, NY: W. H. Freeman and Company.

Keller, E. F. (1985). *Reflections on gender and science*. New Haven, CT: Yale University Press.

Longino, H. E. (1989). Can there be a feminist science? In N. Tuana (Ed.), *Feminism and science* (pp. 45–57). Bloomington, IN: Indiana University Press.

Longino, H. E. (1990). *Science as social knowledge: Values and objectivity in scientific inquiry*. Princeton, NJ: Princeton University Press.

Longino, H., & Doell, R. (1987). Body, bias, and behavior: A comparative analysis of reasoning in two areas of biological science. In S. Harding, & J. F. O'Barr (Eds.), *Sex and scientific inquiry* (pp. 165–186). Chicago, IL: The University of Chicago Press.

National Science Foundation (2008). *Women, minorities, and persons with disabilities in science and engineering*. Retrieved February 22, 2010, from http://www.nsf.gov/statistics/wmpd/figh-2.htm.

Rosenberg, A. (2005). *Philosophy of science: A contemporary introduction*. London & New York: Routledge.

Rosser, S. V. (1989). Feminist scholarship in the sciences: Where are we now and when can we expect a theoretical breakthrough? In N. Tuana (Ed.), *Feminism and science* (pp. 3–14). Bloomington, IN: Indiana University Press.

Rosser, S. V. (2000). Toward inclusionary methods. In J. McErlean (Ed.), *Philosophies of science: From foundations to contemporary issues* (pp. 394–406). Belmont, CA: Wadsworth Publishing. (Original work published in 1991)

Rossiter, M. V. (1982). *Women scientists in America: Struggles and strategies to 1940*. Baltimore, MD: Johns Hopkins University Press.

Sayers, J. (2000). Feminism and science. In T. Schick (Ed.), *Readings in the philosophy of science: From positivism to postmodernism* (pp. 230–235). Mountain View, CA: Mayfield. (Original work published in 1986)

Sayre, A. (1987). *Rosalind Franklin and DNA*. New York, NY: W.W. Norton & Company.

Schiebinger, L. (1987). The history and philosophy of women in science: A review essay. In S. Harding, & J. F. O'Barr (Eds.), *Sex and scientific inquiry* (pp. 7–34). Chicago, IL: The University of Chicago Press.

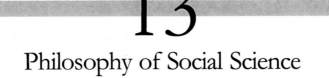

Philosophy of Social Science

Perhaps social science has not yet found its Newton but the conditions are being created in which such a genius could arise.

Peter Winch

INTRODUCTION

There are a great variety of sciences, studies we group under the broad heading "science." We also commonly divide science into two categories, placing the many different sciences under one or the other—though perhaps some do not fit cleanly into one category or the other. Such is often the way with attempts at categorization. These categories are most commonly referred to as natural and social science, though they have gone by other names. The terms "hard and soft science" used to be common. This terminology is considered biased toward the natural sciences. "Hard" implies strength and rigor. "Soft" implies weakness and carelessness. Social sciences are also sometimes called "human" sciences. There seems little biase regarding this terminology. Both "social" and "human" seem appropriate and neutral. "Social" evokes the element of human interaction that is central to many of these sciences. "Human" implies that the human being is the center and focus of this category of sciences, whereas for the natural sciences the focus of study is the natural (nonhuman) world. Natural sciences are also sometimes referred to as "physical sciences," implying that their focus is the physical world and its operations, the realm of physical matter. Although "physical science" might more narrowly refer to the specific science of physics as well. For simplicity's sake we will utilize the terms "natural science" and "social science," regardless of whatever vague or misconceived implications might be involved with such terminology. As noted, the natural sciences are called such for focusing study on the natural world. The commonly accepted natural sciences include physics, chemistry, astronomy, and biology. Social sciences include psychology, economics, sociology, and anthropology. This simple dichotomy implies that there is also a clear distinction between the human and the nonhuman, in terms of the subject–object distinction. As suggested in the previous chapter, there may not be so clear a distinction. Feminists (and others) have argued that there may not be a clear line between what is human and what is nonhuman. To begin with, all that we descry as "natural," is so and in itself interpreted by humans—indeed, even interpreted as "natural" by humans. But we will for now work within this presumed distinction for the sake of the study.

THE CENTRALITY OF HUMAN ACTION

The simple claim that social sciences study humans and that natural sciences study nature (nonhumans) has deeper implications that are more interesting and help define presumed natural sciences like biology and medicine (which also study humans) more clearly as natural sciences. The study of social science, more specifically, is directed at human action. Such action includes eating habits, responses to danger, bad habits (smoking, excessive drinking), good habits (exercise, healthy eating), and social action (practices, rites, etc. attributable to groups of people). What is left out of this list is what can be called mere behavior. "Human action" is human behavior that is (presumably) under our control. Mere behavior includes reflexes and involuntary biological functions. Such behavior is not the focus of social science; human action is. As human action presumes some degree of volition, it also presumes what philosophers call "intentionality." Here we do not mean the colloquial sense of the term that an action is "intentional" if it is goal-directed. "Intentional" in the philosophical sense is related to human minds. There is a difference between saying, "Humans and apes evolved from common ancestors" and saying, "I *believe* humans and apes evolved from common ancestors." The first is not an intentional statement. Its reference or predicate is a state of the external (natural, physical) world. The second *is* an intentional statement. Its reference or predicate is not a state of the external world but a state of mind (the *internal* world you might want to call it). Intentional statements then refer to the content of minds. The difference is more than just one of sentence form. Intentionality is a property of human consciousness, which is, philosophically and scientifically still a supremely mysterious realm, seemingly utterly distinct from the physical realm—yet mysteriously related.

Consider this further example. The ancients identified two distinct bodies in the sky referred to as the "morning star" and the "evening star." The appellations are self-explanatory. However, these were not distinct bodies. They were in fact the same body appearing once in the morning and once again in the evening. In fact, the body was not a star at all but the planet Venus—but that is less important to us at the moment. When someone said "I see the morning star,"[1] this was an intentional statement referring to a mental/perceptual condition: seeing the "morning star." When that same person said twelve hours later, "I see the evening star," that was a distinct intentional statement referring to a distinct mental event. The objects of their perceptions were also distinct: the *concept* of the morning star and the *concept* of the evening star. Thus, if this person were to say in the morning, "I see the evening star," she would

---

[1]To make this statement more consistent with the previous example of intentional statement, we might revise it to "I am having the experience of seeing the morning star," or "I am having the perception of the morning star." These statement forms are clumsier and more awkward, but more clearly express the intentionality of the statement itself.

be confused. Perhaps a bout of sleeplessness led her to confuse morning for evening. If the morning star and the evening star are really the same object (Venus), then in a non-intentional sense, we could use any one of those three terms at any point in time to refer to that one object. Thus, the seemingly counterintuitive statement, "The morning star is the evening star" can make sense, for nonintentionally they both refer to the same thing: Venus.

What does all this mean for social science and its possible distinction from natural science? Human action is intentional action. It has lying behind it mental states (most notably, beliefs and desires) that are integral to its essence and meaning. According to many social scientists, we cannot understand human action without reference to these mental states. The natural world, as commonly accepted, is composed of nonintentional phenomena—phenomena which are simply *there* regardless of specific mental states. Venus simply *is* the morning star and the evening star regardless of what anyone believes. As a statement of astronomical science, one could substitute the terms "morning star" or "evening star" for the term "Venus" in a true statement (or false statement) about Venus (e.g., "Venus' orbit is within that of the Earth's") and a true statement (or false statement) would result—in formal logic this property is referred to as logical equivalence. Such substitution may not work from an intentional perspective because of the influence of intentional states like belief and desire. Intentionally speaking then, predicating the same properties of "Venus," "the morning star," and "the evening star" may not result in logically equivalent statements. Because intentional states seem central to social science, it appears to many social scientists and philosophers of social science that the element of consciousness, of mental states like beliefs and desires, are unavoidable, whereas such concerns may be irrelevant in the natural sciences. What this means further is that if intentionality is central to social science, then social sciences are interpretive sciences. For the inclusion of intentional states like beliefs and desires brings an unavoidable need for interpretation. A state of affairs in social science is not just a state of affairs but a state that is meaningful to and interpreted by a mind (or minds).

Social sciences then are, in philosopher Charles Taylor's term, "hermeneutic" sciences (1971/1994). "Hermeneutic," though, is an equivocal term. At its most basic it simply refers to interpretation. On this level, any act of interpretation can be referred to as a hermeneutic act. Any practice or study that has an essential interpretive element would be a hermeneutic practice or study. Originally this term referred to the study of Biblical interpretation but has been broadened in use over the years. At the same time it has narrowed in use, as it is used also to refer to specific schools of philosophy and of social science which emphasize the interpretive aspect of human existence and the use of interpretation to understand humans and human existence. We will explore that use of the term in the next chapter. Right now we are using the term in a relatively broad sense. In this sense human actions are what Taylor (1971/1994) calls "text-analogues" (p. 181). In the most literal sense when we use the term "interpret" we mean it in reference to a text—a written document. Until a human reads the document, it is but marks on paper (or a computer screen). Once it is read, it must be interpreted in order to be meaningful. Thus, as a matter of intention, it becomes more than marks on paper. But even before then it is more than marks on paper, because a human placed those specific marks due to intentional states of mind. So the marks themselves are intentional in their essence. Otherwise, they are nothing more than marks on paper. Analogously, human actions are like texts. They cannot be understood separate from the intentional states behind them. It is the difference between one's arm raising and raising one's arm. To say "one's arm is raising" (note the use of passive voice) describes a mere movement (behavior). There is no meaning to it. We really do not understand it. To say "raising one's arm" implies intentionality: a conscious mind behind the action that has a reason for acting. This reason (itself implying beliefs and desires) affects the essence of the action, and we can only fully understand the action once we understand (interpret) the intentional states (reasons, beliefs, and desires) behind the action. One might raise his hand because he is in class and knows the answer to a question posed by the teacher. One might raise his hand in salute to a leader. One might raise his hand to hail a cab. Each of these provides different descriptions for the same behavior and implies not only a background of individual beliefs in the actor but also a complex matrix of social rules and practices that help guide the action and give it meaning. The student understands the customs and mores of the classroom setting that gives raising one's hand the meaning he intends. The action implies the proper respect due to teachers, it implies belief of the student that he has the knowledge being sought. Outside the classroom, this movement would not generally have this meaning. The subject who salutes the leader understands that in his society, this motion is a sign of respect and one that is expected of certain persons toward certain other persons. The pedestrian seeking a taxi understands that the gesture he is making is one accepted on the streets as one that taxi drivers respond to. It *means* "I want a taxi." That is its interpretation. That is the interpretation a taxi driver (or any other pedestrian who happens to see him) likely will have of his action. The taxi driver will likely not interpret his action as saying, "I have the answer" or "I salute you." Intentionality, then, can make the same apparent behavior have different meanings. And without these meanings human action may not be properly understood.

For Taylor and others then a clear distinction can be made between natural and social science as the former is not hermeneutic, whereas the latter is. However, recalling the postpositivist critiques we surveyed in earlier chapters (Hanson, Quine, Feyerabend, postmodernists, feminists, and especially Kuhn), the nonhermeneutic quality of natural science may not be so clear. Even in natural science, perceptions are more than (or less than?) brute data. Scientific observations, judgments, testing all imply background knowledge and assumptions—not all of which can be tested. In other words, it is impossible to escape interpretation in even the natural sciences. In Kuhnian terms any scientific investigation (natural or social) exists within and is defined and limited by a paradigm. This paradigm provides a background of beliefs, values, and practices through which facts, justifications, and methodologies must be interpreted. Although even admitting this, one can still identify a principal difference between natural and social science. The natural sciences are hermeneutic in the sense that the objects of study and even the study itself are open to some degree of interpretability. The social sciences are also hermeneutic in this sense. However, the social sciences are hermeneutic in a second sense: that which is being interpreted (human action) is a product of interpretation for the actor. The interpretation of an observation in the natural sciences—for example, markings on photosensitive paper—is not a product of interpretation by the subatomic particles that leave those traces. But the man who raises his arm to hail a taxi does so as an intentional act—as an interpretation of his own that this gesture means, "I want a taxi." As Kuhn explains it, "The natural sciences ... though they may require ... a hermeneutic base, are not themselves hermeneutic enterprises. The human sciences, on the other hand, often are, and they may have no alternative" (1998, p. 133). Whereas the natural sciences require a hermeneutic base, social sciences might be described as "doubly hermeneutic" (Giddens, 1993). They not only have a hermeneutic base but have as their object of study phenomena which are hermeneutic in themselves—meaning they exist *only* as interpreted phenomena, whereas stars, rocks, and matter in general presumably have an independent existence external to human minds.

This recognition of the interpretive (double-hermeneutic) aspect of social science leads us to a general methodological split regarding social science. Interpretivists, as the name suggests, focus on the centrality and inevitability of interpretation in social science. They follow the general line of argument laid out above that humans are in essence self-interpreting beings and this self-interpretation informs how science which aims at humans as intentional beings can be done. Naturalists—also called "correlators" by Taylor (1985a), "empiricists" and "positivists" by others—take natural science as their model for how social science should be done. Naturalists, then, attempt to explain away or set aside this seemingly intractable element of human nature in order to achieve a degree of epistemic objectivity and certainty similar to that of natural science. The double-hermeneutic seems to place serious limitations (beyond the "hermeneutic base" of natural science) on the attainment of objectivity—or even intersubjectivity—in scientific study. So, for naturalists data and results must be understood to be as free of interpretation as the data and results of the natural sciences. Along with that rejection of the double-hermeneutic, comes a neglect of mental states as mental states due to a focus on physical realities, empirical evidence. The only scientifically relevant data is that which can be empirically perceived. Interpretivists refer too much to nonempirical mental states for the comfort of naturalists. Human actions informed by intentional states are acts done for a purpose: to achieve a desire, to conform to a value or custom. This understanding is a form of teleological thinking: phenomena are to be understood through their purposes. Naturalists criticize this type of thinking as premodern and unscientific. Premodern science understood the natural world as a meaningful, purposeful world. Events occurred in relation to some future purpose. Physical objects fall to the earth in order to be with the earth. Rain falls in order to nourish plants and animals. Modern science overturned this view of the world and replaced it with a causal/mechanistic view. In this causal/mechanistic view purposes do not fit. A future purpose cannot be a mechanical cause—causes must precede their effects. In the 19th century, Darwin replaced the last vestige of teleological thinking in natural science (biology) by theorizing a mechanistic process to explain the variety and change of species. This left social science as the only area of science which accepted teleological thought. For the naturalists, this teleological commitment is an obstacle to progress in social science. In order for social science to progress to the same degree as natural science, social science must give up this commitment and adopt the purely empirical, mechanistic views and methodologies of natural science.

Interpretivists, on the other hand, might find the naturalist approach too reductive. It appears to equate humans with mere natural phenomena: stars, rocks, and chemical bonds. But humans are much more than any of these. Humans, interpretivists would say, cannot be understood in their full richness from a purely empirical approach. For social scientists to adequately understand human (or social) action, the inner life (intentionality) must be taken into account. It can be tempting, however, to overstate this division. Most social scientists employ some mixture of the two approaches. But most schools of study tend toward one or the other, and philosophical analyses of social science are often predicated upon this distinction.

THEORY AND SOCIAL SCIENCE

Theories (or the construction of theories) in social science face problems not found in theory construction in the natural sciences. Once again, many of these problems stem from the intentionality of human actions. The social sciences are largely seen as focused on providing an understanding of *particular* actions, which is at odds with the orientation toward the general and universal in natural science and natural scientific theories. The intentionality of human actions creates practical and theoretical obstacles to forming laws in social science. Explaining social action also faces the problem of relating these social explanations back to the intentional states of individual actors. A more detailed analysis is possible if we look at some of the specific purposes of theory we identified in natural science: prediction, description, and explanation.

Prediction

Prediction has been a highly controversial topic in social science. In natural science it appears perhaps the least controversial function of theories—most of the limited criticism there has been coming from feminist philosophers. The main reason, though, that prediction has been such a controversial issue in social science is that social science has not fared well in this regard—especially as compared to the natural sciences. The ability to predict phenomena has been one of natural science's great successes, allowing for important technological advances in engineering, aeronautics, medical science—even in just making daily life easier. Social sciences have not had comparable success in prediction. Psychologists and psychiatrists take great risks in judging which of their patients are dangers to themselves or others. The uncertainty of such judgments comprise a serious criticism of what's known as the *Tarasoff* rule, which holds that a therapist may break confidentiality to warn a specific third party of a mortal threat from a patient. The ability to predict whether a patient is truly a threat to another is so questionable, that it would be ill-advised and maybe unfair to hold a therapist responsible for such predictions. Economists are legendary in their failed predictions—as the many unforeseen recessions and depressions throughout modern history are testament to. For many this inability to consistently predict phenomena is a sign of the inferiority of the social sciences. Naturalists hope to improve this inadequacy; while interpretivists view this "inadequacy" as a sign that prediction is not the appropriate function of social science. It may be appropriate for the natural sciences but, due to the interpretive nature of human intentionality, it is not appropriate for the social sciences.

Several reasons are given for this apparent failure of social science to achieve the predictive powers of the natural sciences. One reason sometimes given is that the social sciences are younger than the natural sciences. Thus, in criticizing the social sciences for not achieving the same predictive successes of the natural sciences, we are not being fair to the social sciences. They have not had the opportunity to develop the mature methodology that natural science has. The problem with this claim is that determining the comparative ages of natural and social sciences, is extremely complex. Such a determination depends on when we mark the beginning of natural science and of social science. Natural science may be said to begin with the scientific revolution in the 17th century. Or, it may date to the work of Aristotle, or to the time of the pre-Socratic philosophers of the 5th and even 6th century B.C.E. The question of social science's beginnings is even more difficult. One might point to the 19th century work of Emile Durkheim or Auguste Comte (who coined the term "sociology"), which were possibly the first instances of social scientific study expressly identified as such. One might go back further to the 17th century work of Thomas Hobbes who utilized (possibly introduced) the central concepts of what would later be called rational choice theory in the social sciences (especially economics). Or one might go as far back as Ancient Greece to the historical studies of Thucydides (460–395 B.C.E.) or Herodotus (484–425 B.C.E.), or the political science of Plato and Aristotle. Without a clear, unequivocal agreement on the beginning of natural science and, especially, of social science, it is difficult to evaluate, to confirm or deny this claim as a reason for the lack of predictive success in the social sciences.

Another common reason given for social science's lack of predictive success is the comparative complexity of the subject matter of social science and natural science. The subject matter of natural science is everything nonhuman: animals, inanimate matter, and human bodies (presumed distinct from human minds). These are subject to physical forces almost exclusively. Humans (*qua* humans), however, are subject to physical forces and to psychological and social forces as well. This fact increases the variables an indeterminate amount. The implication here either is that, following from the previous paragraph, given enough time predictability should improve—possibly to a comparable level as in the natural sciences. Or, this complexity is insuperable and social science will never achieve predictive success comparable to that of natural science. This latter interpretation may be better described as the distinct reason for social science's lack of predictive success that social reality is far more changeable than natural reality, due to the self-interpretation of humans. As soon as we think we have a handle on who we are and how we will behave (a predictive theory), our self-understanding may change, changing predictability based on that theory.

A final reason also points to our intentionality. As self-interpreting beings we can be affected by the very theories we create. Knowledge of those theories can change our view of ourselves, change our reactions; once again affecting the predictability of those theories. Natural objects are not affected by the theories we create about them. They are what they are regardless of our understanding of them or predictions we try to make about them.

A more general reason these other reasons may point to is the difficulty of generating laws in social science. Laws are a necessity for accurate predictions. They are in natural science the engine for generating predictions. If social science cannot generate laws, it will likely not be able to make consistent and accurate predictions. If it is unable to do that, the status of social science as a science may be dubious in the eyes of many. It is largely held that human action follows from rules and reasons, not laws as they are understood in natural science. Reasons are based on those intentional beliefs and desires. According to the interpretivist view, our actions are understood through an understanding of the reasons we do things. Part of the problem with describing these reasons as laws is that they seem to lack the necessary connection (causal or deductively logical) that is typically conceived as part of "law," as we saw in Chapter 11. For any action there can be many reasons and which reason is effective for any individual may depend on a number of particularized factors. Reasons are also seen as an influence on choice, whereas laws determine in a strong sense what event will occur. Choice adds another intentional (and controversial) element, which makes prediction of human action that much more difficult. And further, reasons, unlike natural laws are intentional in that reasons must make sense (be meaningful) for the agents who act upon them—whereas the inverse square law of gravity determines but is not meaningful to a ball rolling down an inclined plane. In the words of anthropologist Roy D'Andrade, the model is one of "'imposed' order based on 'meaning' rather than on natural or physical order" (Bishop, 2007, p. 51). Suppose we ask an alcoholic why he drinks, he would likely answer in terms of reasons expressed as desires and beliefs. "I enjoy the taste." "I enjoy the inebriating effect of alcohol." "I am depressed." None of these statements explicitly refer to desires and beliefs but to other intentional states that implicitly refer to desires and beliefs: "I enjoy the taste or inebriating effect of alcohol, so I want to experience that and believe drinking alcohol will provide me with that." Or, "I am depressed but don't want to be depressed and believe that drinking alcohol will alleviate that state of mind." As reasons, though, these are not determining laws or causes. They are intentional conditions that may lead one to a choice. A *cause* of addiction might more clearly refer to physiological processes and changes that occur in the alcoholic's brain, which is what *really* drives them toward addictive behavior. Here we see a further complication and illustration of the interpretability of reasons. Any one or none of these may be the alcoholic's real reason for drinking. We have to interpret our own reasons for acting and may not always be clear about such things for ourselves. Those on the outside may similarly have to interpret our real reasons (which may or may not be an intentional reason but a physical cause)— for example, a therapist who brings the alcoholic to the realization of his addiction.

Reasons are constructed not only according to beliefs and desires but according to different forms of rules: accepted means of acting and achieving goals within a social group. The student who raises her hand in order to answer a question knows (has been socialized into this body of knowledge) that raising one's hand is a proper and effective gesture for being heard in class. This is a rule in schools in our society in general and in her classroom in particular. The pedestrian who raises his hand to hail a taxi is not following a rule in the formal sense that the student is, but in a more informal sense it is a rule in our society that such a gesture in that context is a call for a taxi. Knowing these rules and having the desire to answer the question or hire a taxi leads these agents to do what they do. But this model, again, is distinct from the use of laws in natural science. Laws cannot be contravened. If they could be, they would not be laws. Rules, however, can be contravened. People can act contrary to social rules. The student can speak out of turn. The pedestrian can jump in front of a taxi in order to stop it.

The examples of the student and the pedestrian above, like most examples in books of this sort, are eminently simple, mundane examples. These types of simple, mundane examples are common for their pedagogical advantage of being relatable to a broad array of readers. Their "everydayness" makes them easy to understand, thus fulfilling their purpose of making a complex or abstract concept or issue more comprehensible. But in this case the mundanity of these examples itself illustrates another important concept. No formal psychological or sociological theory is appealed to in identifying the reasons for these actions. What is appealed to is what philosophers and social scientists call "folk psychology." Folk psychology is little more than a common sense understanding of why people do what they do. Folk psychology draws upon social rules and elements of human nature that people (not philosophers or social scientists specifically) know—at least implicitly. This allows everyone—not just philosophers and social scientists—a limited ability to predict the actions of others. For example, everyone knows that when an auto accident occurs, passersby in cars will turn to look. Not only can that be predicted but we can also predict that traffic will slow down, even if the accident is not blocking or physically impeding the flow of traffic, as individual drivers slow down to get a better look. This phenomenon is so common, so expected that TV and radio traffic reporters have coined the term "gaper delay" to refer to it.

Folk psychology, of course, has severe limits in regard to predicting human action. We can mostly predict in the most general of senses and situations—and cannot predict for all individuals. Naturalists believe that we can improve on folk psychology, develop it into a formal theory that will provide for more accurate predictions. In order to do this, we would have to make explicit the law or principle that connects beliefs and desires to action. Such a principle might be expressed as, "When an agent, desires x and believes y will bring about x, then that agent will do y." As a law, this principle appears to have the appropriate form as a general claim. And it does appear to connect beliefs and desires to action. And the action "y" seems to imply social rules that might be followed. But there are some problems with it. While it may be generally true, on the face of it, it does not seem to be necessarily true. It does not take into account multiple or competing desires and how those would be dealt with by any individual. It does not take into account multiple (and perhaps better) means of achieving x, or whether doing "y" might have other (undesirable) consequences than x. Thus, within this "law" there are many variables that will affect its effectiveness—especially as a means of prediction. One can suggest amending the law to provide for these exceptions. The danger with that strategy is making the law so complex or so particularized that it no longer has the form of a general law. As suggested in Chapter 11 for laws in natural science, one might suggest that an implicit *ceteris paribus* clause be read into the law. Yet, again the "all things" that need to be assumed equal may be so many and so various that the law becomes too vague to be useful for predictions.

Many forms of naturalist social science fall under the heading of behaviorism. Although forms of behaviorism can be found in political science and economics, the most well-known form is found in psychology, following the work of B. F. Skinner (1904–1990). Skinner's behaviorist theory of operant conditioning sets aside explicit concern for intentional states like belief and desire, for a focus on behavior, as behavior is empirically observable. The distinction between behavior and action is dissolved. From a behaviorist perspective all human action, including cognitive processes and consciousness, is indistinguishable from mere reflex. All human action is understood in the same manner as a reflex action: stimulus, response, and reinforcement. By manipulating the environment in order to positively reinforce the behavior of subjects, behavior can (theoretically) be predicted. Specific laws regarding the response of agents can (theoretically) be generated. Behaviorism, as a naturalist approach, takes prediction as a central goal in scientific investigation. Rejecting a focus on intentional states orients social science around causality rather than a (premodern) teleological view suggested by a focus on intentional states. If a social scientist can determine what causes behaviors, then those behaviors can be accurately predicted.

Description

As we saw in Chapter 10, theories in natural science can become controversial when they assert the existence of theoretical, unobservable entities, such as electrons and other subatomic particles. This problem arises in the social sciences as well. Intentional states, being states of mind, are by definition unobservable and often a source of intense controversy in both social science and philosophy. Another problem arises regarding the social sciences that focus on social as opposed to individual human action. If action is meaningful, for whom is *social* action meaningful? And a related problem is the concept of "social facts," the proposed existence of forces that operate on individuals from a social level.

The inclusion of intentional states in scientific investigation requires some appeal to introspection and a further inference (or assumption) that other people's minds are generally similar to what we each discover through introspection. Otherwise, no general claims about these intentional states can be made. This is a species of a classic philosophical problem known as the "other minds" problem. The issue is that you may have direct access to your own mind, but you do not have such direct access to anyone else's mind and thus do not have direct knowledge of other minds. Indeed, the argument often goes further in saying that I cannot know that any other persons have minds at all. You may be the only conscious, mind-possessing creature in a world of mindless automatons for all you know. This raises a problem if empirical evidence is held as a strong requirement for knowledge. Behaviorists resolve this issue by ignoring or redefining folk psychology references to intentional states. Embracing these archaic, nonscientific concepts is what naturalists believe keeps social science from making progress as a predictive science. Assuming the reality of these intentional states makes it difficult to develop empirical laws. Redefining intentional states like belief and desire as empirically observable behaviors in terms of operant conditioning would theoretically allow for the construction of social scientific laws that can be used to accurately predict behavior. The problem behaviorism faces, however, is that a theoretical connection is needed between behavior and the concept of reinforcement. Working just from what is directly empirically observable, all that behaviorism can say is that behaviors that are positively reinforced are more likely to occur in the future and behaviors that are punished are less likely to occur in the future. In order to make a deeper statement about how or why this occurs would require either (1) some theoretical appeal to unobserved, perhaps intentional, concepts or (2) hope that a neurological mechanism will be discovered to explain this. The first option contradicts the naturalistic, empirical commitments of behaviorism. The second option is vacuous until such a discovery is indeed made. It begins to seem unavoidable that in the scientific investigation of human action some appeal to intentional states will play a part.

Certain social sciences, like sociology and anthropology, do not study individuals and individual actions but study societies instead. But what is a society? Is there even such a thing as a "society" in the same sense that there is such a thing as an individual person? A simple definition of a society might be "an aggregate of persons." But this is too simple. "Society," as sociologists understand it, is more than this—that is, a society is more than the sum of its parts. This is why a distinct science of sociology is needed. If society were no more than the sum of people who comprise it, psychology would be adequate to understand social action and social institutions. But it is believed by sociologists that life in a society in general and in particular societies specifically affects the behavior of the individuals who comprise societies. Yet at the same time "society" is highly abstract and conceptual. One can orient oneself toward and point toward an individual. The same cannot be done regarding a society. One point that seems to make the existence of societies as entities that transcend the sum of its individuals is that the rules that govern behavior of the individuals of a society are rules that extend beyond any single individual and may be more effectual and helpful for society as an entity than any particular individual. Most societies, for example, have quite specific and highly regimented rules regarding marriage. And the practice of marriage, guided by social rules, can be beneficial to many individuals in a society. Yet these rules are not the rules of any individual. They extend beyond any individual, and no individual can change them on her own. And beyond the benefits marriage may have for any individual, it is largely accepted that marriage is good for society as a whole. It is meaningful to society. Now that is an odd locution. It makes sense to say that a rule that benefits an individual is meaningful to him. But does a society have intentional states just as individuals do? Emile Durkheim, often referred to as the father of modern sociology, referred the meaning of these rules to an "entity" he called "collective consciousness" or "collective mind" ("*âme collective*" in the original French). Scare quotes are used around "entity" because it is unclear how literally he took this concept to be an entity. He defined it as "the totality of beliefs and sentiments common to the average members of the same society" (Durkheim, 1933/1964, p. 38). This definition sounds more like an abstract concept than a real entity. But even accepting collective mind as an abstract concept is problematic within an empirical approach to science. Yet, without such a concept social rules seem to exist on their own, without relation to an identifiable subject for which it has meaning and for which it functions.

Durkheim further theorized that within societies there was what he called social facts. These are forces, structures, and regulatory concepts (like social rules) that have meaning independent of any individual but influence, guide, even cause, individual action. Durkheim explains, "When I perform my duties as a brother, a husband, or a citizen and carry out the commitments I have entered into, I fulfill obligations which are ... external to myself and my actions" (Durkheim, 1895/1982, p. 50). These duties, commitments, and obligations draw on the individual, guide his actions and give them meaning, but they are not of the individual's own making. The classic argument for the existence of social facts comes from Durkheim's books *The Rules of Sociological Method* (1895/1982) and *Suicide* (1897/1951). In *Suicide*, Durkheim wrote of his studies of the fluctuating suicide rates in 19th-century Europe. He argued that sharp changes in suicide rates could not be explained by the specific causes attributed to these suicides—that is, individual psychological causes. Rather, he pointed to social changes which correlated with the fluctuation of suicide rates. The presumed psychological causes appeared to remain constant through the changes in rates, whereas the social changes he pointed to did not. This fact made it seem more likely that the real cause behind these suicides was sociological, not psychological. In other words, these forces that appear to cause people to commit suicide are just as real, if not more real, as the psychological forces we typically attribute to such behavior. He attributed these differences to religious differences. Catholic societies tend to have lower rates of suicide than Protestant societies. This difference he attributed to a greater sense of individualism within Protestantism and a greater sense of community within Catholicism. One implication of this idea that we will explore further in a later section of this chapter is that our actions may not be due to the reasons we often attribute to them. We may think we are acting out of certain mental, psychological dispositions (i.e., intentional state of belief, desire, etc.), but our actions may be largely influenced by social forces beyond us and beyond our control.

The position that Durkheim is developing here came to be referred to as a form of "methodological holism." The term "holism" here refers to the thesis that society is more than the sum of its constituent individuals. It is an organic whole with its own facts, rules, and forces that needs to be treated methodologically independent of the individual psychology of its members. Durkheim's conclusion that the variation in suicide rates can only be explained through social facts is an argument in favor of this view. Methodological holism defines then sociology as an autonomous science, distinct and independent of psychology. Social facts, as facts about societies, can be used to generate sociological laws that can be used to predict social behavior. This places Durkheim and other methodological holists in the naturalist camp.

The contrary thesis to methodological holism is methodological individualism (Weber, 1956/1978), developed by another pioneer of modern sociology, Max Weber (1864–1920). According to this view, social phenomena can be traced back to the beliefs and desires of individuals. In other words, social forces can be reduced to psychological influences or intentional states. Weber develops a methodology that includes both interpretivist and naturalist approaches. Sociology, according to Weber, is a science of "the interpretive understanding of social action" but is also concerned "with a causal explanation of its course and consequences" (1956/1978, p. 4). He accepts that action is intentional, both individual and social, with social action being that in which "its subjective meaning takes account of the behavior of others and is thereby oriented in its course" (Weber, 1956/1978, p. 4). Yet this intentional action, being a social action, can also be placed within a causal nexus. What makes action social, then, according to the methodological individualist view is that it is behavior that occurs within a social context—in recognition of the intentional states of other psychologically driven beings around one. The intentional states of individual actors are affected by but not independently caused by the social situation. Social facts themselves are reducible then to psychological facts. The problem for sociology this view raises is that if social forces and social facts are reducible to psychology, then sociology may lose the autonomy as a science that holism provides for it. Sociology would appear, at best, a derivative science, at worst, not a real science at all. But there is an aspect of methodological individualism which seems counterintuitive, thereby placing it into question. We commonly refer to forces of an economic, religious, or political nature. Individualism would deny, to some degree, the reality of these forces. These words would be at best shorthand descriptors for complex interactions between individuals. Yet intuitively at least these seem like real forces in society. To remove these—or reinterpret them as shorthand descriptors—would seem contrary to commonsense views of society.

Explanation

The interpretivist view of social science downplays the importance of prediction and is not concerned with the predictive success of social science. To be overly concerned with the predictive success of social science, interpretivists hold, is to misunderstand social science. The primary purpose of social science is not to predict human action but to understand human action, according to interpretivists. This view defines social science as separate and independent of natural science. The naturalist view defines social science as methodologically and epistemologically consistent with natural science. Indeed, the naturalist approach may even lead to a reduction of social science to natural science. The methodological individualists mentioned above would hold that sociology is reducible to psychology, and a broader naturalist view might also imply that social science is reducible to natural science. The intentional terminology of social scientists in reality refers to physiochemical processes of the brain. A more exacting science would eliminate this intentional language in favor of more precise, more "scientific" terminology that refers to brain states not states of mind. In the philosophy of mind these theses are called "reductive materialism" and "eliminative materialism." Reductive materialism is the philosophy of mind thesis that all intentional states can be reduced to physiological brain states. The memory of the smell of a rose is nothing more than a set of firing neurons. Eliminative materialism takes a step further: reference to immaterial, mental states needs to be eliminated in scientific language and replaced with reference wholly to material entities—entities that can be empirically observed. The problem is that neuroscientists have yet to clearly translate physiological brain states to states of intentionality. A set of firing neurons just does not seem the same as the smell of a rose. That rose-smelling experience and the beliefs and desires we have been referring to seem to transcend a mere physiological brain state.

Interpretivists, then, not willing to give up intentional states as central to social science, view the primary role of social science to *understand* human action (to provide explanations) not *predict* it. This further leads to a clear distinction between social and natural science. If intentional states have a reality their own and cannot be reduced to physiological states, then social science cannot be reduced to natural science. It is an approach to science wholly distinct and makes discoveries that a natural science could not. Thus, it has its own value, not one derivative of natural science. The goal of understanding human action means explaining human action. A successful interpretive social science will allow us to explain the individual and social action of human beings. It will bring a deeper understanding of why people act the way they do—even though it may not provide an accurate framework for predicting that action.

The obvious next question is, then, in social science, with an emphasis on interpretation, what makes a good explanation? Many of the natural science models we explored in Chapter 11 will not work with an interpretive framework as the inclusion of laws is a bit at odds with an interpretive framework, as we have seen. The standard for a good interpretation or explanation in social science is typically put in relatively simple even common-sense terms. "A good interpretation," writes Fay and Moon (1977/1998), "... is one which demonstrates the coherence which an initially unintelligible act, rule, or belief has in terms of the whole of which it is a part" (p. 183). Or, in the more direct language of Charles Taylor (1971/1994), "what is strange, mystifying, puzzling, contradictory is no longer so, is accounted for" (p. 182). Put simply, we see someone acting in an initially incomprehensible manner. We then naturally ask, "Why is she doing that?" Or in the case of social action, "Why do they do that?" Social science then takes it upon itself to answer such questions. It does a good job when we are no longer puzzled, when the action referred to makes sense to us. Fay and Moon above use the term "coherence." This term has two related meanings. First, it suggests logical consistency. To understand something, illogic (in the form of inconsistencies and contradictions) must be accounted for— shown to be only apparent illogic or a misperception or misconception. Second, it suggests a form of unification, of all parts sticking together. The Latin root, *cohaerere*, means to cling, embrace or be in harmony. Thus, this term suggests that understanding comes out of a type of logical unification. The action in question is brought under some larger interpretive principles. The incoherent does not fit, falls outside of our understanding. The most interesting action to explain is that which appears (*appears*) irrational. Here irrational may have several interpretations itself. For simplicity's sake we will take the view that rational action is self-regarding, self-interested action. Thus, irrational action will bring some form of harm to the actor. The social scientist will take this apparently irrational action and make sense of it, rationalize it, bring it within the coherent whole of our picture of the world and of human action. Addictive behavior appears irrational. Most addictions harm the addict physically and further prevent the achievement of short-term and long-term goals which would presumably provide for a happy life. A person acting against the achievement of their own happiness seems irrational given the model of rationality adopted here (and adopted by many social scientists) and probably intuitively irrational for most readers also. It seems natural to ask why someone would live their lives in such a way. Social science aims to give us an insight, an understanding of this social phenomenon—to make it make sense to us. Once we can bring it within our general understanding of human action, it is no longer incoherent. Logical inconsistencies are resolved and such behavior is part of a larger, unified view of human and social action.

However, this description of social science explanation is very formal and runs up against some serious problems. One problem concerns the question of what recourse we have when someone does not accept that our explanation for some human or social action is adequate. To make our case, we can only appeal to related interpretive claims, to "a common understanding of the expressions of the 'language' involved" (Taylor, 1971/1994, p. 183). For an interpretive explanation of ours to be meaningful for another, we must share a language. Our explanation only makes sense within the structure of that language. So, for anyone for whom we try to communicate our explanation we must presume we share a language with them. Otherwise we would not share an interpretive framework which would make our explanation intersubjectively meaningful. Here is where we run into our problem though. To understand any "part" of a language, such as an interpretive explanation, one has to understand the language it is expressed in as a whole. To defend our explanation as adequate we can only refer to other expressions within the same language. If our interlocutor does not accept our interpretive framework he will never understand our explanation. But if he does not accept our language, our interpretive framework, he will never see our explanation as adequate. We cannot defend our explanation in isolation but only as part of a larger interpretive framework. This problem is a species of what philosophers and literary theorists refer to as a hermeneutic circle. The part cannot be understood without understanding the whole, and the whole cannot be understood without understanding constituent parts. Being trapped in this circle limits the confidence and certainty of our claims. However, there appear to be only two not very promising strategies for breaking out of this circle (Taylor, 1971/1994). First is a Hegelian approach. Ideally, our understanding would reach an "absolute" position, in which everything is coherent. Our understanding of human action would be completely logical and inclusive—everything hangs together in a logical whole. In such a state what we know would be so clear and evident as to be undeniable. The problem is that it would seem impossible to know when we have reached this point—to know that there is nothing more that is incoherent that needs to be made coherent. Second is a more empirical approach in which we would set aside or redefine intentional states as empirical realities—as brute facts, empirical facts that are simply "there," not ethereal phenomena open to interpretation. This again is the naturalist and reductionist approach outlined above. And the problem with it is that it neglects what seems so intuitively true, that we have beliefs, desires, and other intentional states that are distinct from any external, empirical descriptions of the functions of our brain, and influential on our actions. This makes the identification of mere "brute facts" seem impossible and beside the point. Even in natural science we saw how difficult it can be to make an unproblematic appeal to brute facts.

The idea that a social science is needed to understand human and social action implies a certain opacity to our actions. If our actions were to be explained simply in reference to our intentional states, each of us could simply understand our actions through an act of introspection. Social action could be understood through an act of intersubjective comparison. We would merely discuss our individual intentional states and construct a social explanation through a logical deduction of what motives are intersubjectively common. If this is all there was to understanding human and social action, complex social sciences would not be needed. The problem, though, is that, according to many social sciences, the real explanations for our actions are opaque to us individually, and sometimes socially. Let us return to Durkheim and suicide. Those persons who comprised the statistical reality of suicide as a social phenomenon that he studied presumably had in their minds some understanding of why they were committing suicide. That understanding may have been consistent with the reasons attributed postmortem that Durkheim critiqued, but they were very likely not the socio-religious reasons that Durkheim hypothesized. Indeed, Durkheim's reasons were likely not those of any other observer prior to his work but required formal, structured observation and a theoretical framework. Without these "scientific" techniques these reasons—and thus perhaps the correct explanation—would remain opaque to all who considered the phenomenon of suicide. The broadest concept of this opacity is found in Marxian influenced approaches such as critical theory. Here the Marxian concept of false consciousness defines the presumed understanding of human action that must be pierced through by a presumably better positioned interpretation. According to Marx, the capitalists who own the means of material production (natural resources, factories, etc.) utilize the power this material wealth provides to create a state of mind among the lower classes. This is a false state of mind, a manipulation of people's beliefs and values. The purpose of this manipulation is to keep the working classes in line, keep them complacently working and increasing the wealth of the capitalists. The capitalists use their power to control dissemination of information (newspapers), education, and religious institutions, all to foster a state of mind in the working class that they are in the position that they belong in, that they will be happy if only they work harder, become more productive and don't challenge the system. Social scientists, influenced by this Marxian view, have generalized and broadened this thesis to encompass the hegemonic power structure in general and any oppressed, disempowered class. Potentially, one's whole worldview could be wrong, could be an artifice constructed by another in order to keep people "in their place." A social science would be needed then to pierce through this false consciousness to the reality of human existence and action.

This opacity is manifested in sciences of individual action (psychology) as well. Freudian psychoanalysis overturned centuries of thinking about the human mind. At least since Descartes (and dating back probably to the Greeks, but in Descartes we have a clear, explicit and unequivocal statement of this thesis) the mind had been seen as eminently transparent. To understand oneself or the workings of one's mind, all that is needed is appropriately focused and rational introspection. All is clear. All is there to be "seen" without interpretation. This transparency allowed Descartes to theorize the working of the mind and the brain in his *Meditations*. Immanuel Kant also used introspection similarly, but had to employ as well some degree of logical deduction. All may not have been immediately observable but what was not could be logically derived from what was. Freud, however, theorized a mind that was in need of interpretation to be understood—both generally and particularly. The tripartite structure of the human mind (id, ego, and superego) is not immediately observable. It needs to be drawn out through interpretation to understand how the human mind in general works. Individually, according to psychoanalysis, our actions are affected by desires in our subconscious—a part of our mind below awareness. This subconscious is structured by long-forgotten experiences and psychological traumas—failures to meet the demands of the id, for example. Although far below awareness, the subconscious, according to psychoanalytic theory, influences our actions and choices. It is so far below awareness that introspection is not enough to unearth the real explanations of our actions. Self-interpretation is not enough either. What is needed is an external interpreter, a therapist who can take a noninvested, scientific point of view that will allow her to pierce through the illusions and rationalizations of the conscious mind to the dark truths beneath.

However, this leads us back to the problem of the hermeneutic circle. The explanations of sociology or psychoanalysis can only be understood and evaluated from within a hermeneutic context that presupposes the theory (language) from which the explanation comes. Self-critique, then, becomes impossible for interpretive social sciences, according to Fay and Moon (1977/1998). Yet naturalism, as it follows the critical analysis of the natural sciences, while it would provide this level of self-critique that would better insure the validity of theoretical frameworks, would entirely neglect the intentional states that make this a problem to begin with. What may be needed then is a model for social science that transcends this dichotomy, bringing together the strengths of each model and eliminating the weaknesses of each.

One more specific type of explanation found in the social sciences can also be found in the natural science of biology. This is the functional explanation in which a practice, action, or event is explained in regard to the function it serves for an individual or society. When discussing body parts we commonly understand them in terms of function. The heart pumps blood. The liver filters contaminants. The long neck of the giraffe allows it to eat the leaves at the tops of trees. Functional definitions in biology, however, are somewhat archaic. The teleological presuppositions of such explanations have been overturned by the mechanistic views of Darwinian evolution. In the social sciences, functional explanations are still common and potentially enlightening. Although functional explanations can be found in many areas of social sciences and many theoretical approaches to social science, they also comprise the central concepts of the approach called functionalism. We will cover functionalism and give functional explanations a closer look in the next chapter.

ETHICS AND SOCIAL SCIENCE

Research Ethics in Social Science

In the 1960s, social psychologist Stanley Milgram performed a series of experiments meant to test obedience to authority of ordinary people. Milgram was inspired by the defense of Holocaust architect Adolf Eichmann that he was merely "following orders." Could this be a legitimate defense or even explanation for many of the horrors that occurred during the Second World War? The experiment included pairs of people, one of whom was a "teacher" and the other a "student." The students were actually actors in on the experiment. Milgram told the "teachers" that this was an experiment regarding learning and memory. The student and the teacher would be separated into different rooms with audio communication (or at least apparent audio communication) between the two. The teacher was to give the student pairs of words that the student was supposed to remember. When students failed to remember a pair the teacher would press a lever that would deliver an electric shock to the student. The shocks ranged from 15 to 450 volts. In reality, though, there were no shocks. The true purpose of the study was to see how far an ordinary person would follow an authority figure (a scientist in a white coat) who was telling him to harm another person. The results varied, but 25 out of 40 subjects in the first experiment delivered shocks up to the 450 volt extreme—marked "Danger: Severe Shock" (Milgram, 2010). Some of the 25 may have demurred at points during the experiment, but with a little coaching from the white-coated investigator, they continued.

In 1971, psychologist Philip Zimbardo conducted an experiment at Stanford University in which he took a group of volunteer college students (all male), designating some prisoners and some guards and placed them in a makeshift "prison" in the basement of the Stanford Psychology Department building. The purpose of the experiment was to study "the psychology of prison life," to answer questions such as "What happens when you put good people in an evil place? Does humanity win over evil, or does evil triumph?" (Zimbardo, 2009). The experiment was planned to run for two weeks but had to be halted after 6 days, as the "guards became sadistic and . . . prisoners became depressed and showed signs of extreme stress" (Zimbardo, 2009). One "prisoner" even had to be released after 36 hours due to signs of emotional stress. The guards quickly fell into their role as authority figures to the point of abusiveness. And the prisoners quickly became submissive and obedient.

Ethics is a greater concern for social science than natural science. Certainly ethics is not irrelevant to natural science. There are some serious ethical concerns in the study and results of natural science. Weapons research, for example, raises ethical concerns—particularly weapons of mass destruction. Robert Oppenheimer, so-called "father of the atomic bomb," after seeing the destructive force of that weapon, resisted research into the more powerful hydrogen bomb. And similar debates and controversies have surrounded the development of chemical and biological weapons due to their potential for massive destructive force and particularly torturous means of killing. The branch of natural science that probably raises the most ethical issues is medical research, due to the possible harmful effects on animals and people—and such effects include not only physical harm but moral harm in possibly violating basic rights and dignity. Like weapons research, much of the attention to the ethics of medical research can be traced to events of WWII. The atrocious actions of medical researchers within the Nazi regime are well-known. Persons (especially, such persons not perceived as real or full persons by Nazis) were studied with no regard for their well-being or natural rights. The first major ethical response to these acts was the Nuremburg Code of 1946, which established two basic principles, that research subjects should provide voluntary informed consent and that a research study must be justified by a positive benefit to risk ratio (Glannon, 2005). Other events that raised the visibility of the ethical issues of medical research in the mid- to late 20th century include the Tuskegee syphilis experiment, the development of life-saving technologies and the development of new contraceptive methods. The statement of the Nuremburg Code was later developed and added to by the Declaration of Helsinki in 1964 and in the U.S., the Belmont Report in 1979 (Glannon, 2005).

Social science research raises at least as many, if not more, ethical concerns as medical research. In order for medical research to produce new effective therapies and justified, reliable knowledge claims, humans must be involved as subjects at some point. Once humans are involved, ethical concerns are understandably inevitable. Since humans (or more accurately the actions of humans) are the focus of the social sciences, research will similarly involve human subjects. The two experiments outlined above are illustrative of some of the basic ethical problems that can arise in social science research. For each, it is easy to get lost in the intriguing results, but that simply exemplifies another problem. The Milgram experiment seems to reveal an ugly side of human nature. First, ordinary people seem much more capable of horrific acts than most would assume. Indeed, Milgram notes that the many people, including students, middle-aged lay people, *psychiatrists and students of behavioral science*, he questioned prior to the experiment predicted that most people would not obey the experimenter (Milgram, 2010). These data may also be seen as yet more evidence against the predictive success of the social sciences. The psychiatrists and students of behavioral science apparently had no better insight into the future actions of the subjects than those with no experience in or expert knowledge of those sciences. Second, we typically think of ourselves as autonomous, in control of our own actions. What the results of this experiment suggest is that we are more susceptible to the control of authority and recognized authority figures (such as scientists in white coats) than we think we are. Of course, the immediate reaction of most persons upon hearing of this study is, "That's awful. I would never do that!" But of course we have to consider that those subjects in the experiment would likely have said the same thing beforehand.

But of course these seductively interesting results are not our primary concern here, the research design is. First, there is a concern of deception. The real subjects of this experiment were deceived on to their role in this experiment and the purpose of the experiment. This deception means that voluntary informed consent was not obtained. The subjects were used as objects of scientific experimentation without respect to their rights to know truly what they were entering into. The dilemma that arises, however, is that it does not seem likely that the information obtained could have been obtained without deception. If they had been told the true purpose of the study and their true part in it, they would not have reacted as they did; their reactions would not have been sincere responses to the authority represented by "science" and the white-coated experimenter. So, when deception is necessary for such knowledge, one has to deliberately weigh the value of the knowledge to be obtained against the moral harm of deception. Second, there is a concern of psychological harm to the subjects. Discovering that they are capable of inflicting such harm and unthinkingly following a recognized authority could be emotionally traumatic to some subjects. One of the subjects, after having been told the true purpose of the experiment, suggests such psychological trauma in his reflections on the experiment: "There was I. I'm a nice person, I think, hunting somebody, and caught up in what seemed a mad situation . . . and in the interest of science, one goes through with it" (Milgram, 2010, p. 51). And in a one-year post-study questionnaire this same subject wrote, "What appalled me was that I could possess the capacity for obedience and compliance to a central idea, that is, the value of a memory experiment . . . at the expense of another value, that is, don't hurt someone who is helpless and not hurting you" (Milgram, 2010, pp. 51–52).

The Zimbardo experiment similarly resulted in seductively interesting results. It demonstrated the degree to which our behavior and actions are influenced and even controlled by our environment. Again, seemingly ordinary individuals (this time male college students, a sample of the population with far less variety than Milgram's study) seem to change in character. The "guards" became authoritative to the point of abusiveness, and the prisoners became obedient and compliant to the point of submissiveness. Even Zimbardo admits that he got caught up in the fantasy and confused his dual roles of investigator and warden, to the possible emotional detriment of his subjects (Zimbardo, 2009). Unlike the Milgram experiment, there was no deception in the design of Zimbardo's study. However, deception arose as the experiment played out, particularly in relation to Zimbardo's confused roles. The primary ethical concern here is psychological harm to the subjects. As noted above, that harm became so apparent and possibly serious that the two-week study had to be aborted after only 6 days.

Again, the results of these experiments are so seductively interesting that it is easy to get caught up in the insights into human nature and ignore the ethically questionable methodology. There is possibly much knowledge that can be attained if we neglect any concern for ethics, any concern for the rights and well-being of subjects. The trouble is that respecting such rights is somewhat at odds with traditional standards of justified objective knowledge. The concept of objectivity implies an ontological distinction between the knower and the known, the subject and the object. The object is a thing to be known, separate and distinct from the subject (the knower). This separation preserves the integrity of knowledge. Without it, the knower can be implicated in the known. Such intermingling can result in bias, a slanted, invested perspective that may reduce the quality of the knowledge obtained. This view is relatively unproblematic when that which is being studied is stars or trees or tectonic plates. But when that which is being studied is human beings, problems will arise. The problem patent from this analysis so far is that humans are not just objects, not just stars or trees or tectonic plates. They are living, feeling beings with commonly recognized rights. To treat them like objects, then, undermines this recognition of humans as persons. A deeper problem is that the knower in social science research is not ontologically distinct from the known. They are both in the category of humans, which some would argue, negates the possibility of a true objective attitude. Social science is reflective. Any knowledge gained by the investigator reflects back on the investigator (clearly illustrated by Zimbardo getting caught up in his own study). So, investment of the knower in the known cannot be completely removed. Thus, true objectivity cannot be attained.

Other Ethical Issues

Some ethical issues arise particularly from a naturalist approach to social science. Recall that behaviorism, as a more fully developed theory, would require some deeper understanding of the mechanism that connects reward and punishment to action or behavior. One possibility would be to discover a neurological mechanism to make this connection. The existence of such a mechanism would provide a deep challenge to the concept of free will. The theory of behaviorism as it stands challenges that concept, but if some such mechanism were to be discovered, that challenge would be more serious. Even presuming the theory of behaviorism seems to, at least hypothetically, deny free will. Free will is of course a prerequisite for moral action. With free will denied, hypothetically or in fact, the predictive possibility of social science begins to look morally dangerous. If social scientists were to develop the reliable ability to predict behavior, such knowledge could be engineered toward controlling behavior, with the clear possibility of controlling behavior in a malicious or self-serving manner.

Similar and further ethical problems may arise with other attempts to reduce human and social action to physiological explanations. Attempts to provide such a reduction have been made through genetics and sociobiology. The science of genetics has been around since the work of Gregor Mendel (1822–1884) on pea plants. Although on a broad view of "science" genetics may be said to far pre-date this period as farmers have been hybridizing and crossbreeding plants and animals for centuries or even millennia. But of course Mendel brought to this practice a formal and theoretical knowledge. It wasn't until well into the 20th century that biologists developed an understanding of the molecular function that underlay Mendel's observations and theories. The ultimate development of this science was the Human Genome Project, which ran from 1990 to 2003 and mapped the human genome in order to identify the genes that make up a human being. One possible future application of genetic knowledge might be the development of pharmacogenomics to the point of designing treatments engineered toward the DNA of specific persons (Borém, Santos, & Bowen, 2003). Yet, there is a dark side to all this newfound knowledge and technology. With it has come the concept of genetic reductionism, the idea that we, as humans and as individuals, can be wholly reduced to our genetic makeup. Once again this presents a limitation on the concept of free will. We have seen in our culture the proliferation of single-gene theories for various behaviors. The presumption that there is a single gene (or indeed even combination of genes) for a trait like violence could undermine attempts to punish and control violent behavior in our society. If there is a genetic basis for violent criminal behavior, we would not morally be able to hold the criminal responsible for his behavior. The concept of a "gay gene" has also entered public consciousness. Some gay rights advocates might welcome such an idea as establishing homosexuality to be on an equal ontological footing with race or gender and thus, worthy of the same principles of equality and nondiscrimination. Yet, the results might not be that simple. Such a discovery could lead to recognition of a greater separation (a genetic separation) between heterosexuals and homosexuals. Also, if prenatal detection of this gene were to become possible the abortion of potentially gay babies could result. Or, if *in utero* genetic manipulation were possible, the "fixing" of these gay genes could become common. Research projects intended to study valued traits like intelligence across gender or racial lines could be inspired by or reinforce preexisting stereotypes. In 1994, psychologist Richard Herrnstein and political scientist Charles Murray caused a firestorm of controversy with the publication of their book, *The Bell Curve*, which seems to argue in part that both race and intelligence are genetically determined and correlated with whites being intellectually superior. Herrnstein used the information they gathered to further argue for policy changes such as the elimination of welfare that encourages women of lower socioeconomic classes to have babies they cannot financially care for. Critics charged the authors with basing their study on unproven and even false assumptions about genetics and race and ultimately perpetuating stereotypes rather than contributing to social knowledge.

The previous section alluded to a deeper problem that was developed more in the context of natural science in Chapter 12. It seems even clearer in social science that the goal of attaining a value-free or value-neutral science is not desirable or not even possible. What Longino (1989) identified as contextual values in science seem even more unavoidable in the social sciences. Given the apparent reflective and intentional nature of social science, such values would be inherent. We are studying ourselves, a subject for which we recognize intrinsic value. The choices we make in these sciences will affect us, making the social sciences ineluctably value-laden. Social sciences were once named the moral sciences, possibly in recognition of this value-ladenness. Everything we do with the social sciences has moral implications and should be guided by clearly understood ethical principles. Attempting to ignore the value-ladenness of social sciences in order to pursue a pure, naturalist, value-neutral science may or may not leave us with immoral results but could leave us with a science unguided by values and open to the manipulation of whomever is in power.

CONCLUSION

We are probably in no position to choose between a naturalist and an interpretivist social science. We can recognize values in both approaches: some strengths, some limitations. And indeed in practice social scientists typically do not choose but employ methodologies that are a mixture of the two. We have surveyed a variety of approaches to prediction, description, and explanation in the social sciences and some of the problems that come with those basic goals. And finally, we looked at some of the ethical issues that can arise in social science. In the next chapter, we will continue our study of social science looking at several broad philosophical approaches in both the naturalist camp and the interpretivist camp.

CRITICAL THINKING QUESTIONS

1. Economics is considered a social science. According to interpretivists, this means that it is an intentional science. Demonstrate how or why economics specifically is an intentional science.

2. In your nursing education, which sciences have you studied that might be considered intentional sciences. Demonstrate why they should be considered intentional sciences.
3. Are social sciences teleological sciences?
4. If social sciences *are* teleological sciences what problems might follow?
5. Should social sciences be taken as predictive sciences?
6. Can you think of any successful instances of prediction in social science?
7. Research what is called the Tarasoff Rule in many states' laws. Does this requirement depend too strongly on the capacity for prediction in psychology and other social sciences?
8. Is sociology reducible to psychology? Or are these completely distinct and independent sciences?
9. What basic moral principles should underlie research in social science? Why would these be the most appropriate principles?
10. Do you find the Zimbardo and Milgram experiments morally problematic? If so, what about them is morally problematic? Do they not meet the principles indicated in your answer to Question 9? Why would Zimbardo and Milgram engage in such morally questionable science?

REFERENCES

Bishop, R. C. (2007). *The philosophy of the social sciences: An introduction.* New York, NY: Continuum International Publishing Group.

Borém, A., Santos, F. R., & Bowen, D. E. (2003). *Understanding biotechnology.* Upper Saddle River, NJ: Prentice-Hall.

Durkheim, E. (1951). *Suicide: A sociological study* (J. A. Spaulding, & G. Simpson, Trans.). New York, NY: The Free Press. (Original work published in 1897)

Durkheim, E. (1964). *The division of labor in society* (G. Simpson, Trans.). New York, NY: The Free Press. (Original work published in 1933)

Durkheim, E. (1982). *The rules of sociological method and selected texts on sociology and its method* (S. Lukes Ed., & W. D. Halls, Trans.). New York, NY: The Free Press. (Original work published in 1895.)

Fay, B. & Moon, J. D. (1998). What would an adequate philosophy of social science look like? In E. D. Klemke, R. Hollinger, & D. W. Rudge (Eds.), *Introductory readings in the philosophy of science* (pp. 171–189). Amherst, NY: Prometheus Books. (Original work published in 1977)

Giddens, A. (1993). *New rules of sociological method.* Stanford, CA: Stanford University Press.

Glannon, W. (2005). *Biomedical ethics.* Oxford, UK: Oxford University Press.

Kuhn, T. S. (1998). The natural and the human sciences. In E. D. Klemke, R. Hollinger, & D. W. Rudge (Eds.), *Introductory readings in the philosophy of science* (pp. 128–134). Amherst, NY: Prometheus Books.

Longino, H. E. (1989). Can there be a feminist science? In N. Tuana (Ed.), *Feminism and science* (pp. 45–57). Bloomington, IN: Indiana University Press.

Milgram, S. (2010). The perils of obedience. In C. H. Sommers, & F. Sommers (Eds.), *Vice and virtue in everyday life* (pp. 46–56). Belmont, CA: Wadsworth.

Taylor, C. (1985a). *Human agency and language: Philosophical papers 1.* Cambridge, UK: Cambridge University Press.

Taylor, C. (1994). Interpretation and the sciences of man. In M. Martin, & L. C. McIntyre (Eds.), *Readings in the philosophy of social science* (pp. 181–211). Cambridge, UK: The MIT Press. (Original work published in 1971)

Weber, M. (1978). *Economy and Society.* In G. Roth & C. Wittich (Eds.); E. Fischoff, H. Gerth, A. M. Herderson, F. Kolegar, C. W. Mills, T. Parsons, M. Rheinstein, G. Roth, E. Shils & C. Wittich (Trans.). Berkeley, CA: University of California Press. (Original work published in 1956)

Winch, P. (1958). *The idea of a social science and its relation to philosophy.* London, UK: Routledge & Kegan Paul.

Zimbardo, P. G. (2009). *Stanford prison experiment: A simulation study of the psychology of imprisonment conducted at Stanford University.* Retrieved April 16, 2010, from http://www. prisonexp.org/

14

Philosophies of Social Science

*Man, who desires to know everything, desires to know himself. Nor is he only one ...
among other things he desires to know. Without some knowledge of himself,
his knowledge of other things is imperfect: for to know something without knowing
that one knows it is only a half-knowing, and to know that one knows is to know
oneself. Self-knowledge is desirable and important to man, not only for its own
sake, but as a condition without which no other knowledge can be critically justified
and securely based.*

R. G. COLLINGWOOD

INTRODUCTION

Now that we have some of the basics of social science down and the problems that
inhere in its study, we will look at some of the major movements in modern social
science. Most of these range over the many social sciences—that is, are manifested
in sociology, psychology, and so forth. Most can clearly be placed into the naturalist
or interpretivist camp—although a close look may find elements of both views. And
all presume a theory of human nature that itself needs to be unearthed in order to
fully understand the broad theoretical structure of the movement.

RATIONAL CHOICE THEORY

Rational choice theory is a naturalist approach found most prominently in economics
and political science. It presumes a particular view of reasoning, already alluded to in
Chapter 13 as self-regarding, self-interested action, known as instrumental reasoning
or instrumental rationality. According to instrumental reasoning, to be rational is to
employ a means-end strategy. You have a goal (an end) in mind (determined by
needs, desires, etc.) and you choose the most efficient strategy (means) to attain it.
The most efficient means will provide you with the most of what you want with the
least expenditure (of work, money, time, or other personal and social goods). Rational
choice theory also presumes a theory of human nature consonant with this concept of
rationality. Humans are in essence rational beings, rational in the sense of instrumental
rationality. Thus, humans are primarily (if not solely in more extreme views) self-
interested beings. The interests of others may come into play at times but primarily

it is one's own interests that define and determine one's actions and choices. Humans are also, in this view, free and autonomous beings. We may not choose all of our needs and desires (some seem thrust upon us) but we do choose how we pursue those needs and desires, how we prioritize them. As long as we identify with those needs and desires, own them as our own, then in following them we are free. And finally, humans are essentially individuals. We form societies and other groups of people out of individual needs, to better meet those needs. It follows further then that rational choice theorists tend also to be methodological individualists.

The beginnings of rational choice theory can reasonably be pinpointed in the work of Thomas Hobbes, especially his seminal book, *Leviathan*. Following tendencies in natural science in his day, Hobbes viewed humans as purely material beings, driven by desires and aversions. Our actions/behaviors can simply (too simply?) be explained as oriented toward our desires and away from those things to which we are averse: pains, frustrations, and so forth. This all occurs due to certain, but not understood certainly in Hobbes's day, physical activities within the brain. As we all have a similar physical nature we have similar physical needs and desires, which would, at least theoretically, lead to common rules or even laws of action or behavior. The next major development came from the utilitarian ethical theory of Jeremy Bentham (1748–1832) and John Stuart Mill (1806–1873), which held that we are utility-maximizing creatures. Here, "utility" encompasses the concept of being useful but also being a human want, which fulfilled will contribute to happiness. Bentham opened one of his most important works, "Nature has placed mankind under the governance of two sovereign masters, *pain* and *pleasure*. It is for them alone to point out what we ought to do, as well as to determine what we shall do ... every effort we can make to throw off our subjection, will serve but to demonstrate and confirm it" (Bentham, 2000, p. 14). The subjective experience of pain dissuades us from certain activities. For example, once a child touches a hot stove, that child will likely not repeat that act. The experience of pleasure leads us toward performing other acts. The rewards we receive from hard work encourage us to continue to work hard. Bentham's statements above are both descriptive claims about human nature and normative claims about morality. His language is somewhat fanciful and poetic. We are slaves to the masters of pain and pleasure. This is human nature. Thus, pain and pleasure "determine what we shall do." We cannot escape that inevitability. Even when we voluntarily endure pain, we do so for some further pleasure in the future. As a matter of ethics, pain and pleasure also define "what we ought to do." Since people in general enjoy pleasure and suffer from pain, we should seek to increase pleasure and decrease pain.

The next major step forward in the development of rational choice theory involves a development in economics by a school of economic theorists in the 19th century known as marginalists. Marginalists also viewed humans as utility-maximizing creatures but went further in claiming that people could rank their pleasures. This process, called cardinal utility, would entail assigning a quantified number of utility units to any proposed pleasure received from a good. A night out with friends might be given 5 units. A meal at a fast food restaurant might be given 2 units. A meal at a four-star restaurant might be given 10 units. In this way, we can quantify desire and satisfaction. The naturalism here is coming clear. Although marginalists (following Hobbes and the utilitarians) still used the language of intentional states, they were progressively attempting to remove the presumed intentionality behind that language and conceive desires, beliefs, and so forth from an external, objective, natural scientific point of view. Desires and pleasures for them were not intentional, experiential, phenomenological states but objective realities that could be measured. This further would allow for interpersonal comparison of utilities. We could accurately understand how much one another desire the pleasure received from specific goods. From this we could construct social, political, and economic policies which would benefit people in general, which could distribute social goods in the most efficient manner and a manner which would provide the most benefit. It could also, theoretically, allow us to predict the actions of others. Although such predictions require a dubious assumption about rational agents, that they always have clear and accurate information about the world in which they live. This is clearly not the case. But without an assumption about what agents know, we cannot accurately predict how they are going to act to fulfill their desires.

Cardinal utility, however, assumes that we can clearly rank all our pleasures when in reality such objectified ranking seems dubious. Compare it to the nurse who asks a patient to rate his pain on a scale of 1–10. Any such judgment will be extremely limited in quantified objectivity because there is no real objective scale for pain. This limitation may not completely devalue this health-care tool, but it does limit the amount and degree of clear, objective information that can be inferred from it. But to base all of economic theory on such a dubious process was too much for the science. Cardinal utility eventually gave way to ordinal utility, in which, instead of placing quantified values to various pleasures, people are only expected to order their preferences. This seems a bit of a slide back from quantification to qualification. The assumptions regarding to what degree we could quantify our intentional states was moderated. However, this meant that we could no longer compare desires and pleasures between people, reducing the predictive application and making policy determinations more difficult.

In order to get back on a naturalist track, economics took a more behaviorist turn (Szenberg, Ramrattan, & Gottesman, 2006), eliminating reference to intentional states and applying mathematical tools such as statistics and game theory. A desire becomes no more than a "revealed preference" (Varian, 2006), a term that refers to no more than one's behavior as evidence of choice. No assumptions are made about what intentional states might underlie that behavior. This behavior takes the place of assumed intentional states. This stripping down of human action/behavior to its purely empirical manifestations allows for the mathematization of economics and other social sciences and the development of game theory as a central tool in contemporary social science.

Game theory (von Neumann & Morgenstern, 2007) arose in the 1940s as a tool for economics originally but has been adopted by many other social sciences and philosophy as well. Game theorists hypothesize situations in which an agent's behavior is constrained by the presence, choices, and behaviors of others. Game theorists hold that these strategic games reflect real life. They are composed of hypothetical situations analogous to situations we face every day. In the words of game theory founder John von Neumann, "Real life consists of bluffing, of little tactics of deception, of asking yourself what is the other man going to think I mean to do. And that is what games are about in my theory" (Poundstone, 1992, p. 6). The most well-known example is the Prisoner's Dilemma (PD). This game is immediately relatable to anyone who has watched a television crime drama. In this game you are arrested for a crime. Simultaneously your partner is also arrested. Whether you and/or your partner are actually guilty is not relevant to the game. The presumptions about self-interested human nature, instrumental reason, and the determination of your captors to convict *somebody* make guilt and innocence beside the question. The police place the two of you in separate interrogation rooms. They offer you a deal with several alternatives, which they tell you your partner is also being offered. (a) If you confess and testify against your partner but she does not confess, then you will go free and she will be sentenced to 10 years in prison. (b) But in the reverse situation, you will go to prison for 10 years and your partner will go free. (c) If you both confess, you will each receive five years of imprisonment. (d) If neither of you confesses, they will charge you both with a lesser crime and you each will receive a year in prison. As noted above, guilt and innocence are irrelevant here, because it is assumed you (and your partner) are wholly concerned with getting as little prison time as possible—maximizing your utility—not with defending one's integrity. Game theorists don't accept that an innocent rational person would take a stand on principle. Similarly, loyalty is not a relevant consideration. First, loyalty is emotion based and not rational. Further, in such a blind situation, a suspect will only be as loyal as she can assume (trust) her partner will be. Assuming her partner is also a self-interested rational chooser, she will infer certain limits to loyalty. The question then is whether or not you should confess in order to pursue your self-interest: to spend as little time in prison as possible. A little rational analysis will provide a clear answer. If your partner confesses (option b or c), then you will receive 10 years if you do not confess and 5 years if you do confess. If your partner does not confess (option a or d), then you will receive 1 year if you do not confess and go free if you do confess. In either situation, you will receive less (or no) time in prison *if you confess*. However, here is where things get tricky. Remember that your partner is a self-interested rational chooser just as you are. Therefore, she will employ the same analysis. Therefore, she will most likely confess. You both confess; you both receive 5 years in prison. However, if you both had refused to confess, you would have each received only 1 year in prison. If the two of you had been allowed contact, you might have been able to make an agreement not to confess. But without such contact it seems impossible to rationally reach either what is optimal for you alone (going free), or what is optimal for the two of you together (1 year in prison). You might "take a chance" and refuse to confess. However, that is a big chance. If your partner similarly does not confess, then you will each receive only 1 year. But if your partner *does* confess, then you will receive 10 years. That is too big of a gamble to be considered "rational" by most people—especially considering that your partner, as a self-interested, rational chooser, would likely confess.

As noted above, if you and your partner could communicate, the two of you might agree not to confess in order to ensure a mere 1 year sentence for each of you. However, it's not that simple. Even with such an agreement, each of you would still have to trust that the other would honor the agreement. If your partner goes back on the agreement and confesses, she will go free (a better result than 1 year in prison) and you will receive a 10-year sentence. Knowing this, you might also go back on your agreement and confess. In which case both of you confess and we're back to 5-year sentences for each of you. Part of what a game like this demonstrates is how our actions and choices are constrained by others. All things being equal, we would all prefer to go free. However, given the circumstances of the PD, it does not seem possible to achieve that goal through a rational process. The only way to do that is through an irrational "bet" on an unlikely outcome. We may never find ourselves in exactly this situation, but as von Neumann says, we do find ourselves in analogous situations quite commonly. It is amazing, especially in some cities, that in maneuvering through traffic there are as few auto accidents as there are. A large part of the reason may be that in recognizing our own goals of rational self-interest and inferring that thought process is active in other drivers we fairly accurately predict the actions and movements of other drivers. In other PD-like situations in which we find ourselves we may not act according to what rational choice theory might predict. In any transaction of goods, the "rational" thing to do (that which will increase your utility the most) would be to cheat: take the goods and keep your money. Since we live in a complex society in the midst of traditional social structures, a singular PD game may not accurately reflect our experiences and the rational thinking that must go into those experiences. Rather, what might be a more accurate reflection of our life experience is what is called an "iterated dilemma" (Poundstone, 1992). An iterated dilemma is a repeating game. Since we rarely are in unique, never to be repeated situations (like the one the PD sets out), it makes more sense to recognize that our rational reactions may be geared toward the realization that you will find yourself in this position again. Long-term self-interest may then trump short-term self-interest.

Even given iterated dilemmas and other complex developments of game theory, there are clear examples in life that seem to contradict the assumptions of game theory and rational choice theory in general. These examples are likely due to elements of human nature not recognized by the presumptions of rational choice theory, elements that are not rational—at least in terms of instrumental rationality. Take the example of another game, the ultimatum game (Lehrer, 2009; Ruffle, 1998). This game involves two players: an allocator and a recipient. The allocator has a sum of money, say $10. The allocator then is given the power to give a portion of that $10 to the recipient. But the recipient can choose to accept the deal, in which case both players will receive the amount agreed upon, or refuse the deal and neither player will receive any money. Theoretically, from a rational choice perspective, the likely outcome would seem to be that the allocator would offer the recipient a small amount of money, say $1, leaving the allocator with $9. That would seem to follow from rational self-interest. And from rational self-interest it would seem that the recipient would accept such a deal rather than reject it and receive nothing. Yet when this game is played with actual people, it rarely follows that pattern (Lehrer, 2009; Ruffle, 1998). When the allocator offers a "fairer" amount, say around $5, the recipient is more likely to accept the deal. In fact, allocators typically tend toward this "fairer" amount either out of a sense of fairness, altruism, or perhaps expectation of the rejection of an unfair proposal. It seems then that making decisions may involve more than a consideration of self-interest. It may involve moral feelings of fairness and altruism, which are in principle inconsistent with naked self-interest. There is further evidence that cultural differences may also play a part in how one responds to the ultimatum game (Oosterbeek, Sloof, & van de Kuilen, 2004).

Or take an example from history. Following a survey of thousands of American troops in WWII, Brigadier General S. L. A. Marshall discovered that less than 20% of soldiers shot at the enemy when under attack (Lehrer, 2009). In dangerous combat it would seem rational to do everything possible to preserve one's own life. Killing the enemy before they kill you seems unavoidably rational. Yet there seemed to be something preventing many soldiers (the vast majority in fact) from actually shooting at other human beings—even though they are marked as "enemies" and likely a mortal threat. Again, there seems to be some element of human nature in the way of moral feelings, a connection with others (even if they are "enemies") that gets in the way of doing the "rational" thing. Following WWII, the army adopted new training techniques that drew from behaviorist sciences. Soldiers were trained with human-shaped targets (Lehrer, 2009). The idea was that once in actual combat they would not see the enemy as humans but simply respond, as per their training, shooting at the human-shaped targets. The enemy soldiers were no longer humans but merely targets—dehumanized humans. Likely due to this training, that 20% figure rose to 55% in the Korean War and almost 90% in the Vietnam War (Lehrer, 2009).

Another problem, which will be developed in a later section, is that the view of rationality assumed in rational choice theory is too narrow and is tacitly normative. Rationality includes more, say critics, than simply attempting to maximize one's utility. This view is tacitly normative in that it is presumed to be a neutral, descriptive concept of rationality but is in fact a view of what rationality *should be*. Any actions or choices that run counter to this view of rationality are simply dismissed as irrational. Given the existence of other plausible models of rationality, this judgment moves from the descriptive to the normative. These two problems and the empirical problems raised above lead to a further, more general problem. Realizing that rational choice often does not manifest as expected in real-world examples or even in laboratory settings such as the ultimatum game, we might see rational choice theory as an ideal. In Chapter 11, we saw that this strategy may be used in regard to natural scientific laws. Newton's laws of motion, for example, do not take account of all possible variables regarding the motion of any piece of matter—say a ball rolling down an inclined plane. As such Newton's laws are ideal laws, specifically about ideal situations but still applicable to real-world situations—as has been shown through centuries of practice. Similarly, in regard to rational choice theory not all people may act and react in the manner that is consistent with being a rational self-interested chooser, but given a large enough sample, the theory may accurately (enough) predict how a society will respond, what political or economic trends may be on the horizon. Underlying this "ideal" view is either the assumption that, although people individually do not always act "rationally," their actions collectively average out to this view of rationality, or that this "ideal" view is a form of instrumentalism. The presumptions of the theory may not accurately depict reality but predictive success allows the theory to be used as a reliable tool or instrument. Either way, it becomes an empirical question whether rational choice theory is adequate.

FUNCTIONALISM

Functionalism developed from Durkheim's methodological holism as a theory which holds that all or most social practices and institutions can be explained by or even exist because of some function they serve in society. And further, these practices and institutions continue to exist because they aid in maintaining "'social equilibrium' or societal survival" (Kincaid, 1994, p. 417). This way of thinking is found not only in macrosocial sciences such as sociology, economics, and political science but is common in folk psychology and in biology. If you were to ask any nonscientist (or scientist) why people go to work every day, the likely answer would be that they work in order to make money to live. This is a functionalist explanation. It explains this activity in reference to what the activity provides for individuals. On the other hand, a less likely nonfunctionalist explanation might be that they have been socialized into this repetitive behavior. If you were to ask a biologist why rabbits have long ears, the answer would likely be along these lines: "The rabbit's ears allow it to detect and avoid predators. As prey for many predators, rabbits need to be on constant alert. The size and shape of their ears capture many sound waves that would elude the ears of most animals. By capturing sounds early rabbits increase their chance of eluding or escaping an approaching predator." This is an explanation anyone can understand and almost anyone can accept. The problem is that, according to modern biological science, it is false, or at best inaccurate. This is a functionalist explanation. It explains the particular structure of rabbits' ears according to what they are supposed to *do* for the rabbit as an individual or as a species. However, such an explanation is too teleological given the state of modern biology. Rather, the biologist really means a more complex answer, such as: "There was a time in which not all rabbits had long ears—possibly even a time when no rabbits had long ears, or were some other, proto-rabbit type animal. Then, due to a random mutation likely caused by ambient radiation, a few larger eared rabbits were born. These rabbits were better able to hear approaching predators because of their larger ears. Thus, they were better able to survive, reproduce and pass on this genetic mutation for large ears. Over time small-eared rabbits, being less able to detect predators, eventually disappeared. So today all rabbits have long ears and what was once a mutation is a 'normal' part of genetic makeup." This more complicated explanation employs, instead of teleological thinking, mechanistic thinking, appealing to evolutionary theory for an impersonal, material mechanism to explain this biological phenomenon. Yet, as noted in the previous chapter, teleological explanations have not disappeared from the social sciences as completely as they have from the natural sciences.

Functionalism is intuitively appealing because it seems consistent with a natural way of thinking or looking at the world. We assume that things and activities exist and occur for a reason (a purpose). This assumption helps us to make sense of our world, to bring together disparate parts and events under a relatively small number of principles. It is also intuitively appealing because when presented with a new and mysterious phenomenon (physical, psychological, or social), the easiest first question to investigate is often what purpose it serves. The history of its development may be obscure, the inner structure of the phenomenon may be hidden in a proverbial "black box," but usually a function can be easily identified. Identifying functions can also allow us to make unexpected and possibly revealing and insightful connections between seemingly disparate activities and practices. One might understand the American educational system by its function to ensure and perpetuate democracy. An educated public is necessary to ensure participatory democracy. Voter registration campaigns also function to ensure and perpetuate democracy in our society. Yet these two institutions may not immediately be seen as in the same category. Placing them in the same functional category reveals connections and similarities between them and may also point to deeper values in our society. Along these same lines, a functional analysis can bring out deeper meanings of social practices and institutions. Merton (1973, 1996) refers to manifest and latent functions. Manifest functions are, as the name suggests, obvious and on the surface. Yet for that reason they might not provide much insight or deep understanding. A deeper analysis, or complementary theoretical structure, may reveal an unexpected, unseen function. For example, it is not uncommon for Marxists and critical theorists to find the latent function of maintaining the extant capitalistic power structure in social practices and institutions that on the surface may not seem related to such a function at all. Often these latent functions are identified as the "real" functions. The manifest functions may be not merely superficial but illusory. It takes the observation and study of a social scientist to see through this illusion (false consciousness) to the "truth" of such institutions and practices.

As common and easy to understand as functional explanations seem to be, functionalism as a theory has met with many criticisms. Hempel (1959/1994), for example, rejecting what he calls "functional indispensability" (p. 359), points out that functionalism can only explain that a practice or institution of some type is necessary for the function in question, not necessarily the practice or institution under study. If the rain dance of a society is functionally explained as maintaining and encouraging social cohesion, there may be an indefinite number of ceremonies that could fulfill that function. This functional explanation does not explain why this particular practice developed and continues in a society—that is, why this particular practice is "indispensible" for fulfilling this function. Another problem, raised by functional sociologist Robert Merton (1968) is that not all practices and institutions in societies seem to clearly fulfill some beneficial function for society. Merton, then, proposes a more modest functionalism which affirms a functional explanation only in situations in which a beneficial effect for society is identified. But even this more modest form of functionalism has problems. Recall the problem noted with the more general theory of methodological holism (Chapter 13). When we say that a practice or institution is understood through the function or purpose it serves to society, what is this "society" we refer to? What is the relationship between this practice and society? Does society "cause" this practice to begin and develop? If so, what sort of entity is society? Functionalism raises and largely leaves open these and other fundamental questions. One attempt to answer such questions is to appeal to Durkheim's concept of collective consciousness (Chapter 13). This option, however, is too metaphysical for most contemporary philosophers and social scientists. A more empirical option is to suggest that social development is an analogue of biological development. That is, change in biology is determined not by teleological forces but by the evolutionary mechanism of natural selection (Elster, 1983/1994). To carry through this analogy, however, a similar mechanism is needed in society. Yet no such mechanism has been clearly identified. In addition, in social change and the development of social practices and institutions human consciousness can conceivably play a role that is not conceivable in biological evolution. Societies do not simply blindly develop according to social needs but can in some measure recognize those needs and affect its own development. Of course, now we are again going down the mysterious path of attributing intentionality to aggregates of people rather than individual persons. Moreover, to accept an evolutionary analogue solution would deform the original intent of functionalism and functional explanations. It would turn functional explanations into causal explanations and thus not provide the type of "understanding" originally intended.

Finally, a criticism along moral rather than logical lines is that functionalism may be seen as "an unintended bulwark against social change" (Rosenberg, 2008, p. 163). That is, if a social practice or institution is not only understood but justified through a functional understanding, there is no reason to change. This would be true even if a society were morally repugnant. If the institution performs a necessary function for society—especially doing so in an efficient manner—then that appears to be a justification for it and no good reason can be gleaned from such an analysis to change it. Perhaps one historical example of this problem is the oft-cited claim that Mussolini made the trains run on time. The implication is that fascism is efficient and fulfills the necessary functions for society. Thus, from a functional perspective fascism appears justified as a political system.[1]

HERMENEUTICS

We have already encountered "hermeneutics" as a general term referring to interpretation and noted its original application to the study of Biblical interpretation. "Hermeneutics" also refers to a particular interpretive approach to social science. What distinguishes this use of the term "hermeneutics" from the hermeneutic aspect of interpretivist social science in general is an attention to social context. The two figures most identified with hermeneutics are the German philosopher Hans-Georg Gadamer (1900–2002) and the French philosopher Paul Ricoeur (1913–2005). They both emphasized that understanding human action required looking not only at the individual and the mind of the individual but the social and historical context in which that individual acts. One cannot interpret actions solely from the beliefs, desires, and so forth of an individual. For human actions (and the beliefs and desires that lie behind them) only make sense within a social and historical context of other actions, beliefs, and desires. Nor, of course, can one understand human actions from a naturalist perspective that neglects intentionality.

Let us begin with what is, especially within a modern context, the most counterintuitive and thereby likely the most interesting aspect of Gadamer's thought. Prejudice is typically taken to be a bad thing—both in science and more generally in culture and society. It is widely accepted that prejudices prevent us from proper

---

[1]Of course this example might be weakened when one recognizes the challenges to the claim that Mussolini indeed made the trains run on time. But for heuristic's sake we'll leave the example open at least as hypothetical.

learning, from coming together socially, from understanding one another, from making clear and objective judgments. According to Gadamer, however, prejudice is not only beneficial to these goals but necessary for them (1975/2004). Gadamer emphasizes that we, as humans, are not only social beings but *historical* beings as well. What we are *and* how we understand ourselves is largely determined by our socio-historical circumstances. When we interpret ourselves we are doing so from a particular historical moment. We have reached where we are historically from a particular path. This path imbues us with prejudicial beliefs that structure our thinking in a very deep sense. Without these prejudices our thinking would be unstructured. However, while we are in the historical moment we find ourselves, we cannot identify those prejudices. Only "temporal distance" can provide us with the viewpoint to see these prejudices. We cannot get behind those prejudices as it were, to an objective, or "god's eye view." Since they structure thinking and are part not only of our intentional states but our socio-historical existence, prejudices bring these together, allowing for effective social action. The student who raises her hand in response to a teacher's question does so within a socio-historical context in which that gesture has a specific meaning. More deeply, such a gesture is also a sign of respect for the teacher. This gesture, as a sign of respect, is so only within a socio-historical context. Within another historical moment the gesture might have a different meaning, or respect might be signified by a different action. The woman who requests a breast examination from her physician because of an advisory from the Centers for Disease Control and Prevention does so with a whole slew of prejudicial beliefs regarding the authority of science and the authority of a benevolent democratic government. We may be tempted to say (as a rational choice theorist might) that she is simply weighing the pros and cons, performing a benefit–risk analysis. However, even to perform this analysis requires the structure of prejudices like those mentioned.

Employing a metaphor of Gadamer's, our historical situation is a horizon (Gadamer, 1975/2004). The limits of that horizon are the limits of our understanding. There may be something beyond that horizon, but it is beyond our understanding, beyond the current prejudices necessary for interpretation. Since Gadamer focuses less on individuals than on socio-historical groups, understanding is never an individual act. It is first, as we have been saying, a function (or "effect" to use Gadamer's word) of history and society, and second, a dialectical or dialogical process. That is, understanding and interpretation occur in discursive interaction with others. Language then is central to ourselves as beings and our attempts to understand. Discourse occurs within a language and our being in the world is structured by our language. When we interact discursively we do so because we share a language and to some extent share a horizon. Without this sharing of language we would not be able to create understanding, to fuse our horizons. When we come together in dialogue in an attempt to create understanding, our horizons fuse (Gadamer, 1975/2004). When we come to new understandings we create new horizons. What was strange and unfamiliar becomes integrated into our new horizon. There is no ultimate goal however. There is no point at which we will achieve the broadest, most inclusive of horizons which will provide some absolute or purely objective knowledge. It is an ongoing, never-ending process of understanding and interpretation. However, this need for a common language raises the problem of the hermeneutical circle. The interpretation of any text or action requires understanding its place within the whole of language and understanding the whole of any language implies being able to understand any part (particular text, action) of it. For Gadamer, however, this circle merely provides further support for his view. There is no external, objective perspective to judge or understand from. All perspectives, all attempts at interpretation and understanding, are from within a historical moment.

Since there is no end to human understanding, but a continual process of horizon fusing, the objective, nonintentional knowledge that naturalistic social sciences pursue will not be achieved. Knowledge is always contextual and limited by our historical moment. There seems a clear parallel here to Kuhn's theory of paradigms and scientific change. And indeed, Gadamer's analysis here could apply to the question of natural science as well as it does to social science. That is, even the knowledge gained from natural science is limited by our prejudicial horizons. Although Gadamer's view allows for future historical change in ourselves and our interpretation (i.e., we are not frozen at some historical moment unable to change our way of being), this prejudicial view of his has been criticized as a form of ideological conservatism (Habermas, 1970/1988). The concern is that the apparent championing of prejudice over critical rationality will turn back the advances of modernism and return us to an epistemic and political orientation in which tradition and authority rule. Even though historical change is possible, a clear reason to change (to improve ourselves) is lacking. The view then risks a descent into epistemic, moral, and political relativism.

The concept that most marks Ricoeur's contribution to hermeneutics is "narrative." He shares Gadamer's emphasis on language, discourse, the action/text analogy and the embeddedness of action within a social context, and a universe of other actions. Rather than texts, actually, Ricoeur analogizes actions to discourses (Ricoeur, 1981). Discourses occur within the medium of a language, and actions occur within the medium of social rules. The language as a whole gives a particular discourse its meaning, as do the rules guiding actions. Discourses also are concrete and particular, like actions. Distinct from natural sciences, then, the social sciences do not aim at laws to explain general events but at understanding concrete, particular actions. Another distinction from the natural sciences might be found in the openness of interpretation. One might imagine the study of natural science as finite. There is, presumably, a natural world of limited facts and laws for natural scientists to study. To learn everything may take an extremely long time, but it is at least conceivable that the natural world could be exhausted of facts and laws. Human action, however, like texts and discourses, is always open to new interpretations, new meanings (Ricoeur, 1981). This is especially true due to the open future providing new interpretations. This leaves the full meaning of any action never fully determined, always "in suspense" (Ricoeur, 1981, p. 208). With new meanings and new interpretations possible, there is then always something new to learn about human action. But this does not mean that all interpretations are equal. Interpretations can be evaluated, not in the strict logical sense that claims to knowledge in natural science are evaluated but through a process Ricoeur describes as guessing and validating (1981). We make a guess at what an action means and then in a dialectical process attempt to validate that guess. This sense of validation is "comparable to the juridical procedures of legal interpretation ... a logic of uncertainty and of qualitative probability" (Ricoeur, 1981, p. 212). He brings some sense to this notion of validation by the analogy to legal interpretation, which has a long history in our culture. Legal interpretations, similarly, are rarely final, but they are not simply relativistic or subjective either. They are interpretations within loose bounds of rules, social structure (the legal system, legal academia), and history. And they are interpretations often open to reasonable disagreement. This is why higher courts are composed of multiple judges. Similarly, a text or action exists "in a limited field of possible constructions" (Ricoeur, 1981, p. 213). So, all interpretations are not equal but exist themselves within an open field of discourse, in which we can "arbitrate between them ... seek for an agreement, even if this agreement remains beyond our reach" (Ricoeur, 1981, p. 213).

Just as the meaning of discourses is dependent in part on the relation of a discourse to other discourses, the meanings of actions depend in part on their relationships with other actions. All action is, in essence, interaction. Further, our actions have effects we do not intend. They "escape us" (Ricoeur, 1981, p. 206). That is part of their nature as social phenomena. The student who raises her hand to answer a question may make another student feel inferior for not knowing the answer. The man who raises his arm to hail a taxi may unknowingly receive a taxi whose driver purposely passed by an African-American pedestrian also raising his hand. Therefore, this innocently intended gesture could perpetuate racism. The woman who seeks a breast exam may, in that very action, encourage or inspire other women to be tested. Our actions are of the world, not just of ourselves.

The means of holding together all these elements and all these open and conflicting interpretations is through narrative. Narrative provides direction, order, coherence, and cohesiveness to the interpretations that comprise our understanding of the world and ourselves: "encompassing them in successive totalities" (Ricoeur, 1981, p. 279). The social sciences then become a "literary artifact" (Ricoeur, 1981). As such, the proper tools for studying human action may be found in the humanities (literary studies, semiotics, etc.). This may seem odd to many, as much literature is fictional in nature and social sciences—like natural sciences—presumably aim to discover truth and knowledge. But social science is both a literary artifact *and* a representation of reality. As a "self-sufficient system of symbols," it is a literary artifact (Ricoeur, 1981, p. 291). As it "depicts ... claims to hold for real events in the real world," it is a representation of reality (Ricoeur, 1981, p. 291).

There are two more points worth noting regarding heremeneutics. As an approach to social science, it rarely stands on its own. It more often works in relation to other interpretive approaches, such as the ones to follow: phenomenology, critical theory, and postmodernism. Second, any hermeneutic approach will inevitably have to face a rather intractable problem. The hermeneutic circle that any system of hermeneutics finds itself in makes it difficult to confirm a specific theory of hermeneutics itself. The theory only makes sense within the system which it is describing. So one cannot step outside and evaluate it. But then this goes again for all interpretive/interpretable systems. And if all human life and action can only be understood through an interpretive lens, then the only knowledge we can hope for is that trapped within an interpretive scheme—even if the interpretive scheme we are trapped within tomorrow might be a different one.

PHENOMENOLOGY

Phenomenology is an approach to social science that developed from the work of philosopher Edmund Husserl (1859–1938). His work influenced many other philosophers and social scientists of the 20th century, including Gadamer and Ricoeur. Other important philosophical phenomenologists are the French philosopher Maurice Merleau-Ponty (1908–1961) and the Lithuanian-born French philosopher Emmanuel Levinas (1906–1995). And Alfred Schutz (1899–1959) is the social scientist most recognized for applying the insights of philosophical phenomenology to sociology (1960/1967). The epistemological and metaphysical focus of phenomenology is the "phenomenon." "Phenomenon" is a highly equivocal term. In common parlance it seems to have many meanings, but none of them very clear. Even philosophers and scientists will use the term in a variety of inconsistent manners. Phenomenologists, however, have a specific meaning for the term. For phenomenologists, a phenomenon is anything directly present to one's consciousness. What does this include? First it includes sense perceptions. Like empiricists, then, sense perceptions are epistemically relevant for phenomenologists. However, phenomenologists conceive of sense perceptions differently. Taking sense perceptions as central to epistemology leaves empiricists having to deal with a difficult problem regarding how these sense perceptions relate to the "real" world. Some empiricists (e.g., Locke) respond to this question with what is called a representative theory of knowledge: the perceptions one has directly in one's mind are representations of objects existing in an independent reality external to the mind. This answer follows a trope in Western philosophy that stretches back to Plato and even pre-Socratic philosophy: a distinction between an apparent world and a real world. A representational theory of knowledge runs into certain metaphysical problems of establishing what the nature of that real world is, what the relationship between the apparent and real world is, and how we can claim to know anything of this real world. Pheonomenologists avoid all these questions by not assuming that sense perceptions are representations of anything else and by not accepting the dichotomy between a real and apparent world. For phenomonologists, the only world that matters is the world as it appears to us, a world composed of phenomena—things which appear directly to our mind or consciousness.

Phenomenologists do not actively deny the existence of a world beyond our phenomena (as Berkeley denies the existence of a separate material world) but do not view the existence or nature of any such world epistemically or philosophically relevant. All that is relevant is that which appears directly to our consciousness. Since phenomenologists do not presuppose the relation of sense perceptions to some extramental reality (e.g., material reality), this leaves room for other types of phenomena, including "believing, remembering, wishing, deciding and imagining things; feeling apprehensive, excited, or angry at things; judging and evaluating things; the experiences involved in one's bodily actions, such as lifting or pulling things" (Hammond, Howarth, & Keat, 1991, p. 2). All these mental or intentional states are also phenomena in the sense meant by phenomenologists. Thus, in their metaphysical and epistemological outlook, they are no less real and no less epistemically relevant than sense perceptions. Altogether they compose what phenomenologists call the *lebenswelt* (the lifeworld), the sum total of all phenomena and phenomenal experiences. But they do not generate the type of epistemic testability that it is usually presumed (by various forms of empiricists) that empirical sense perceptions are meant to. The feeling of being angry is no less real or epistemically relevant than the perception of a strip of litmus paper changing color. These two phenomenal experiences both refer to what Husserl (1913/1931) calls intentional objects: that which we are conscious of, without any presumptions of independent reality.

So far this explication may seem to lead to a form of solipsism: a reduction of existence to oneself and one's internal states. Solipsism has generally been eschewed by philosophers because it seems such an epistemological and metaphysical dead end. Phenomenologists also avoid solipsism. For humans, claim phenomenologists, other humans appear not as mere objects but as subjects of their own existence, as "the Other" (Husserl, 1913/1931, 1950/1977; Levinas, 1961/1969; Merleau-Ponty, 1945/1962). The Other is to us not just another object but is experienced phenomenally by us as a subject of phenomenological experience. This perception of the Other is not based upon an inference of the subjectivity of others but something more immediate, more intuitive. Our very being and activity in the world (the lifeworld) presupposes this perception; it does not infer it. In the words of Levinas, "Doing, labor, already implies the relation with the transcendent [the Other] ... the social relation is experienced preeminently, for it takes place before the existent that expresses himself, that is, remains in himself" (1961/1969, p. 109). This recognition of the Other provides the basis for intersubjective experience (Husserl, 1913/1931; Schutz, 1960/1967). Thus, we are not bound up in ourselves in a solipsistic manner. Even to have and conceive of an individual self, rather, requires a perception of a world of Others. The streams of consciousness of I and the Other intersect. The Other, explains Husserl, is a "modification" of myself (1950/1977). I see "my own stream of consciousness and yours in a single intentional Act which embraces them both" (Schutz, 1960/1967, p. 103).

Schutz (1960/1967) defines a taxonomy of Others that we experience phenomemologically, though not always empirically. Consociates are those we experience physically because they share the time and space we inhabit. Contemporaries share our time but not our space. From a merely empirical standpoint it might be said that we have no experience of contemporaries, but our knowledge of them presupposes a phenomenological experience of them. The same goes, if somewhat more abstractly for Predecessors and Successors—those who came before and come after us. Although we have no empirical experience with contemporaries, predecessors, and successors, we do have phenomenological experiences of them in relation to our understanding of them and the manner in which they (or more accurately, our phenomenological experience of them) may affect our actions. And even when it comes to consociates our experiences of them cannot be reduced to that which is directly empirical. They are more than aggregates of sensations; they are human beings like me.

One should not confuse phenomenology with what is known as psychologism: the thesis that all experience can be reduced to and explained through psychological principles, that all studies are psychological studies. One important distinction to be made here is that, according to Husserl (1950/1977), logic cannot be reduced to psychology. Logic is an independent theoretical study which allows for a deeper, *a priori* understanding of psychology and other means of bringing meaning to human action, thought, and intentionality. The phenomenologist is not a psychologist but studies the grounds of such studies as psychology.

A phenomenological study requires a certain "distancing" from one's subjective experience, what phenomenologists call a phenomenological reduction. In this process one "brackets" a particular experience (intentional, not empirical) in order to set aside the prejudices and theoretical commitments typically associated with it and get to the essence of the experience, "to elucidate and render explicit the taken-for-granted assumptions of everyday life and, particularly, to bring to the fore one's consciousness of the world" (Toombs, 2001, p. 2). An implication of this is that not all experience is meaningful for phenomenologists. We live much of our lives in what phenomenologists call the "natural attitude" with little attention to our experiences. Our experiences themselves have no inherent meaning. It is only when we reflect upon them through bracketing that these experiences become meaningful. When we stop and think about these experiences we give them meaning, lifting them out of the stream of consciousness and identifying them as experiences "constituted in such and such a way and in no other" (Schutz, 1960/1967, p. 215). In the normal course of events, our experiences just happen. This bracketing can also illuminate the nature of our actions. In Schutz's (1960/1967) analysis when we plan an action we project into the future based upon intentional, reflective acts. These intentional acts are the motives for our actions. The outcomes of our actions are not their motives. This analysis addresses the charge of teleology often leveled against social sciences. The outcomes of our actions are not their "cause" or motive. The motive exists intentionally, prior to the act. This analysis seems reasonable when we realize how often the outcomes of our actions are not what we originally had in mind. When facing obstacles to our goals, we often have to adjust our motives to fit reality. Therefore, there can be a clear distinction between the outcome and the motive of the action.

Phenomenology does not dispute the existence of a material world or present itself as an alternative to (or try to supplant) the empirical sciences that typically study the supposed material world. Rather, it is conceived as more fundamental than the empirical sciences, whether natural or social. The empirical sciences presuppose the phenomena under study by phenomenology. "Empiricism begins where phenomenology leaves off" (Natanson, 1973, p. 33). In a sense then phenomenological study gets behind the experiences that are the focus of empirical sciences, identifying and setting aside the prejudices and theoretical commitments that color those experiences in order to reach the essence of those experiences. At the heart of this study is the intentionality of those experiences (whether empirical or not) because before we can empirically theorize, test, or confirm an experience "we must be directed toward, we must intend, some object" (Natanson, 1973, p. 33). The point is not to set an inner intentional world against an external, material world. That is the dichotomous manner in which human experience has been conceived for hundreds of years—at least since Descartes. The point is to challenge and break down this distinction—itself a prejudice to be set aside. Phenomenology attempts a *rapprochement* of these two traditionally separate worlds in order to effect a more holistic view of human experience (Natanson, 1973). For example, in the medical and health sciences a phenomenological approach may contribute "in furthering our understanding of the relation between medical science and clinical practice, as well as in recognizing the differences between, say, the immediate experience of illness versus the conceptualization of illness as a disease state, and the body-as-experienced versus the body as the object of scientific inquiry" (Toombs, 2001, p. 2).

Phenomenology does, however, suffer from a possible charge of circularity: "its method and its object are continuous because they constitute the circumference of one mode of pure reflection" (Natanson, 1973, p. 36). The object of phenomenology's study exists within a phenomenological field which provides the methodology for its study. The defense to this charge is that though phenomenology may be circular, its circle is not a vicious one.[2] A vicious circle is one in which no new knowledge can be obtained, one element is completely defined in terms of the other and vice versa. The claim that phenomenology has provided us with new knowledge must itself then be evaluated in order to judge this criticism. Another possible problem is with our knowledge of the experience of others. Despite (or because of) the presumption of intersubjectivity we can never be sure of our comprehension of another's intentionality, action, and lifeworld. As Schutz explains, "The very postulate of the comprehension of the intended meaning of the other person's lived experiences becomes unfulfillable. Not only this, but it becomes in principle doubtful whether the other person attends to and confers meaning upon those of his lived experiences which I comprehend" (1960/1967, p. 107). This problem may not be enough to bring down the approach as a whole but may reduce the confidence we can have regarding phenomenological conclusions.

CRITICAL THEORY

Critical theory grew out of the founding of the Institute of Social Research at the University of Frankfurt in 1923—also known simply as the "Frankfurt school." The group of philosophers and social theorists associated with this school came together with a common interest in Marxist critique of society and a resistance to positivist (naturalist) approaches to social science. Members of the Frankfurt school include the economic historian and founder of the Institute Carl Grünberg (1861–1940), philosopher/ sociologist Max Horkheimer (1895–1973), philosopher/sociologist Theodor Adorno (1903–1969), psychologist Erich Fromm (1900–1980), and philosopher Herbert Marcuse (1898–1979). Later theorists associated with the school and credited with developing critical theory further include philosopher/sociologist Jürgen Habermas (1929–), sociologist/political scientist Claus Offe (1940–), and philosopher Albrecht Wellmer (1933–)—these last two both former students of Habermas.

Critical theory embraces, more than any other theoretical approach to social science, the value-ladenness of social science by instituting a more prescriptive than descriptive approach. In a 1968 lecture, Adorno defined sociology as "insight into society, into the essential nature of society ... insight into what is, but it is a critical insight, in that it measures that which 'is the case' in society ... by what society purports to be, in order to detect in this contradiction the potential, the possibilities for

---

[2]Natanson (1973) also cleverly asserts that "it is important not to relinquish a position because of a geometric slur" (p. 36).

changing society's whole constitution" (1993/2000, p. 15). Following this definition it is the nature of sociology not merely to describe or understand the world but to reveal problems and provide solutions, which of course presumes a value-laden view of science, as problems and solutions can only be meaningful against a background of values. This prescriptive view follows from the two streams of thought most influential on the movement: Marxism and Freudianism, although the influence of Kant, Hegel, and Weber can also be found in much critical theory. From Marxism they draw a concern for social/economic critique that the real social meanings of actions, practices, and institutions are often hidden beneath a superficial or constructed meaning that functions to keep the masses content and productive for the benefit of those in power (the capitalists). Uncovering these real meanings then can *emancipate* people, allow them to achieve their potential as humans rather than existing under the control of powers they may not even recognize. And from Freudianism they draw a similar notion on a more individual level. Individually, we hold illusory beliefs that also entrap and ensnare us. Psychoanalysis can *emancipate* us from these illusions. The prescriptive goal of critical theory, then, is ultimately *emancipatory*. By breaking through illusions to reality critical theorists hope to emancipate or free ordinary people, to contribute to "the development of a non-authoritarian and non-bureaucratic politics" (Held, 1980, p, 16).

According to Adorno, only an approach that appeals to both micro- and macro-social science (psychology and sociology) can provide an analysis of the "social whole" (Held, 1980, p. 110). Critical theory, following this understanding is then neither methodologically holist nor methodologically individualist. The individual and social spheres are "interdependent but irreducible to each other" (Held, 1980, p. 110). So a study on both levels is needed, both to address the issues of both levels and to ferret out the specifics of this interdependence. In Adorno's powerful words,

> there is nothing under the sun ... which, in being mediated through human intelligence and human thought, is not also socially mediated. For human intelligence is not something given to the single human being ... Intelligence and thought are imbued with the history of the whole species and ... with the whole of society.
> — *Adorno, 1993/2000, pp. 15–16*

Further, there is no one relationship between the social and the individual. This relationship varies by culture and by history. It is a relationship open to historical change, which then allows for the emancipatory changes critical theorists seek but also means an ever-present risk of losing freedom.

Critical theorists see us as individuals *in* a society, not individuals who comprise a society or individuals as mere determined elements of a society. As individuals we have specific interests that must be met. These interests are plural and complex but the most central are based upon our nature as rational and autonomous beings. Social institutions that inhibit our reason or freedom, then, are in need of change. Reason provides the basis of our freedom as human beings. Reason allows us to make rational choices and not simply follow little-understood urges in our psyche or mindlessly, uncritically follow rules set by our society. At the center of critical theory then is an investigation and critique of the concept of rationality. This critique drew in part on an analysis of rationality by Weber (1956/1978). Specifically, critical theorists were critical of the rise of what Weber called *zweckrational* thinking (instrumental or purposive rationality) in the modern world. The secular political, economic, scientific, and even to some degree ethical/philosophical advances of the modern era is largely characterized by this type of thinking, a type of means-end rationality. This type of reasoning was raised in relation to rational choice theory earlier. It presumes we are self-interested individuals and defines rationality against that presumption: rational decisions are self-interested and self-regarding. According to critical theorists, this reduction of reasoning brought about a reduction of the personal, social, and physical worlds "to mere raw materials for an individual's manipulation in order to achieve some pre-selected purposes ... [implying further] ... that other people are eventually reduced to being mere means for domination and manipulation to meet an individual's needs or desires" (Bishop, 2007, p. 91). This modern concentration on instrumental rationality then leads to a diminution of the human being, an alienation from the deeper aspects of the human and ourselves: our "spirit." Naturalist social science is characterized by instrumental rationality which makes it, according to Adorno, merely "a stock-taking and a reflective form of spirit rather than its proper life; it wants to come to know spirits as something dissimilar from itself and elevates that dissimilarity into a maxim" (1969/1998, p. 38). In the study and practice of science as based on instrumental rationality what is lost is "[s]pontaneity, imagination, freedom toward the subject matter" (Adorno, 1969/1998, p. 38). A restriction to instrumental rationality then limits the productivity and creativity of social science. Also, Adorno alludes to the presumed subject–object division that is part of a modern sense of objectivity. This sense of objectivity, rather than enhancing knowledge and the justification of knowledge claims leads to an alienating separation from that which social scientists study—the problem being that they are intrinsically part of their object of study. Thus, we become alienated from ourselves and our own humanity.

Zweckrational thinking is opposed to *wertrational* thinking or value-rationality: "the rationality of values, ends and possible attitudes towards life" (Held, 1980, p. 67). Value-rationality addresses not just our goals in acting but the source of those goals: the values that are part of our personal and social lives and part of our conception of a good life. Instrumental rationality assumes the propriety of goals and does not question them, does not address the deeper issues of our values and humanity:

> Propositions concerning production, effective organization, the rules of the game, business methods, use of science and technique, are judged true or false according to whether or not the "means" to which they refer are suitable or applicable (for an end which remains, of course, unquestioned).
>
> —*Held, 1980, p. 67*

With no questioning of the ends or goals toward which means are engineered the status quo is maintained, progress and emancipation become impossible. And on the individual level, critical thought is quashed. Life becomes mechanical rule following. Because of the ability to follow these rules and attain ends individuals may feel free but without a critical evaluation of these ends, freedom and autonomy are restricted. As the mind and rationality are not fully developed, neither is human freedom and autonomy. Human life and society become, to use Herbert Marcuse's metaphor, "one-dimensional" (1964). Modernism viewed itself as a beacon of rationality and freedom.

Part of the project of critical theory is to reveal the illusion that this view is. The rationality and freedom supposed in modernism represents really a more subtle form of restriction and control—so subtle that people do not even understand the reasoning or freedom that they lack. A critique of social structure and a critique of one's own thinking, values, and so forth provide a means of attaining a broader sense of freedom.

Criticisms of critical theory, beyond the general criticisms of Marxism which it faces, largely charge that the theory is not as practically oriented as its proponents would claim. Common criticisms are that science and politics are reduced to philosophy, that it does not connect theory to praxis as is typically required by Marxist approaches, that it lacks "economic concreteness," and that its theorists were (ironically) alienated from "working-class politics" (Held, 1980, pp. 354–356). Karl Popper more pithily merely accused the critical theorists of "simply talking trivialities in high-sounding language" (Held, 1980, p. 380). As a practical method, it is clearly limited. But its importance may lie in its prescriptive, emancipatory focus, to recognize that the intentionality of social science demands a recognition of the values implied by that science and a goal of improving society and our individual lives.

POSTMODERNISM

We have already encountered postmodernism in our study of natural science, but this movement is arguably more influential in the social sciences. It would be good then to begin with a clearer definition or explication of just what postmodernism is. The problem with that as a starting point, however, is that, due to the variable, fragmented nature of the movement, a singular, consensual definition is difficult to locate. Another problem is that postmodernism is largely a critical, negative view with few positive characteristics. A decent starting point might be the definition proffered by French philosopher Jean-François Lyotard: "incredulity toward metanarratives" (1979/1984, p. xxiv). By "metanarrative" he means a totalizing story or theory which could provide a framework or methodology for understanding everything, "such as ... the hermeneutics of meaning, the emancipation of the rational or working subject, or the creation of wealth" (Lyotard, 1979/1984, p. xxiii). Metanarratives, by implication of the term postmodern, would characterize modernism. It was always at least a tacit belief of Enlightenment modernism that through free and rational application of the human mind the one and proper means of understanding and achieving all could be found: in politics, in the sciences, and in the arts. This sort of presupposition can be found in all the views of natural and social science we have surveyed so far. Indeed, in the above quote, Lyotard identifies some of these: hermeneutics, rational choice theory, Marxism/critical theory, and liberal economics. The reason postmodernists take an incredulous view toward metanarratives is that, according to these theorists, there is no external, objective position to view and evaluate these metanarratives—no "view from nowhere" to borrow a term from nonpostmodernist Thomas Nagel (1986). All views, rather, are views from *somewhere*. All thinking, critique, and criticism takes place *within* and *bound by* a socio-historical view. All metanarratives then are social constructions built up by no particular person but through a complex history of discourse, rhetoric, and power. With no common metanarratives to hold everything together, to provide a coherent view of the world or a coherent method for coming to understand the world, we are left with a fragmented world and fragmented knowledge. We are left with distinct, conflicting even incommensurable views, theories, and methodologies, none of which can be shown as superior to the others. Epistemic and ethical relativism then become basic to postmodern views and their primary source of controversy within the broader intellectual world.

One central figure in this school of thought is French philosopher Michel Foucault (1926–1984) who maintained that all knowledge was a result of power relations within a society. On the surface this may sound like Marxism—and indeed Foucault once identified as a Marxist—but he left Marxism behind early in his career as a flawed view. One flaw is that Marxism assumes there is a truth, but the "powers that be" obscure this truth in order to maintain their position of power. Foucault argues, however, there is no truth to be uncovered. There is in society simply a complex structure of discourse and power that produces what is accepted as knowledge at any one time in culture, in politics, and in the sciences (Foucault, 1972). "It is a question of what *governs* statements," says Foucault in an interview from 1977, "and the way in which they *govern* each other so as to constitute a set of propositions which are scientifically acceptable and hence capable of being verified or falsified by scientific procedures" (1977/1980, p. 112).

Another common theme in postmodernism is antihumanism—the "death of man" in Foucault's terminology (1966/1994). Modernist views are typically humanist: the idea that the individual (the human subject) is the source of human thought and action. Rather, our thought and action are the result of the complex matrix of socially constructed knowledge and power we find ourselves enmeshed in. Thus, the freedom and autonomy that have been central to modernist views of the human subject are just an illusion. There is no human subject to be freed from the power of the king, the state, or the capitalists. In fact, our very notion of having such a subject is in part due to the existence and influence of such power, but not in the devious sense a Marxist or critical theorist might think when proclaiming something similar. This points to another way in which Foucault separated himself from Marxist views: a reevaluation of the concept of power. Power, for Foucault, is not some oppressive force keeping us down and all we have to do is remove it and we will be able to be our free, full, and real selves. There is no self beneath power. There is a self, in fact, *due* to these power relations. Power relations define us as subjects and formulate our social and individual identities. Yet these power relations are radically fluid. So change is possible. But any change replaces one set of power relations with another. For example, employing a Foucaultian analysis to analyze the experience of gays in the late 20th century, literary theorist Eve Kosovsky Sedgwick (1950–2009) argues that the experience of "coming out of the closet" does not simply and unproblematically "free" a gay person from oppression (Sedgwick, 1990). In the closet there is clearly a sense of oppression and suppression, a lack of freedom and sincere expression. That is one set of power relations. But out of the closet is to be found another set of power relations the newly "out" gay person will have to navigate.

In addition to knowledge and methodologies of knowledge acquisition being fragmented, we are also left with a fragmented sense of self. Concepts and theories of human nature and psychology have become fragmented. There is no one accepted view but a constellation of incommensurable views. Modern views (following the anthropologies of Descartes, Kant, Hegel, and others) assumed that there was some coherent, cohesive "self" underlying our fluxive appearance. Postmodern views see the self as one radically historically and socially constructed. For example, in his first volume of *The History of Sexuality*, Foucault argues against the common knowledge that we have some buried, essential sexual self that Victorian era conservative mores have suppressed, and that since then we have been trying to break through these oppressive mores in order to be our true sexual selves (1976/1990a). This view can be found in much psycho-sexual study from Freud to Kinsey and beyond. Part of this oppression is the myth that we have not been allowed to speak about sex, that we have suffered an imposed silence on matters of sex. The types of censorship we see on television and in the movies and laws against prostitution, homosexuality, and other "deviant" forms of sex seem consistent with this myth. However, it is Foucault's contention that there has rather been a vast proliferation of discourse on sex for the last 200 years. On a personal level there may be some suppression of sex discourse, but on the level of scientific and social scientific study there has been an explosion of it, almost a compulsion to discuss sex:

> It may well be true that adults and children themselves were deprived of a certain way of speaking about sex ... as being too direct, crude, or coarse. But this was only the counterpart of other discourses ... discourses that were interlocking, hierarchized, and all highly articulated around a cluster of power relations.
>
> —*Foucault, 1976/1990a, p. 30*

It is the scientific, social scientific (but also political and legal) discourses of sex that have socially constructed the knowledge we have of sex today. This discourse in a sense "invented" the homosexual—although this claim is often overinterpreted and overstated by both Foucault's critics and his followers. He compares our concept of homosexuality to that of the ancient world and the Medieval and early modern world. Before this post-Victorian explosion of discourse on sexuality, there were of course people who engaged in homosexual activity, but it was not until the late 19th century that people became defined as this or that type of sexual being. Defining a class of beings as homosexuals had both positive and negative consequences for those identified in that class. On the one hand, this classification provided a label, a simultaneous concrete and conceptual target for oppression and marginalization. On the other hand, more positively, this identification provided a seemingly coherent, cohesive definition of self to draw on in seeking liberation. There cannot be "gay rights" or a gay rights movement without social identification and recognition of "gays" as a class themselves.

In Foucault's first major work, *Madness and Civilization*, he develops a powerful criticism of psychology, psychiatry, and the presumptions of modern concepts of mental illness. Modern views of psychology and psychiatry see the developments of these practices as civilizing and humanizing as compared to how the mentally ill were treated in the premodern world: merely shut away, shunned, or tortured. But Foucault argued that the truths and treatments of modern psychology and psychiatry are largely social constructions and not discoveries of natural causes and kinds. The concept of madness becomes a subtle means of social control to perpetuate conventional morality. He makes a thematically similar argument in the later *Discipline and Punish* (1975/1995) but in a more general manner about modern society and politics. It is often presumed that the modern world provides us with greater personal and political freedom than political and social structures of the past. But, Foucault argues, we are just as under the control of power in the modern world. That power simply operates in a more subtle manner. He uses the metaphor of a prison design by 18th century philosopher Jeremy Bentham called the panopticon. The panopticon is a circular or semicircular prison design in which a guard tower is at the hub and cells are placed along the spokes. Pictured is Bentham's original design (Figure 14.1).

The guard tower in the middle radiates light. This allows the guards to see the prisoners but does not allow the prisoners to see the guards. The prisoners know the guard tower is there but because of the light they can never know at any particular time that the guard is looking at them. Thus, they always have to behave. Eventually, this good behavior becomes part of the character of the prisoner and prison becomes a form of rehabilitation, not mere punishment. Foucault claims that all of modern society is like this. We think that we are free but indeed we are being watched and controlled in this manner in a variety of ways by governmental forces. The proliferation of security cameras, metal detectors, and other countless means of observation in our society lend

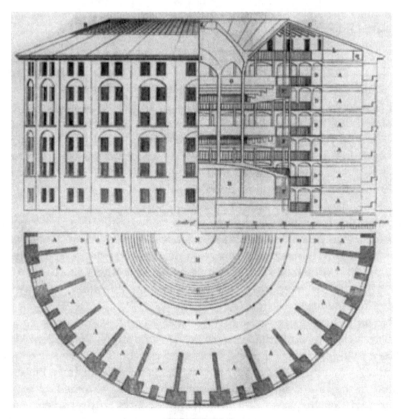

FIGURE 14.1
Jeremy Bentham's Panopticon Design. (Crime and punishment, 2009)

support to Foucault's arguments. The government collects information on us in a variety of ways. In a health care context public health authorities gather information about the health of individuals and communities. Social workers operate as arms of the state to surveil women and those of lower socioeconomic classes in order to ensure the adherence to accepted social and family values.

Foucault and postmodernism in general have been criticized for encouraging epistemic and ethical relativism, which, critics say, may lead to the justification of horrific systems and acts. If there is no truth (epistemic, political, or moral), if there is no one right system to be found tyranny may be seen as good as democracy. A related, more specific charge often leveled at Foucault is that of political quietism. If we are forever enmeshed in power relations and no matter what we do we cannot escape, what is the point of doing anything, particularly of trying to fight for political liberation? On the surface, this seems like a reasonable charge. What makes it ironic, though, is the reputation Foucault had during his lifetime for political activism. Foucault's stated defense to this charge is that his point "is not that everything is bad, but that everything is dangerous" (1982, p. 232). There is no perfect system, no perfect theory, and no perfect freedom. We need to continually fight and work to attain as much freedom as possible, because, though we are enmeshed in this matrix of power relations, we too are nodes in this matrix and thus sources of power as well. So his theory, rather than political quietism, leads, he argues, to a continuing political activism.

A similar criticism of postmodernism, alluded to before, is that it is completely critical and provides no positive notions of self, knowledge, or reality. Late in his career Foucault attempted to develop a more positive philosophy based upon a concept of aesthetics of existence. "By resisting the forces that created us (our selves, our consciousness, our souls, if you will) and forming and re-forming who we are we employ a type of aesthetic freedom and life itself becomes a creative act, a creative, artistic, subjective, aesthetic act" (Dahnke, 2007, p. 110). Through acts of transgression and self-transformation we do not seek to conform to some preconceived theory of what we should be as humans or individuals or human subjects but seek to make our life "into an *oeuvre*" (Foucault, 1984/1990b, p. 10). Unfortunately, Foucault died before he fully developed this line of thought.

CONCLUSION

This chapter does not of course exhaust the philosophical approaches to social science. It is merely introductory in that regard and introductory regarding the various approaches addressed here. There is much more to be studied for each of these and students are encouraged to pursue any of these they find particularly interesting.

This chapter closes this section on the philosophy of science. We are perhaps left with more questions than answers. Such is the nature of philosophy. Does this mean that there are no answers to these questions or that we need to study further to find these answers? That is a question each student has to answer on his own. Our hope is that you will accept the latter answer and the puzzles, problems, and questions presented here will inform your later studies and practice. Perhaps we might think of ourselves in a similar position as is presented at the end of the *Euthyphro*. And we have to ask, are we going to be like Euthyphro and run off in the face of uncertainty, or like Socrates in moving forward in inquiry and investigation?

CRITICAL THINKING QUESTIONS

1. Are humans rational in the sense rational choice theory assumes? What evidence can you provide for your answer?
2. Is the sense of rationality presumed by rational choice theory normative or is it merely descriptive?
3. Is real life, as John von Neumann asserts, like the games in game theory?
4. Formulate a functional explanation for nursing that identifies both manifest and latent functions.
5. What is the "hermeneutic circle"? How do we deal with the problem that circle presents?
6. According to phenomenologists, what is the difference between mere perception and phenomenal experience?
7. Should social science be "emancipatory," as critical theorists contend?
8. Should natural science be "emancipatory"?
9. What does Foucault mean by the "death of man"? What significance does this concept have for social science?
10. Do we live in a disciplinary society, as Foucault avers? Are we freer in our being and actions than he suggests?

REFERENCES

Adorno, T. W. (1998). *Critical models: Interventions and catchwords* (H. W. Pickford, Trans.). New York, NY: Columbia University Press. (Original work published in 1969)

Adorno, T. W. (2000). *Introduction to sociology* (C. Gödde Ed. & E. Jephcott, Trans.). Stanford, CA: Stanford University Press (Original work published in 1993)

Bentham, J. (2000). *An introduction to the principles of morals and legislation.* Kitchener, Ontario: Batoche.

Bishop, R. C. (2007). *The philosophy of the social sciences: An introduction.* New York, NY: Continuum International Publishing Group.

Collingwood, R. G. (1946). *The idea of history.* Oxford, UK: Clarendon Press.

Crime and Punishment in 18th and 19th Century England. (2009). Retrieved April 2, 2010, from http://www.deakin.edu.au/alfreddeakin/spc/exhibitions/candp/candp.php.

Dahnke, M. D. (2007). *Film, art, and filmart: An introduction to aesthetics through film.* Lanham, MD: University Press of America.

Elster, J. (1994). Functional explanation: In social science. In M. Martin, & L. C. McIntyre (Eds.), *Readings in the philosophy of social science* (pp. 403–414). Cambridge, MA: The MIT Press. (Original work published in 1983)

Foucault, M. (1972). *The archaeology of knowledge & the discourse on language* (A. M. Sheridan Smith, Trans.). New York, NY: Pantheon Books. (Original work published in 1971)

Foucault, M. (1980). Truth and power (A. Fontana, & P. Pasquino, Trans.). In C. Gordon (Ed.), *Power/knowledge: Selected interviews & other writings, 1972–1977* (pp. 109–133). New York, NY: Pantheon Books. (Original work published in 1977)

Foucault, M. (1982). The subject and power. In H. Dreyfus, & P. Rabinow (Eds.), *Michel Foucault: Beyond structuralism and hermeneutics* (pp. 208–228). Chicago, IL: Chicago University Press.

Foucault, M. (1990a). *The history of sexuality: An introduction (Vol. I)* (R. Hurley, Trans.). New York, NY: Vintage Books. (Original work published in 1976)

Foucault, M. (1990b). *The use of pleasure: Volume 2 of the history of sexuality* (R. Hurley, Trans.). New York, NY: Vintage Books. (Original work published in 1984)

Foucault, M. (1994). *The order of things: An archaeology of the human sciences.* New York, NY: Vintage Books. (Original work published in 1966)

Foucault, M. (1995). *Discipline and punish: The birth of the prison* (A. Sheridan, Trans.). New York, NY: Vintage Books. (Original work published in 1975)

Gadamer, H. G. (2004). *Truth and method* (J. Weinseimer, Trans.). London: Continuum Books. (Original work published in 1975)

Habermas, J. (1988). *On the logic of the social sciences* (S. W. Nicholson, & J. A. Stark, Trans.). Cambridge, MA: The MIT Press. (Original work published in 1970)

Hammond, M., Howarth, J., & Keat, R. (1991). *Understanding phenomenology.* Oxford, UK: Blackwell Publishers.

Held, D. (1980). *Introduction to critical theory: Horkheimer to Habermas.* Berkeley, CA: University of California Press.

Hempel, C. G. (1994). The logic of functional explanation. In M. Martin, & L. C. McIntyre (Eds.), *Readings in the philosophy of social science* (pp. 349–375). Cambridge, MA: The MIT Press. (Original work published in 1959)

Husserl, E. (1931). *Ideas: General introduction to pure phenomenology* (W. R. Boyce Gibson, Trans.). New York, NY: Humanities Press Inc. (Original work published in 1913)

Husserl, E. (1977). *Cartesian meditations: An introduction to phenomenology* (D. Cairns, Trans.). The Hague: Martinus Nijhoff Publishers. (Original work published in 1950)

Kincaid, H. (1994). Assessing functional explanations in the social sciences. In M. Martin, & L. C. McIntyre (Eds.), *Readings in the philosophy of social science* (pp. 415–428). Cambridge, MA: The MIT Press.

Lehrer, J. (2009). *How we decide.* Boston, MA: Houghton Mifflin Harcourt.

Levinas, E. (1969). *Totality and Infinity* (A. Lingis, Trans.). Pittsburgh, PA: Duquesne University Press. (Original work published in 1961)

Lyotard, J. F. (1984). *The postmodern condition: A report on knowledge* (G. Bennington, & B. Massumi, Trans.). Minneapolis, MN: University of Minnesota Press. (Original work published in 1979)

Marcuse, H. (1964). *One-dimensional man: Studies in the ideology of advanced industrial society.* Boston, MA: Beacon Press.

Merleau-Ponty, M. (1962). *Phenomenology of perception* (C. Smith, Trans.). New York, NY: Routledge. (Original work published in 1945)

Merton, R. K. (1968). *Social theory and social structure.* New York, NY: The Free Press.

Merton, R. K. (1973). *The sociology of science: Theoretical and empirical investigations.* Chicago, IL: The University of Chicago Press.

Merton, R. K. (1996). *On social structure and science.* Chicago, IL: The University of Chicago Press.

Nagel, T. (1986). *The view from nowhere.* Oxford, UK: Oxford University Press.

Natanson, M. (1973). Phenomenology and the social sciences. In M. Natanson (Ed.), *Phenomenology and the social sciences* (Vol. 1) (pp. 3–44). Evanston, IL: Northwestern University Press.

Oosterbeek, H., Sloof, R., & van de Kuilen, G. (2004). Cultural differences in ultimatum game experiments: Evidence from a meta-analysis. *Experimental Economics, 7*(2), 171–188.

Poundstone, W. (1992). *Prisoner's dilemma: John von Neumann, game theory, and the puzzle of the bomb.* New York, NY: Doubleday.

Ricoeur, P. (1981). *Hermeneutics and the human sciences: Essays on language, action and interpretation* (J. B. Thompson, Trans.). Cambridge: Cambridge University Press.

Rosenberg, A. (2008). *Philosophy of social science*. Boulder, CO: Westview Press.

Ruffle, B. J. (1998). More is better, but fair is fair: Tipping in dictator and ultimatum games. *Games and Economic Behavior, 2*(23), 247–265.

Schutz, A. (1967). *The phenomenology of the social world* (G. Walsh, & F. Lehnert, Trans.). Evanston, IL: Northwestern University Press. (Original work published in 1960)

Sedgwick, E. K. (1990). *Epistemology of the closet*. Berkeley, CA: University of California Press.

Szenberg, M., Ramrattan, L., & Gottesman, A. A. (Eds.) (2006). *Samuelsonian economics and the 21st century*. Oxford, UK: Oxford University Press.

Toombs, S. K. (2001). Introduction: Phenomenology and medicine. In S. K. Toombs (Ed.), *Handbook of phenomenology and medicine* (pp. 1–26). Dordrecht, Boston: Kluwer Academic Publishers.

Varian, H. R. (2006). Revealed preference. In M. Szenberg, L. Ramrattan, & A. A. Gottesman (Eds.), *Samuelsonian economics and the 21st century* (pp. 99–115). Oxford, UK: Oxford University Press.

Von Neumann, J., & Morgenstern, O. (2007). *Theory of games and economic behavior*. Princeton, NJ: Princeton University Press.

Weber, M. (1978). *Economy and society*. In G. Roth, & C. Wittich (Eds.). Berkeley, CA: University of California Press. (Original work published in 1956)

15

The Path to Nursing Science Today, 1910–2010

Nursing education is undergoing drastic changes.
ANNIE W. GOODRICH (1936)

INTRODUCTION

In this chapter, we will attempt to frame at least a rudimentary picture of how nursing science has evolved in the last 100 years and pose questions for classroom discussion about an evolving discipline. We will frame these developments in the nursing profession in a very unique way by also placing them into their historical context. Events shape history. We hope this will help the reader better evaluate nursing's disciplinary developments as they were impacted by events in contemporary society. For five years, the first author of this text (a philosophy professor) has taught *Nurs 700: Philosophy of Natural and Social Science: Foundations for Inquiry into the Discipline of Nursing*[1] in the first quarter of our doctor of nursing practice curriculum. For the last meeting of this course each quarter, the second author of this text (a nursing professor) has joined the class to help cofacilitate the following question: *Now that you have learned some basic principles of philosophy of science, do you think nursing is a science?* It has been an enormously effective critical thinking exercise and very popular with the first quarter doctoral students. However, the question is posed, not because the students have had content in nursing epistemology (actually they have not), but because now they have been exposed to the principles related to the question of *what is science?* This allows them at least to ponder the question and have some informed (but certainly preliminary) discussions about the legitimacy of the scientific underpinnings of the nursing discipline and to explore the extent to which nursing is a science. In many ways, we have written this text with the introductory and concluding chapters on the discipline of nursing to enhance this discussion.

Because we estimate only 25% of current doctor of nursing practice curricula have explicit content on nursing epistemology, in Chapter 16 we will at least tie this content to an emerging practice epistemology for nursing—a discussion of possible next steps

---

[1]We have included our 5-year philosophy of science syllabus in Appendix A. We have also adapted the syllabus using this new published text in Appendix B for both semester and quarter system use.

toward practice knowledge development. Reed calls this the "practice turn in nursing epistemology," but Reed does not necessarily tie this turn to the contemporary practice doctorate movement (2006, p. 36). We will, however, attempt to do this. This chapter concludes with a description of how our final critical thinking module exercise is conducted. We encourage faculty using this text to consider this a pedagogical exercise. We have identified three primary articles we have employed in the last 5 years. They are used not because they are necessarily the most current (alas they are not), but because over time they have been very instructive at differentiating the debate and discourse among students and faculty when asking—*is this article nursing science?* Course faculty are free to choose different articles and still employ the same pedagogical techniques and questions. Alternatively, you may want to use these three articles as an example of the exercise and then add three new ones so the student and faculty generated questions and commentary (the most important!) are fresh.

A 100-YEAR HISTORY OF NURSING SCIENCE: WHAT WAS BEING PUBLISHED?

The Nursing Field Circa 1910

In order to best appreciate where we are in 2010, we begin our roughly 100 year retrospective with a period around 1910 which nurse historian Patricia Donahue terms "the era of the rise of organized nursing" (1996, p. 318). Ten years after the turn of the century, William Howard Taft was the 27th President[2] of the United States What was American life like in 1910?

> The average life expectancy in the U.S. was 47 years. Only 14 percent of the homes in the U.S. had a bathtub. Only 8 percent of the homes had a telephone and a three-minute call from Denver to New York City cost eleven dollars. There were only 8,000 cars in the U.S., and only 144 miles of paved roads. The maximum speed limit in most cities was 10 mph. Alabama, Mississippi, Iowa, and Tennessee were each more heavily populated than California. With a mere 1.4 million people, California was only the 21st most populous state in the Union. The tallest structure in the world was the Eiffel Tower! The average wage in the U.S. was 22 cents per hour. The average U.S. worker made between $200 and $400 per year. A competent accountant could expect to earn $2000 per year, a dentist $2,500 per year, a veterinarian between $1,500 and $4,000 per year, and a mechanical engineer about $5,000 per year. More than 95 percent of all births in the U.S. took place at home. Ninety-percent of all U.S. doctors had no college education. Instead, they attended so-called medical schools, many of which were condemned in the press and by the government as "substandard."[3]

The developments in nursing at this time, which included the 1910 timeline of accomplishments mentioned in Chapter 2, would culminate with and then initiate the rise of nursing as a profession in the United States. As Donohue (1996) and others have noted "nursing has made its greatest advances and notable achievements in connections with wars" (p. 352) and WW1 broke out in June 1914 in Sarajevo, Serbia

---

[2]William Howard Taft (b. 1857, d. 1930), a Republican, was defeated after one term in 1912. He later served as the 10th Chief Justice of the United States and is the only person to have served in both offices (Bromley, 2003).

[3]These 1910 statistics have been pooled from a number of open-source citations.

TABLE 15.1
Table of Contents April 1910, *10* (7) *American Journal of Nursing*

Editorial Comment

The Confusion of Existing Conditions—Sophia F. Palmer, Editor-in-Chief

Articles

The Moral Influence of Superintendents and Head Nurses Elisabeth Robinson Scovil

Hook-Worm Disease—Harriet B. Gibson

An Obstetrical Case at Home—Jennie M. Putnam

A High Caloric Diet in Typhoid—Mary E. Thornton

Suggestions for What is Required in Building a Nurses' Home—Agnes S. Ward

Diet Lists for Obstetrical Patients—F. Christie & V. Jessie

Nursing in Mission Stations

Foreign Department—Lavinia L. Dock

Department of Visiting Nursing & Social Welfare—Harriet Fulmer & Mabel Jacques

Letters to the Editor

Entertainment for Sick Children

Private Duty for Pupil Nurses

"The Ideal Nurse"

Operations on Male Patients

Better Nursing for Children in Public Orphanages

A Successful Central Registry

Private Duty Problems

A Prayer for Nurses

when the archduke of Austria and his wife were killed (Gavin, 1997; Higonnet, Jenson, Michel, & Weitz, 1987). Nevertheless, just after the turn of the century nursing was very difficult work and wages were variable. The average salary was about $1,000–$1,500, although some private duty nurses took work at whatever price they could get (Sussman, 1999; Wickwire, 1937).

The *American Journal of Nursing* (*AJN*), founded in 1900 with Sophia F. Palmer[4] as its first editor, was the leading nursing journal at that time and still continues today (Mason, 1999). Here is the table of contents from April 1910 Volume 10, Issue 7. By examining the journal articles (see Table 15.1), what kinds of assumptions about nursing and the nursing discipline might you make?

The following excerpt is from the 1910 editorial comment:

No group of educators and workers has been more subjected to criticism than the teachers and graduates of schools of nursing. Some of it is undoubtedly sincere, much of it suggestive and helpful, but a great deal comes from those who see in the movement for higher education for nurses the cutting off of a means of revenue which threatens to destroy

---

[4]This book's second author had never heard of Sophia Palmer until research for this text. Her death on April 27, 1920 at the age of 67 due to a severe cerebral hemorrhage and the rather fascinating details of her life were published in an April 1920 editorial in *AJN* (Volume 2, No. 7) in just over three pages. The idea for state registration of nurses was first proposed by Miss Palmer.

their business. Such criticisms are especially prominent in commercial magazines, and are made by those connected with short-course and correspondence schools and by the proprietors of hospitals who have found in the maintaining of a training school without standards a means of increasing the dividends on their investments, or by ill-trained physicians who fear a competitor in the competent nurse.[5]

—Palmer, 1910, pp. 451–452

What we find most interesting about this early issue of *AJN* is that already we have evidence of one of the earliest iterations of *practice inquiry* which has reawakened in a new framework in the nursing literature almost 100 years later by nursing scholars at the University of Washington, one of the leading Schools of Nursing in the United States (Magyary, Whitney, & Brown, 2006). Thorton's article on typhoid is a representative example. Typhoid fever was still a serious illness in 1910. It was an acute, life-threatening bacterial illness contracted by ingesting contaminated water or food. It was one of the most serious health problems in the 19th-century and early 20th-century America particularly because the universal water supply in America was not adequately filtered and safe (Gaspari & Wolf, 1985). With an estimated population of 22,573,435 in the United States in 1910, there were 4,637 recorded deaths (there were likely many more undocumented) or a death rate of 20.54 per 100,000 from typhoid (*American Journal of Public Health*, 1940).[6] Walton and Connelly (2005) describe the very expert care by trained nurses in the care of children with typhoid at the Children's Hospital of Philadelphia between 1895 and 1910. They conclude "Then, as now, expert nursing care and collaboration with medical colleagues ensured optimal outcomes. A better understanding of the historic importance of the professional bedside nurse may improve our ability to attract and retain nurses—so important today" (p. 74). These comments may also be apropos today as we prepare for a more highly educated advanced practice nurse workforce. Finally, these early writings also indicate that nurses were inquisitive and sought answers to the nursing and health issues of the day. Most importantly, by publishing their work so others might benefit, they were demonstrating scholarly inquiry and a commitment to the improvement of the field of nursing.

Nursing: A "Field" Technically Becomes A "Profession" Circa 1935

Some 25 years later in 1935, America was slowly emerging from the ravages of the 1929–1933 depression (Friedman, 2008). Despite the election of Franklin Delano Roosevelt in 1933 and the first real economic plans to defeat the depression (e.g., the 1935 Social Security Act), the aftereffects would last until the end of WWII (Goodwin, 1995). In 1935, American nursing also found itself ramping up for WWII. Japan invaded Manchuria in 1931[7] and China later in 1937, and WWII exploded with the German invasion of Poland in September 1939 (Maddox, 1992). The United

---

[5]Palmer, S. (1910). The confusion of existing conditions. *American Journal of Nursing, 10*(7), 451–452. Reprinted with permission by Wolters Kluwer Health.

[6]By 1939, with a larger population of 37,112,665, the death rate from typhoid had plunged to 0.65 (*American Journal of Public Health*, 1940).

[7]Since health research must be funded by some source in order for a health professions discipline to mature, it should be noted that the National Institutes of Health (NIH) was created in 1931.

States would join WWII with the bombing of Pearl Harbor in December 1941. The national unemployment rate was 20.1%; among nurses (graduate, registered, and licensed), it was not until 1937 that nurses (those fortunate to be employed) would be relieved from working 12 hours a day and up to 70 hours per week to working only 8 hours a day and limited to 6 days a week (Byers, 1999; Kangas, 1997). This was the landscape that American nursing found itself in 1935.

In 1934, the final report by the grading committee *Nursing Schools Today and Tomorrow* was published and it reported on the state of nursing and nursing schools in the United States at the time (*AJN*, 1934).[8] In describing findings from the document, Goodrich[9] later wrote:

> It is not necessary to discuss in detail the defects revealed in the present system of nursing education. The number of schools still existing, approximately 1,500, is suggestive of the situation, without the very definite evidence of inadequate instruction, inadequate clinical experience, and hours of physical and mental output generally conceded as detrimental to health—in short, an educational interpretation out of step with present-day social conditions, educational methods, and scientific conclusions.[10]
>
> —*Goodrich, 1936, p. 766*

Goodrich further indicated that the League of Nursing Education in 1934 identified only 136 schools of nursing that were fully connected with universities, although many others (particularly Catholic affiliated schools) had very loose connections [to colleges or universities] that she criticized as "but in name" (p. 767) only. She also envisioned the "field of nursing" (p. 768) moving quickly away from the outmoded classification of nursing as private duty, institutional, and public health nursing and more toward specialization in, for example, pediatrics and obstetrics (1936).

On October 7, 1935, in a memo written by Harry L. Hopkins of the federal Work Progress Administration (WPA), nurses were reclassified from "skilled nonmanual workers" to "Class 4 professional and technical workers" (*AJN*, 1935). While nursing leaders had been working behind the scenes for years to accomplish this, this federal reclassification elevated the status of nursing and made nurses eligible for many federal WPA health projects (Lusk, 1997). In many ways, this important date has been lost in history, but it remains a landmark in the quest for nursing to be fully recognized as a profession, independent and away from the oppression of medicine. Among the most vocal and visible advocates for nursing at this time were two of nursing's most important pioneers of the 20th century—Lavinia Lloyd Dock[11] and Isabel

---

[8]This influential report was preceded by the landmark Goldmark Report of 1921 that became the first national survey of the nursing profession in the United States and which made the first national policy suggestions for the improvement of nursing education.

[9]Annie W. Goodrich, R. N., D.Sc. was the founding Dean of the Yale School of Nursing in 1923, the first independent university-based School of Nursing. It was established with funding from the Rockefeller Foundation.

[10]Goodrich, A. A. (1936). Modern trends in nursing education. *American Journal of Public Health, 26,* 764–770. Reprinted with permission by the American Journal of Public Health Association.

[11]Lavinia L. Dock's (b. 1858, d. 1956) impressive contributions to nursing are too numerous to cover in this text. But one notable accomplishment is that in 1899 she cofounded the International Council of Nurses (ICN) with an English nurse, Ethel Gordon Fenwick. An excellent dissertation of her life and social activism was written in 2002 by Soledad Smith.

M. Stewart.[12] In a confrontational way, almost unheard of due to the social mores still expected of women in the 1930s, they both wrote that nursing is not:

> ... a subordinate or 'satellite' vocation ... nursing is as old if not older than medicine and has had an independent existence for hundreds of years ... nursing was not that of a sub-caste of medicine or a 'handmaid of medicine'
>
> *—Dock and Stewart, 1938, p. 365–366*

They both further stated that:

> "... nursing flourishes best when it is directed and controlled by skilled and experienced nurses and given the largest possible measure of freedom for the exercise of its particular functions"
>
> *—Dock and Stewart, 1938, p. 367*

With a general worldview of the events of and around 1935, we examined the February 1935 issue of the *AJN—still* considered the leading journal for American nursing in this period (see Table 15.2). What kinds of topics were covered in comparison to the previous 1910 issue?

One observation we made is that there does not appear to be any significant movement to publishing research studies, which in many ways is further evidence that nursing was still a maturing field, and not yet a discipline. This will be discussed forthright in this chapter. In 1935, the Association of Collegiate Schools of Nursing was founded with a mission to promote nursing education in the collegiate/university environment and away from the hospital-based programs (Williams, 1945). The principle aims of this new organization were (1) to develop nursing education on a professional and collegiate level; (2) to promote and strengthen relationships between schools of nursing and institutions of higher education; and (3) to promote study and experimentation in nursing service and nursing education (Goodrich, 1936). This may have been the first highly visible policy record to encourage nursing research. You can see for yourself whether the research goals of nursing in 1935, "To promote study and experimentation in nursing service and nursing education" (Goodrich, p. 767) are the same or different today.

On the Precipice of a "Discipline" and the Rise of Modern Nursing Circa 1960

Twenty-five years since 1935, America was about to undergo a decade of immense, significant social change. On November 8, 1960 John F. Kennedy[13] was elected at age 43 as the youngest President in a very narrow election. The Vietnam War, unlike previous

---

[12]Isabel M. Stewart (b. 1878, d. 1963) was a 1902 graduate of Winnipeg General Hospital (WGH) Training School for Nurses in Canada. In 1913 she became the first nurse to receive a masters degree from Teacher's College, Columbia University. She became assistant professor there in 1917 and succeeded Dr. Adelaide Nutting as chair. She was a prolific writer, authoring several books on nursing history and education, 123 articles and 20 monographs. She was the driving force behind the preparation of the 1917, 1927, and 1937 NLN curriculum guides (Winnipeg General Hospital/Health Sciences Centre Nursing Alumnae Association Archives, 2001).

[13]John F. Kennedy (b. 1917, d. 1963) was the 35th President of the United States, serving from 1961 until his assassination on November 22, 1963. He was also the first Catholic to serve as President (Dallek, 2003).

TABLE 15.2
Table of Contents February 1935, *35*(2) *American Journal of Nursing*

Editorial Comment

Who Should Hold Office?

No Stars?

Department of Nursing Education

A Tentative Program for Curriculum Reconstruction—Isabel M. Stewart

Let us Look at Our Clinical Services—Blanche Pferfferkorn & Claribel E. Wheeler

Articles

What Registries Are Doing: Seventy-Four Registrar's Report for November 1934

Department of Red Cross Nursing—Clara D. Noyes

Notes from Headquarters American Nurses' Association

Student Nurses' Page: Residual Paralysis Following Poliomyelitis—Gwen Barnett

What Equipment Should a Student Bring to Her School?—Helen John

The Open Forum

The "New" Journal—K.D., W.

The Florence Nightingale Memorial—Jessie Shaw Coman

Joy and Psychiatric Nursing—J. P., W.

A Study Club—M.S.R., N.

Private Duty Records—R., N.

Pertinent Questions—Ella Best

Improvised Equipment—L.E., Y.

Warning—T.C. Edwards

In a Mental Hospital—Zella Nicholas

Journals Wanted—

International Nursing Review Wanted

wars, had no definitive beginning, but the United States gradually began its involvement between 1950 and 1965 and America's involvement escalated further during the early Kennedy administration (Rotter, 1999). Some 7,484 women (6,250 or 83.5% were nurses) served in Vietnam and eight nurses died in that war, including one killed in action (Veterans Administration, 2010). While nurses, such as Margaret Sanger[14] and her sister Ethel Byrne, were involved in the earliest movements to support birth control and the rights of women, it would not be until 1965 that the Supreme Court would finally legalize birth control in all 50 states (Hampton, 2004; Reed, 1978; Sanger Katz, Hajo, & Engelman, 2002).

---

[14]Margaret Higgins Sanger Slee (b. 1879, d. 1966) was a trained nurse, feminist, and social activist and founded the American Birth Control League in 1921 (Sanger et al., 2002).

In 1960, it was estimated that only 55.4% of the trained nurses were actually employed (approximately 504,000),[15] and it was surmised that a large number of qualified nurses were therefore married and actively not seeking employment (Cleland, 1967; U.S. Dept of Health, Education, & Welfare, 1970). At this time, it was generally assumed that new professionals [nurses] who invested in professional education and training would remain an active part of the workforce (Bishop, 1970). But these labor statistics indicated something very different for nursing. These qualified, but electively unemployed nurses were actually exacerbating the nursing shortage of the day (Fagin, 1980). But was perhaps marital status not the only factor contributing to trained nurses forgoing full-time employment? Certainly the working conditions of nurses described in 1935 had improved, but evidence suggests not by much (Budd, Warino, & Patton, 2004). Further, the average annual salary for a general duty, hospital-based nurse reported in 1961 was $3,380/year in Atlanta and $4,628 in Los Angeles accounting for regional differences (*AJN*, 1961). It is, however, in this chaotic social climate of nursing in the 60s, that the profession began to modernize itself.

Just about a decade before 1960, this unsigned editorial appeared in the *American Journal of Nursing*:

> One of the most serious handicaps to effective research in nursing . . . has been our failure to make definite plans for scientific investigation. The nursing profession has made no concerted effort to promote, support, direct, or evaluate research in nursing and there has been no central clearing house for exchange of information.[16]
>
> *—1949, p. 743*

Three years later, in 1952, the nursing profession had its first research journal— *Nursing Research*—under the inaugural editorship of Dr. Helen L. Bunge[17] (Notter, 1970). The first issue's main article was a very sophisticated and meticulous report

---

[15]Comparatively, according to 2009 U.S. Dept. of Labor Bureau of Labor Statistics, RNs constituted the largest health-care occupation, with 2.6 million jobs and about 60% of RN jobs in hospitals.

[16]American Journal of Nursing. (1949). Nursing Research [unsigned editorial]. *American Journal of Nursing, 49*(12), 743–744. Reprinted with permission by Wolters Kluwer Health.

[17]Dr. Helen L. Bunge (b. 1906, d. 1970) was Dean of the Frances Payne Bolton School of Nursing of Western Reserve University (founded in 1923) from 1946 to 1953 and Dean of the University of Wisconsin–Madison School of Nursing (founded in 1924) from 1959 to 1969. Signe Cooper, MEd, RN, FAAN, Professor Emeritus at Wisconsin (also a AAN Living Legend) who worked for Dr. Bunge has written: "Although Helen Bunge's contributions to nursing research were often underappreciated, they were recognized by her being named posthumously to the Nursing Hall of Fame in 1984. At that time she was recognized as one 'who contributed significantly to the promotion of research in nursing.' She believed that research was essential to move the profession forward and that nurses must be involved in the systematic study of clinical nursing. As a dean, she encouraged research efforts by her faculty, and her own involvement in nursing research verified her belief in its importance. The periodical *Nursing Research* was proposed by the Committee on Research of the American Association of Collegiate Schools of Nursing, chaired by Helen Bunge. When the publication was undertaken by the American Journal of Nursing Company, she was invited to chair the editorial board, becoming the volunteer editor, a position she held from 1952–1957" (personal communication March 26, 2010).

(23 pages) titled *"The Personal Adjustment of Chronically Ill Old People Under Home Care,"* and was a summary of the PhD dissertation of Margery J. Mack from the University of Chicago in 1951 (1952). The journal was initially an enterprise of the American Journal of Nursing Company and struggled financially for many years. After 10 years of publication, Bunge (1962) reflected on the journal's first decade and made a couple of assessments: (1) "the scarcity and sometimes paucity of manuscripts suitable for publication" (p. 137); (2) "many more manuscripts from the area of psychiatric nursing are submitted than manuscripts from other clinical fields"[18] (p. 137); and (3) persistent questions over who should be the journal's audience, writing "Shall it aim to appeal to students, to persons engaged in and sophisticated in research, or to persons comparatively unknowledgeable in research?" (p. 137).

Nevertheless, returning to 1960, we have earlier detailed in Chapter 2 how many modern developments in nursing took place as the decade of the 60s progressed. But in 1960, nursing appeared to still be on the precipice of a discipline. Only one doctoral nursing program, a PhD in Nursing at the University of Pittsburgh in 1954, had been added since 1935, and by the end of the 1950s only 39 doctoral degrees in nursing had been awarded (Nichols & Chitty, 2005; Parietti, 1990). Since the conduct of research in any discipline requires financial resources, without a source of funding nursing could not advance its scientific basis. One major development during this era was the founding of a research and fellowship branch in 1955 within the federal Division of Nursing Resources (founded in 1948), with the first applications received, reviewed, and first federal grants for nursing research awarded that fall (Gortner, 1986; Gortner & Nahm, 1977; Stevenson, 1987). The year 1960 also pre-dated the majority of the early nursing theorists; although Dr. Faye Abdellah[19] and colleagues published *Patient-centered Approaches to Nursing* that year and Abdellah's very influential list of "21 nursing problems" were described (Abdellah, Beland, Martin, & Matheney, 1960). An examination of the published titles in the Fall 1960 issue of *Nursing Research* in Table 15.3 reveals what new trends from 1935?

With a new research journal in the field of nursing, it is interesting to note that these were the featured articles some eight years into the journals history. Bunge's (1962) earlier comment about the problem with publishing nonresearch articles in a *research journal* is evident here. There was great debate on the editorial board about this, but remember that there was still a dearth of qualified submissions in the early days of the journal, is evident here. Nevertheless, the idea that nurses could be scholars, conduct experimental research, have scholarly discourse, and critique another's published work, are clearly advances for the scientific development and maturation of a slowly emerging discipline. Nursing appears to be at nexus here in 1960— perhaps no longer just a field, but not quite a fully fledged discipline.

---

[18]This may be partly due to the significant influence of Hildegard Peplau's work and book *Interpersonal Relations in Nursing* and its impact on psychiatric nursing (1952).

[19]Faye Abdellah, RN, Ed.D., Sc.D., FAAN (b. 1919) was the first Deputy Surgeon General of the U.S. Public Health Service.

TABLE 15.3
Table of Contents Fall 1960, *9* (4) *Nursing Research*

Editorial

U.S. P. H. S. Division of Nursing

ANA Conference on Research

Articles

Myocardial Infarction: Stages of Recovery and Nursing Care— Harriet M. Coston

Discussion of Paper Presented by Harriet Coston—Rena Boyle

Nursing Needs of Chronically Ill Ambulatory Patients—Doris Schwartz

Discussion of the Paper Presented by Doris Schwartz—Louise C. Smith

The National League for Nursing—Its Role in Research

The International Seminar in Delhi—Rena E. Boyle

Comparative Ratings of Medical and Surgical Nurses—Edith M. Lentz & Robert G. Michaels

Experimental Design in Nursing Research—Eugene Levine

Published Research Reports

Published Research Reports

Research Reporter

Tracking Down Lost Patients

Community Nursing Services for Discharged Psychiatric Patients

The Psychiatric Nurse as Ward Therapist

An Evaluation and Study of Faculty Research Potential

The Role of the Nurse in the Preventive Services of a Student Health Service

The Role of the Nurse in the Follow-up of Children From a Psychiatric Service

Uninterrupted Patient Care and Nursing Requirements

Status of Prediction Studies in Nursing

Essentials for Public Health Field Experience

The Scientific Discipline of Nursing Emerges Circa 1985

The 25-year span of nursing between 1960 and 1985 represented nursing's definitive emergence as a discipline, even if there are retrospective analyses that question the overall contribution the voluminous early nursing theorists have made to the science of nursing today. The trajectory of what took place during the modern era of nursing (1960–1985) is far too extensive to cover in this chapter, but some important landmarks in nursing did occur that set nursing on a different course. In January of 1985, Ronald Reagan[20] began his second term as President. In his first term, he slowly guided the country out of a short, but severe recession that lasted from 1981 to 1982 with a peak unemployment rate of 10.8% in November–December 1982

---

[20]Ronald Wilson Reagan (b. 1911, d. 2004) was the 40th President of the United States and served two terms 1981–1989.

(Bandyk, 2009).[21] Reagan's second term had more emphasis on foreign affairs and included the end of the Cold War, the bombing of Libya, and the Iran-Contra Affair. With the AIDS epidemic beginning in 1981, Reagan was criticized for being slow to respond to the epidemic at the federal level and for not mentioning the epidemic publically until 1985 (Stinson, 2004).

As the decade began, the ANA published in 1980 its inaugural and highly controversial *Nursing: A Social Policy Statement* (ANA, 1980). Hobbs (2009) has written a marvelous paper on the prickly constituents who fought and debated the language of this document, especially since many of them feared the impact of its codification at all levels of nursing oversight. Hobbs describes how the primary debate was not over the odd language of the newly revised definition of nursing[22] (though this was indeed one of the document's controversies), but a debate over the definition of *specialization*. The burgeoning nurse practitioner movement in particular voiced displeasure about the final document permitting *specialization without an advanced nursing degree* and failing to be more explicit about the scope of the advanced practitioner to diagnose and treat disease and illness (Cronenwett, 1995; Hobbs, 2009).

Despite advances in the nursing profession, struggles to enact a minimum educational requirement for professional nursing continued by the ANA without much success. The ANA's 1965 statement on the education of nurses called for a minimum of a bachelor's degree for entry into professional nursing. But this call largely fell flat due to rising enrollments in Associate Degree nursing programs and the burgeoning political power and influence of those involved in ADN nursing education (Donley & Flaherty, 2008). In 1978, the ANA House of Delegates reaffirmed the 1965 statement and endorsed two levels of nursing practice—professional and technical, but in 1982 the move to formalize the BSN as minimum entry level to professional nursing was rebuffed permanently (Nelson, 2002). Joel has aptly written "The health care industry has traditionally ignored the advice of the nursing profession" (2002, p. 1) and this statement reflects the many congealed forces that have successfully defeated a universal upgrade in basic nursing education in the United States since the 1960s. As a consequence, one reason for nursing's historical lack of influence, despite the modernization of the profession and the growing numbers, can be attributed to Domino's assertion that nurses are the least educated of all the major health-care professionals (2005). Sadly, the nursing workforce in 2010 still resembles the landscape in 1985, as even today, while there are certainly fewer nurses prepared at the diploma level, the average RN still does not have a baccalaureate degree (Dreher, 2008).

The formal recognition of advanced nursing practice was also quickly progressing. The advanced practice nursing movement first began in 1965 at the University of Colorado with the first pediatric nurse practitioner certificate program established

---

[21]Comparatively, what is now termed "The Great Recession" and global financial crisis of 2008–2009 is more severe than the 1981–1982 recession (Karabell, 2010). But as of the writing of this text, unemployment peaked at 10.1% in October, 2009 (U.S. Dept of Labor, 2010). Between June 2007 and November 2008, Americans lost an estimated average of *more than a quarter* of their collective net worth (Luhby, 2009)!

[22]ANA revised definition of nursing as "The diagnosis and treatment of human responses to actual and potential health problems"(1980, p. 9).

by Dr. Loretta Ford and Dr. Henry Silver, a pediatrician (Hoekelman, 1967). Congressional legislation enacted in 1971 provided federal support for primary care intervention recommendations for which nurses and physicians could share responsibility, thus job opportunities for nurses as primary care providers grew (Sherwood, Brown, Fay, & Wardell, 1997). The Rural Health Clinic Services Act of 1977 was another important landmark piece of legislation that permitted reimbursement to nurse practitioner and physician assistants for federal Medicaid and Medicare reimbursement to patients in underserved, rural areas, and this move helped further progress the nursing primary care movement (Silver & McAtee, 1978; Wriston, 1981). It would be several decades, however, before the MSN would be required for advanced nursing practice for all four primary advanced practice specialties (Dreher, 2009). Now we have a new movement by the AACN to require the doctorate instead (AACN, 2004). How long do you think this will take?

During this period, immense lobbying was taking place at the highest levels of nursing in the Washington, DC, and in April 1986 the first National Center for Nursing Research at NIH was founded. Interestingly, the first Acting Director was a physician (Schlepp, 1987). While not a full research institute, "Center" status was considered the first step to an ultimate National Institute of Nursing Research (NINR) (Merritt, 1987). In Chapter 2, we described the surge of new doctoral nursing programs in the 1970s, and this continued into the 1980s with 34 new doctoral nursing programs established by 1985 (Boland & Finke, 2005). This total also included the first ND established at Case Western Reserve University in 1979 (Fitzpatrick Boyle, & Anderson, 1986). While many today will refer to the ND as the first practice doctorate in nursing, it really was the first professional doctorate and prepared students for entry into the profession[23] in the way the MD degree was intended for entry into the profession of medicine (after first being awarded an undergraduate degree in some field) (Forni, 1989). Historically, this degree model never became widespread and only four programs were ever established.[24] Masters level nursing programs also thrived in the 1980s, although the focus of this text is on the doctoral nursing scholars who are better positioned to advance the practice-oriented and theoretical knowledge of the discipline (Dunphy, Smith, & Youngkin, 2009).

Another sign of the maturing of the nursing discipline was the proliferation of nursing specialty journals, not just in the United States, but worldwide. It is difficult to be precise about the number of nursing journals that began publication since 1960, but the numbers obviously surged chiefly as more nurses sought higher education, and the audience for nursing scholarship grew precipitously. One measure of the growth and impact of nursing scholarship is Garfield's (1984) table (Table 15.4) that identifies the 10 most cited journals in 1983 (and their initial date of publication). The most cited journal article from 1966 to 1983 was Dr. M. V. Marston's (Francis Payne

---

[23]This was a very radical idea, *doctoral level entry* into professional nursing, especially since the profession could yet not agree on whether all nurses should have a BSN for entry level into the profession! One note—if one considers the EdD at Teacher's College in 1924 *technically* a professional doctorate then the ND was actually the "second."

[24]Since 2005, all four programs eventually closed and converted to DNP programs.

TABLE 15.4
Ten Most Cited Nursing Journals in 1983

Rank	Journal Title	Publication Year
1	*Nursing Research*	1952
2	*American Journal of Nursing*	1900
3	*Journal of Nursing Administration*	1971
4	*Nursing Outlook*	1952
5	*Nursing Times (U.K.)*	1906
6	*Journal of Advanced Nursing*	1976
7	*Journal of Nurse Midwifery*	1955
8	*Nursing Clinics of North America*	1966
9	*International Journal of Nursing Studies (U.K.)*	1964
10	*Research in Nursing & Health*	1978

Data adapted from Garfield, G. (1984). Journal Citation Studies. 44. Citation patterns in nursing journals and their most-cited articles. *Essays of an Information Scientist, 7*, 336–345.

Bolton School of Nursing, Case Western Reserve University) *"Compliance with Medical Regimens: A Review of the Literature"* published in *Nursing Research* in 1970 (Garfield).

Finally, one historical landmark that we would remiss if we did not address is the contribution of the nursing theorists to the nursing discipline during this 25-year period. While our purpose in this chapter or text is not to address their epistemological contribution to nursing (many other scholars have covered this topic exceptionally well),[25] our acknowledgement is more their intellectual contribution to framing the theoretical question: *"What is nursing?"* and *"What do nurses do?"* Any discipline, even a practice-oriented discipline such as nursing, cannot avoid completely the theoretical discussions and debates which may not have direct meaning for the common practitioner. To do so would be completely anti-intellectual. However, this is likely one of the faults of the theorists—the inability to convince lay nurses (whether technical, professional, or advanced) that nursing theory has real, direct application to their work. Nevertheless, from a historical perspective, Martha Rogers, Imogene King, Dorothea Orem, Sister Callista Roy, Rosemarie Parse, Jean Watson, Madeleine Leininger, and Helen Erickson (and others) have made a unique contribution to a profession that unfortunately *overvalues* the practical and the concrete and *undervalues* philosophizing, contemplation, reflection, and theorizing. It is quite likely, however, that the theory of transcultural nursing proposed by nurse anthropologist Madeleine Leininger,[26] and

---

[25]We recommend three texts to explore the epistemological contribution of the "grand nursing theories" to the nursing discipline: J. Fawcett's 2004 *Contemporary Nursing Knowledge: Analysis and Evaluation of Nursing Models and Theories, 2nd edition*; A. Meleis' 2007 *Theoretical Nursing: Development & Progress, 4th edition*; and M. R. Alligood & A. M. Tomey's 2009 *Nursing Theorists and Their Work, 7th edition*. Additionally, Reed and Shearer's 2007 *Perspectives on Nursing Theory, 5th edition*, is an excellent text that has combined discussion of philosophy, nursing epistemology, and grand and middle-range nursing theories.

[26]Madeleine Leininger's theory was fully articulated in her book *Culture Care Diversity and Universality: A Theory of Nursing* (1991).

the theory of human caring, chiefly articulated by Jean Watson,[27] may be the grand theorists who will have the most lasting impact on contemporary nursing practice.

Another type of nursing theory, termed *middle range* theory, evolved in the latter half of this 25-year span in nursing. The term was initially coined or invented by Merton, a sociologist in 1964 (Merton, 1964). According to Meleis, "Middle range theories deal with more specific phenomena" (2007, p. 213). One classic example of a middle range theory is Mercer's Theory of Maternal Role Attainment which appeared in the 1985 issue of *Nursing Research* (see Table 15.5) (1981, 1985). These theories may have the most direct impact on nursing practice and practice knowledge development. Examine Table 15.5 and the articles listed for the 1985 issue of *Nursing Research*. What kind of assumptions can you make when comparing *Nursing Research* from 1960?

TABLE 15.5
Table of Contents July/August 1985, *34* (4) *Nursing Research*

Editorial

Unidentified Acceptable Manuscripts—Florence Downs

The Process of Maternal Role Attainment over the First Year—Ramona Mercer

Incoming Mail

Re: 'Nursing Research Published as a Complete Book'

Re: 'The Telephone Survey: A Procedure for Assessing Educational Needs of Nurses'

Re: 'Institutional Sources of Articles Published in 13 Journals 1978–1982'

Re: 'Nursing's Divided House—An Historical Review'

Articles

Mothers' and Unrelated Persons' Initial Handling of Newborn Infants—Lorraine J. Tulman

Development of Infant Tenderness Scale—Deidre M. Blank

Spouse Support and Myocardial Infarction Patient Compliance—Gail A. Hilbert

Nursing Students' Assessments of Behaviorally Self-Blaming Rape Victims—Shirley Damrosch

Types and Sources of Social Support for Managing Job Stress in Critical Care Nursing—Jane Norbeck

Stress in ICU and Non-ICU Nurses—Anne Keane, Joseph Ducette, & Diane C. Adler

Predicting Nurses' Turnover and Internal Transfer Behavior – M. Susan Taylor & Mark A. Covaleski

Determining the Market for Nurse Practitioner Services: The New Haven Experience—Sherry A. Shamanski, Lynne S. Schlung, & Troy L. Holbrook

Professional and Bureaucratic Role Perceptions and Moral Behavior Among Nurses—Shake Ketefian

Methodology Corner

Reliability Estimates: Use and Disuse—Mary R. Lynn

Researcher's Bookshelf

Multivariate Statistics for Nursing Research—Thomas R. Knapp

Introduction to Qualitative Research Methods: The Search for Meaning—Janice M. Morse

---

[27]Jean Watson has continuously updated her work and her most recent work is *Assessing and Measuring Caring in Nursing and Health Science* (2008).

In reviewing these journal titles one very visible sign of the emergence of nursing as a scientific discipline is that there no longer appears to be a scarcity of "true research" articles, an admission of the journal's early editor and editorial board (Bunge, 1962). In great part, this can be attributed to the enormous number of new doctoral programs, an increase in funding sources for nursing research as noted earlier, the growing sophistication of nursing scholars to oversee the conduct of scientific research, and the availability of a new generation of mentors for the new generation of nurse scientists. We suggest you procure one of the research articles in this table. How would you evaluate the researcher's method and findings in 1985 compared to contemporary nursing research found in any leading research-oriented nursing journal today?

A Critical Juncture for Nursing Knowledge Development Circa 2010

We finally arrive at 2010. Historical events since 1985 are more recent and need to be refreshed less. If we focus, however, on global health issues, we have the progression of HIV/AIDS as a global pandemic, and the emergence of new infections like the 2003 Severe Acute Respiratory Syndrome (SARS) and H5N1 avian influenza (World Health Organization, 2004, 2010). SARS conclusively emphasized that the health of a single traveling citizen in one distant country could literally affect the health of anyone, anywhere on the planet and very quickly (Dreher et al., 2004). These events alone indicate the doctoral prepared nurse, no matter the degree, needs more preparation in global health nursing and public health content. We would further suggest they also need real world exposure to international health experiences including study abroad programs at the doctoral level (Dreher, Lachman, Smith Glasgow, & Ward, 2008). Since 1985, nurses also served admirably in the first Gulf War in the 1990s and the current wars in Iraq and Afghanistan (Scannell-Desch & Doherty, 2010; Sheehy, 2007). Nurses and other first responders were also at the forefront of responding to the deadliest terrorist attack on the United States on September 11, 2001 risking their own lives and health (Pak, O'Hara, & McCauley, 2008; Ungvarski, 2002).

Assessing the current landscape of nursing education, the issue of entry level into professional nursing appears to have been abandoned permanently. An alternative movement (to meet some of the original goals) to require instead the BSN after 10 years of having an Associate Degree in nursing, termed *RN + 10* or *BSN in 10* appears to have the most likelihood of entry-level reform. This legislation continues to percolate in New York, New Jersey, and Pennsylvania (Boyd, 2010; Dreher, 2008). The national median salary for the estimated 2.6 million RNs in 2008 was $62,450 (U.S. Department of Labor, 2009). And while the issue of entry level into professional nursing is now only percolating, the move to change the education entry level education for advanced practice nurses has swelled. In October 2004, the AACN voted narrowly to require the DNP degree instead of a masters degree for entry level into advanced practice nursing (the nurse practitioner, nurse midwife, nurse anesthetist, and clinical nurse specialist roles) by 2015 (AACN, 2004). As detailed earlier in this text, while this has been a goal of the AACN, no major advanced practice specialty organization has agreed to this final timetable. Actually, only in March 2010 did the ANA submit a draft statement for public comment on the DNP degree (ANA, 2010).

As of this writing, the draft is only undergoing formal review before a final proposal is approved and then it must go to the full ANA House of Delegates for a vote.[28] Nevertheless, in five short years, there has been explosive growth in new DNP programs. The latest AACN data indicate there are at least 119 DNP and 120 research-focused doctoral nursing programs (mostly PhD) (Fang, Tracy, & Bednash, 2010).[29] Figure 15.1 indicates the projected number of DNP versus PhD program in the near future. Obviously, many current graduate and current matriculating students have opted to not wait for 2015 or *possible* prospective enforcement by leading APRN organizations, nursing accrediting agencies, or state Nurse Practice Acts for a DNP degree requirement to enter Advanced Practice Nursing.

Whatever the consequence, it is not likely that the AACN or other nursing leaders could have projected this momentous rise in enrollment to an alternative to the PhD degree. Moreover, neither did they anticipate the DNP's real impact on nursing knowledge development, particularly with the very labile enrollment and graduation rates from PhD programs that are not keeping pace with nursing faculty retirements. It is not surprising that the PhD degree is in a state of crisis. In the early part of the decade, the University of Washington's sponsored *Re-envisioning the PhD* (Nyquist & Wilff, 2000) project was highly critical of contemporary PhD degree programs and offered solutions for reform. More recently, the Carnegie Foundation for the Advancement of Teaching has affirmed this and called for more PhD degree reform in *Envisioning the Future of Doctoral Education: Preparing Stewards of the Discipline* (Golde & Walker, 2006). In reality, it should not be surprising that the PhD in Nursing/ Nursing Science degree is experiencing difficulty, particularly with all the national

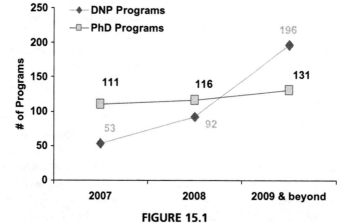

FIGURE 15.1

Projected number of DNP versus PhD programs 2007–2009 and beyond (extracted from AACN data 2007–2009)

---

[28]We must be emphatic that this cited draft *is not final*, and must undergo a lengthy process of public comment, revision, and then final approval. The entire process could take up to 1–2 years. Finally, remember how successful the 1985 ANA position statement on the BSN has been?

[29]While the first DNP program was founded in 2001 at the University of Kentucky, the real growth of doctor of nursing practice programs did not really begin until 2005.

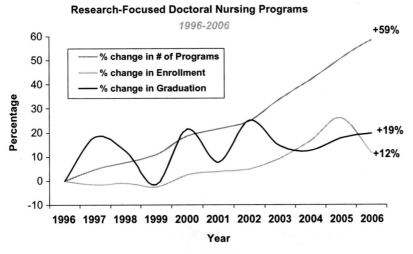

FIGURE 15.2

New programs, enrollments, and graduations in research-focused DNPs, 1996–2006. Table reprinted with permission from F. A. Davis from L. A. Joel's *Advanced Practice Nursing: Essentials for Role Development*, 2nd edition (2009).

attention on the doctor of nursing practice degree (Dreher, 2009; Fontaine & Dracup, 2007; O'Sullivan, Carter, Marion, Pohl, & Werner, 2005). Figure 15.2 indicates the stagnation of the PhD in Nursing over a recent 10 year period (1996–2006), despite the 59% increase in the overall number of PhD programs since 1996.

New 2009–2010 data is mixed with a 5.1% increase in total number of PhD in Nursing students, but only a 2.2% increase in graduations (Fang, Tracy, & Bednash, 2010). Full-time post-doctorate enrollment (a large gauge of the future nurse scientist pool) is down 6.1% (Fang, Tracy, & Bednash). As mentioned earlier, if retirements of senior faculty are factored into this scenario, it is likely even these slightly optimistic numbers are not enough to replace those exiting the profession. Impacting these flat enrollments and graduations is the discouraging, lengthy 8.3 year average it takes a nurse to obtain a PhD post the awarding of the MSN (Valiga, 2004). Part-time PhD enrollment is also problematic, because it contributes to these lengthy times to the award of the PhD degree, but full-time graduate enrollment is usually not an option for working nursing professionals. It is likely that the tensions between the PhD degree and DNP degree will continue as the profession debates what each degree needs to best contribute to the discipline in the next 20 years or more. The profession needs both nurse scientists and doctoral-educated practitioners/clinicians as stewards of the discipline. The debate of today and the future will be around the nature of this stewardship.

The advancement from center status to full institute status at the NIH finally happened in 1993 with the signing of the NIH Revitalization Act of 1993. A longstanding vision to house a nursing research enterprise, the NINR, at the NIH became a reality (Hurd, 1995). In 2000, the Council for the Advancement of Nursing Science (CANS) was formed within the prestigious American Academy of Nursing (founded in 1973) whose mission is to support "the preparation and use of knowledge in guiding nursing practice and shaping health policy" (Hinshaw & Holzemer, 2000,

p. 240). CANS mostly replaced the function of the ANA Council of Nurse Researchers founded in 1971 which disbanded in the 1990s and the ANA Cabinet on Nursing Research founded in 1970 which was phased out in the 1980s (See, 1977). Despite this new support for nursing research (and other private sources), nursing research in 2010 continues to be seriously underfunded, especially considering nursing is the largest health profession and the nursing care needs for America's estimated 308.4 million residents in 2010 are so vast (Schlesinger, 2009).[30] In 2005, Aaronson pointed out that the NINR was the lowest funded of 27 NIH Institute and Centers with only $139 million requested for fiscal year 2006 and remained only slightly more funded than the National Center for Complementary and Alternative Medicine (NIH, 2005). According to more recent data distributed by the AACN:

> NINR's FY 2010 funding level of $145.66 million is approximately 0.47% of the overall $31.247 billion NIH Budget. Spending for nursing research is a modest amount relative to the allocations for other health science institutes and for major disease category funding.
>
> — *AACN, 2010, p. 1*

Further, the NINR indicated to the nursing community that to adequately continue and further its mission, the institute must receive additional funding (AACN, 2010). The nursing research mission of the discipline must continue and be ramped up, especially with some 33 more millions Americans about to enter the health-care system with the passage of health-care reform in Congress in March 2010 (Irving, 2010). Just look at some of the seminal nursing research that has been conducted by nurse scientists in the last decade:

- **Reducing High Blood Pressure (HBP) Among Inner-City Black Men,** *Dr. Martha Hill, The Johns Hopkins University, 2003*
- **The Working Hours of Hospital Staff Nurses and Patient Safety,** *Dr. Ann E. Rogers, University of Pennsylvania, 2004*
- **Transitional Care Improves Outcomes of the Elderly,** *Dr. Mary Naylor, University of Pennsylvania, 2004*
- **Reducing Premature Infants' Length of Stay,** *Dr. Bernadette Melnyk, Arizona State University, 2006*
- **Improving Outcomes for Defibrillator Implant Patients,** *Dr. Sandy Dunbar, University of Pittsburgh, 2009*

In 2006, the Director of the NINR, Dr. Patricia Grady announced the NINR Strategic Plan with an emphasis on the following: (1) promoting health and preventing disease; (2) improving quality of life; (3) eliminating health disparities; and (4) setting directions for end-of-life research (NINR, 2006). We earnestly believe the DNP graduate can be a partner in this mission to improve health through advancing nursing knowledge. It is likely that the only way this kind of meaningful research is

---

[30]The U.S. population in 1985 was approximately 238 million (U.S. Bureau of the Census, 1999) and was 281,421,906 on April 2, 2000 (U.S. Census Bureau, 2009). A new census is being taken now in 2010.

going to increase in breadth is if PhD and DNP grads team up on meaningful translational clinical research teams. This has been suggested recently by Hastings and colleagues (Hastings, Mitchell, & Loud, 2010) and by Cacchione (2007). However, to accomplish this, the doctor of nursing practice graduate is going to have to acquire basic research skills, including a sound grounding in the scientific method. Moreover, this skill set will need to go beyond the evaluation and dissemination of research findings, which has always been a competency required for the baccalaureate[31] and masters-prepared graduate (AACN, 2008; Burke et al., 2005).

Table 15.6 describes the kind of nursing science being published today. A University of Manitoba analysis of the highest nursing journal impact factors for nursing publications 2003–2008 rated *Nursing Research* the third-highest cited nursing journal, after *Birth—Issues in Perinatal Care* and the *International Journal of Nursing Studies* (Plohman, Cepanec, & Heaman, 2008). What visible comparisons can you now make to nursing science in 1960 to 1985 to 2010? Are any of these titles related

TABLE 15.6
Table of Contents March/April 2010, *59* (2) *Nursing Research*

Editorial

The Promise of PROMIS—Molly Dougherty

Features

*Skin-to-Skin Contact After Cesarean Delivery: An Experimental Study—*Gouchon, Silvia; Gregori, Darion; Picotto, Amabile; Patrucco, Giovanna; Nangeroni, Marco; & Di Giulio, Paola

*Measuring the Quality of Care Related to Pain Management: A Multiple-Method Approach to Instrument Development—*Beck, Susan Larsen; Towsley, Gail L.; Berry, Patricia H.; Brant, Jeannine M.; & Lavoie Smith, Ellen M.

*Pain Barriers: Psychometrics of a 13-Item Questionnaire—*Boyd-Seale, Debra; Wilkie, Diana J.; Kim, Young Ok; Suarez, Marie L.; Lee, Hilary; Molokie, Robert; Zhao, Zhongsheng; Zong, Shiping

*Reliability and Validity of the Perspectives of Support from God Scale—*Hamilton, Jill B.; Crandell, Jamie L.; Carter, J. Kameron; Lynn, Mary R.

*Bullying (Ijime) Among Japanese Hospital Nurses: Modeling Responses to the Revised Negative Acts Questionnaire—*Abe, Kiyoko; Henly, Susan J.

*Psychometric Evaluation of a New Instrument to Measure Uncertainty in Children and Adolescents with Cancer—*Stewart, Janet L.; Lynn, Mary R.; Mishel, Merle H.

*Cognitive Deficits in Chronic Heart Failure—*Pressler, Susan J.; Subramanian, Usha; Kareken, David; Perkins, Susan M.; Gradus-Pizlo, Irmina; Sauvé, Mary Jane; Ding, Yan; Kim, JinShil; Sloan, Rebecca; Jaynes, Heather; Shaw, Rose Mary

*Psychological Vulnerability Predicts Increases in Depressive Symptoms in Individuals with Rheumatoid Arthritis—*Sinclair, Vaughn G.; Wallston, Kenneth A.

Method

*A Multilevel Confirmatory Factor Analysis of the Practice Environment Scale: A Case Study—*Gajewski, Byron J.; Boyle, Diane K.; Miller, Peggy A.; Oberhelman, Frances; Dunton, Nancy

Reviewer List

Nursing Research thanks the following for their contributions as reviewers in 2009

---

[31] According to the AACN 2008 *The Essentials of Baccalaureate Education for Professional Nursing Practice,* "Professional nursing practice is grounded in the translation of current evidence into practice" (p. 15).

to your clinical area or your proposed doctoral clinical problem of interest or clinical research question?

We find two very obvious trends in this 2010 issue. First, there are no publications from sole investigators, but that research teams now appear to be the norm. This is actually a trend not just in nursing science today, but in the overall conduct of science. The trend is actually toward interdisciplinary teams where nurse investigators may even lead a team of physician investigators or they may share coprimary investigator status. According to the NIH Roadmap on research teams of the future

> "The scale and complexity of today's biomedical research problems demand that scientists move beyond the confines of their individual disciplines and explore new organizational models for team science. Advances in molecular imaging, for example, require collaborations among diverse groups—radiologists, cell biologists, physicists, and computer programmers. NIH wants to stimulate new ways of combining skills and disciplines in the physical, biological, and social sciences to realize the great promise of 21st century medical research"
>
> —*NIH, 2008, p. 1*

Houldin, Naylor, and Haller (2004) have called for more physician–nurse collaboration in research and the May 2008 issue of *Nursing Outlook* was exclusively dedicated to articles and essays on nursing and interdisciplinary research. In a guest editorial for this issue, Grey and Mitchell (2008) wrote:

> Not so long ago, one of us (PM) asked the question "What's in a name?" in calling attention of the discipline of nursing science to the burgeoning movement of interdisciplinary research. In just a few years, there have been a number of shifts in definition, even within the National Institutes of Health (NIH). The NIH placed interdisciplinary research and development of the interdisciplinary workforce at the core of the Roadmap Initiative. For example, NIH originally defined interdisciplinary as collaborative work on a common problem that maintained several disciplinary foci. More recently, this definition has changed to what others have called transdisciplinary—the emergence of a new discipline, framework and/or methods from the work of researchers who come from the parent disciplines.[32]
>
> —*Grey and Mitchell, 2008, p. 95*

The single investigator is really passé. A team approach where each member can approach a clinical problem from his or her own unique disciplinary perspective and contribute to the overall problem of study has finally been recognized as the best way to conduct scientific inquiry. Ultimately, this trend toward "collaborative and team generated science" may even have an impact on PhD dissertations or DNP practice dissertations (or other common forms of the final doctoral project for the DNP degree). Why should these formal methods of graduate study inquiry be conducted using the "sole investigator model" (e.g., the PhD or DNP student investigator), when this method of isolated scholarly work is the antithesis to how good science is now normally produced? Why could not two or three doctoral students

---

[32]Grey, M., & Mitchell, P. (2008). Guest editorial: Nursing and interdisciplinary research. *Nursing Outlook, 56*(3), 95–96. Reprinted with permission by Elsevier.

collaborate intensely on a research project, or better yet, add a member from another discipline to form a real trasnsdisciplinary research or practice-oriented study? Our historical, very traditional methods of knowledge generation in the nursing discipline are going to need to be examined further. Moreover, it is obvious that the doctor of nursing practice degree is going to put more needed pressure on this analysis.

A second trend we discerned in the titles (and authors) of the 2010 *Nursing Research* issue is the authorship of several articles that were from international nursing scholars. This indicates a maturation of the nursing discipline internationally and also the prestige international scholars attribute to publishing in such a high impact, visible nursing journal. There are now many international nursing journals, and one, *The Journal of Nursing Scholarship*, has a specific international mission detailed on its website:

> "Reaching health professionals, faculty and students in 103 countries, the *Journal of Nursing Scholarship* is focused on health of people throughout the world. It is the official journal of the Honor Society of Nursing, Sigma Theta Tau International, and reflects the honor society's dedication to providing the tools necessary to improve nursing care globally"
>
> *—2010, p. 1*

A 2009 review article described the growth of international nursing research in Mainland China from 1989 to 2007 (Li, Wei, Liu, & Tang, 2009). In this review, these scholars identified 57 English papers in PubMed that were originally conducted in Mainland China during this period. As English still is the international language of science, this is a very visible sign of the global spread of nursing knowledge and the international growth of nursing as a discipline (Falagas, Fabritsi, Chelvatzoglou, & Rellos, 2005; Kvarko, 2008[33]).

Finally, we end this 100-year journey highlighting the very first journal in the nursing discipline devoted to scholarship emanating from doctor of nursing practice scholars, *Clinical Scholars Review*. First published in 2008, it is the first nursing journal to be devoted to publishing various types of scholarship that will promote the doctor of nursing practice degree (see Table 15.7). For that reason, it may be looked at in the same light as the first publication of the *AJN* in 1900 or the first issue of *Nursing Research* in 1952. Therefore, we do not want to be overly critical in our initial impressions here. After all, as we have seen in this chapter, in nursing "everything takes time."

Our quick impressions include the following:

1. As *Nursing Research* initially struggled with submissions that met the true research criteria, it appears that *Clinical Scholars Review* will similar undergo a journey to publishing DNP-authored, featured clinical submissions.

---

[33]This specific citation is a very interesting blog entry that actually describes some of the contemporary limitations of English as the universal language of science. Even so, French in France is under siege by spoken English among not just the French intelligentsia, but among diverse immigrant populations according to a recent *New York Times* article (Kimmelman, 2010).

TABLE 15.7
Table of Contents 2009, *2* (2) *Clinical Scholars Review: The Journal of Doctoral Nursing Practice*

2. As *Nursing Research* struggled with "Who is our audience?" this appears to be a problem for this new journal also. Who is it really for? DNP educators? DNP clinicians? A broader national audience?

3. Columbia University School of Nursing certainly deserves credit for giving birth to this scholarly venture, but the journal has not penetrated into the wider doctor of nursing practice network; Columbia's unique model of DNP education still is a tacit focus.[34]

This raises another important question—are DNP graduates really being uniformly socialized to be *clinical scholars?* Are these graduates going to publish and disseminate their acquired knowledge (so the health of the aggregate may benefit) in larger numbers and with more influence than the average MSN-prepared advanced practice nurse has? Maybe DNP scholarship will not just reside in specific journals as *Clinical*

---

[34]Again, Columbia was at the forefront of the doctor of nursing practice movement with their Clinical Doctorate (Honig & Smolowitz, 2010) which they first described as a *DrNP in Primary Care* degree model (Dreher, Donnelly, & Naremore, 2005). Their very unique second year of intensive residency, however, has not been copied by any other DNP program in the country to our knowledge, despite their changing to a DNP model in 2008.

Scholars Review, but be disseminated throughout all the major clinical specialty journals? However, a review of authors in the March 2010 issue of *Clinical Nurse Specialist: The Journal of Advanced Nursing Practice* found none of the 12 featured articles had DNP educated authors or coauthors. Similarly, the March 2010 issue of the *Journal of the Academy of Nurse Practitioners* also had no DNP educated authors or coauthors, and both of these journals are leading clinical specialty journals indexed by the ISI to calculate impact factor. Again, since the doctor of nursing practice degree has been around substantively since 2005, we hope this is not a publishing trend for the discipline and should be an alert to DNP educators and doctoral nursing education scholars if anything.

SUMMARY

This chapter, we admit was a grand undertaking, and we are certain to have made arbitrary decisions about what to focus on (or omit) from a 100 years of nursing scholarship. Our attempt was not by any means to be comprehensive, but to offer a template by which the historical evolution of nursing from a vocation and field to a discipline, within a historical context, could be traced. Too often in contemporary baccalaureate, masters, and doctoral nursing education there is so little focus on nursing history or nursing sociology; often missing is the societal context in which our discipline's evolution took place. We hope we have accomplished this in some small way—and that you can perhaps better appreciate our journey on this long path to a contemporary scientific discipline. We did not accomplish all that we have, because nurses easily agree. Obviously they (we) do not! Conformity has both helped us and hurt us at different times. From 1910 to 2010, nursing indeed changed, as did the U.S. Doctoral education was very, very revolutionary in 1924 when Columbia started the first EdD. Now we have a relatively new doctoral degree, and again, under great influence from Columbia University School of Nursing, which has served the profession most admirably. We contend that the time for discussions about what kind of knowledge doctor of nursing practice graduates are producing, or *should more comprehensively produce* for the profession and discipline has arrived. As M. Adelaide Nutting said in 1925, "We need to realize and to affirm that nursing is one of the most difficult of arts. Compassion may provide the motive, but knowledge is our only working power" (p. 1).

OPTIONAL SET OF CRITICAL THINKING EXERCISES: IS THIS NURSING SCIENCE?

The following is a classroom exercise that we have used for five years. At the end of NURS 700 the class is cofacilitated by both a philosopher of science and a doctoral nursing professor. The group project has the following guidelines from Appendix A:

Group Project

In the last module of the course, we will be applying what we've learned to some recent examples of nursing science. The class will be divided into three groups and assigned one of three articles from a nursing science journal in order to apply the inquiry learned throughout the course to scholarly example of nursing science. The purpose of the assignment is to engage class discussion, particularly toward the question as to whether and in what way *nursing is a science*. Each group of authors will submit a summary 3–5 page report in APA style, outlining their arguments made in the presentation. An abstract is unnecessary.

We particularly suggest discussing the three articles in the following order.

Article #1

Dixon, J. K., & Dixon, J. P. (2002). An integrative model for environmental health research. *Advances in Nursing Science, 24*(3), 43–57.

CRITICAL THINKING EXERCISE QUESTIONS

1. On what page is the word "nursing" first used? And the second time?
2. Before real discussions of the merits of this article, using your initial instincts, is this article representative of nursing science? Why or why not?
3. Is environmental health research necessarily "nursing research?"
4. Nurses, with their general education, are sometimes criticized for being *all over the place* or having a *lack of focus* in their scholarship. What specific type of environmental health research could be "uniquely within the domain of nursing?"
5. Describe a uniquely nursing-sensitive question within the physiological domain.
6. Describe a uniquely nursing-sensitive question within the vulnerability domain.
7. Describe a uniquely nursing-sensitive question within the epistemological domain.
8. Describe a uniquely nursing-sensitive question within the health protection domain.
9. Conclusively, does this article belong in this journal? Why or why not?
10. Conduct a new research/literature review on Dixon and Dixon's model. Is this nursing science?

Article #2

Morse, J. (2001). Toward a praxis of suffering. *Advances in Nursing Science, 24*(1), 476–459.

CRITICAL THINKING EXERCISE QUESTIONS

1. Is the concept "suffering" important to nursing science and nursing practice?
2. Do psychiatric nurse practitioners diagnose and treat "suffering?" Why or why not?
3. From each specific nursing specialty in class, discuss how "suffering" is or is not an important concept to your practice.
4. Is the concept "suffering" different in (a) middle-class America vs. (b) Baghdad or Kabul vs. (c) contemporary Haiti?
5. The author defines *suffering* by labeling it a component state of both (a) enduring and (b) suffering. Is it not redundant to define a concept by the concept itself? Or is the concept suffering perhaps irreducible?

6. Do you agree with the Figure 15.1 explanation of moving back between "enduring" and "emotional releasing?"
7. Do you agree with the author that individuals who are "enduring" should not receive empathy or be touched?
8. This study (and the supporting studies), were largely qualitative in design. Is this design a limitation to conducting good nursing science? Do you consider this study good nursing science?
9. How might a doctor of nursing practice student extend or improve this study for more clinically clarity? How might a PhD student approach this study differently?
10. Compare articles #1 and #2. Which better represents nursing science knowledge development?

Article #3

Jacobs, B. B. (2001). Respect for human dignity: A central phenomenon to philosophically unite nursing theory and practice through consilience knowledge. *Advances in Nursing Science, 24*(1), 17–35.

CRITICAL THINKING EXERCISE QUESTIONS

1. Nightingale held a view that "men of action" and "men of thought" should not be isolated. How would you trace her view throughout the last 100 years of nursing's history? Is nursing at all anti-intellectual?
2. Schlotfeldt suggested that in 1989 that by "the beginning of the 21st century" nursing's body of knowledge will be identified. Has this happened? Why or why not?
3. Reed suggests that the noun "nursing" and the discipline "nursing" are confusing and detrimental and suggested "nursology" as a better way to describe the study of nursing in much the same way "sociology" or "history" are so identified. What are your thoughts?
4. Fawcett has been criticized for using the concept *"nursing"* as one of the four metaparadigm concepts for nursing (person, environment, health, and nursing)? Do you agree or not, and why?
5. Jacobs suggests that nursing's central phenomenon is *respect for human dignity.* Do you agree or not? Or is it *caring*, or is the central focus of nursing something else? Explain.
6. Do you agree with the principle of consilience? Explain.
7. Is Jacobs' philosophical musing helpful to nursing science? To nursing practice? Explain.
8. How would you compare articles #1, #2, and #3?
9. Jacobs claims practice needs theory? Is this true? Can practice be a-theoretical? Explain.
10. Discuss the value (you can argue for more or less of each) of concrete thinking and abstract thinking to the delivery of nursing practice, in particular, to doctoral advanced nursing practice or doctoral advanced practice nursing?

CRITICAL THINKING QUESTIONS

1. Read an article from 1900 to 1910 in the *AJN* and reflect on the quality of that contemporary scholarship.
2. Pick an early historical nursing leader who you have previously known very little about. Perform a quick literature review and summarize the person's contributions to nursing.
3. Read an account of a nurse at war in WWI, WWII, or the Vietnam War. How has nursing during wartime advanced our profession?
4. Why did nursing have such a hard time historically moving into and being accepted into the university setting?
5. Is nursing more art (practice) or science? Explain.
6. Should nursing embrace or reject its identity as a woman's profession?
7. Select a random article from a 2010 or more recent issue of *Nursing Research* and summarize and critique the article's implication for nursing practice.
8. Should doctoral education be required or an option for advanced nursing practice? Why or why not?
9. Discuss your view of the DNP graduate as a clinical scholar.
10. How will you be more of a steward of the discipline with a doctorate than with a master's degree?

REFERENCES

Aaronson, I. (2005). *The road to interdisciplinary research: NINR and the NIH roadmap.* Paper presented at the 2005 AACN Doctoral Education Conference, Coronado Island, CA.

Abdellah, F. G., Beland, I. L., Martin, A., & Matheney, R. V. (1960). *Patient-centered approaches to nursing.* New York, NY: Macmillan.

Alligood, M. R., & Tomey, A. M. (2009). *Nursing theorists and their work* (7th ed.). St. Louis, MO: Mosby.

American Association of Colleges of Nursing. (2004). *AACN Position Statement on the Practice Doctorate in Nursing October 2004.* Retrieved April 12, 2010, from http://www.aacn.nche.edu/DNP/pdf/DNP.pdf

American Association of Colleges of Nursing. (2008). *The Essentials of Baccalaureate Education for Professional Nursing Practice.* Retrieved March 23, 2010, from http://www.aacn.nche.edu/Education/pdf/BaccEssentials08.pdf

American Association of Colleges of Nursing. (2010). *National Institute of Nursing Research: Promoting America's Health through Nursing Science.* Retrieved March 23, 2010, from http://www.aacn.nche.edu/government/pdf/NINRBrochure.pdf

American Journal of Nursing. (1934). Final report of the grading committee nursing schools—Today and tomorrow. *American Journal of Nursing, 34*(9), 840: Author.

American Journal of Nursing. (1935). The WPA and nursing: The nurse's status; projects; state committees [Unsigned Editorial]. *The American Journal of Nursing, 35*(12), 1154–1156.

American Journal of Nursing. (1949). Nursing research [Unsigned Editorial]. *American Journal of Nursing, 49*(12), 743–744.

American Journal of Nursing. (1961). How much are nurses paid [Unsigned Editorial]. *American Journal of Nursing, 61*(5), 89–92.

American Journal of Public Health. (1940). Typhoid fever in the United States [Unsigned Editorial]. *30*, 957–958.

American Nurses Association. (1980). *Nursing: A social policy statement.* Kansas City, MO: Author.

American Nurses Association. (2010). *Draft ANA Position Statement: The Doctor of Nursing Practice: Advancing the Nursing Profession.* Retrieved March 22, 2010, from http://www.nursingworld.org/DocumentVault/NursingPractice/DNP-Advancing-the-Nursing-Profession.aspx

Bandyk, M. (2009). Is unemployment the worst since the great depression? *U.S. World News & Report.* Retrieved from http://www.usnews.com/money/business-economy/articles/2009/08/27/is-unemployment-the-worst-since-the-great-depression.html

Bishop, C. (1970). Manpower policy and the supply of nurses. *Industrial Relations: A Journal of Economy and Society, 12*(1), 86–94.

Boland, D. L., & Finke, L. M. (2005). Curriculum designs. In D. M. Billings, & J. Halstead (Eds.), *Teaching in nursing: A guide for faculty* (2nd ed.) (pp. 145–166). Philadelphia, PA: Elsevier.

Boyd, T. (2010). New York, New Jersey Educators Debate BSN in 10 Bills. Retrieved March 20, 2010, from http://news.nurse.com/article/20100222/NY01/102220022.

Bromley, M. L. (2003). *William Howard Taft and the first motoring presidency, 1909–1913.* Jefferson, NC: McFarland.

Budd, K. W., Warino, L. S., & Patton, M. E. (2004). Traditional and non-traditional collective bargaining: Strategies to improve the patient care environment. *Online Journal of Issues in Nursing, 9*(1). Retrieved September 5, 2010, from http://www.nursingworld.org/MainMenuCategories/ANAMarketplace/ANAPeriodicals/OJIN/TableofContents/volume92004/No1Jan04/CollectiveBargainingStrategies.aspx

Bunge, H. (1962). The first decade of 'Nursing Research.' *Nursing Research, 11*(3), 132–138.

Burke, L. E., Schlenk, E. A., Sereika, S. M., Cohen, S. M., Happ, M. B., & Dorman, J. S. (2005). Developing research competence to support evidence-based practice. *Journal of Professional Nursing, 21*(6), 358–363.

Byers, B. K. (1999). *The lived experience of registered nurses, 1930–1950: A phenomenological study.* A dissertation in Higher Education for the Doctor of Education Degree, Texas Tech University.

Cacchione, P. Z. (2007). What is clinical nursing research? *Clinical Nursing Research, 16*(3), 167–169.

Cleland, V. S. (1967). The use of existing theory. *Nursing Research, 16*(2), 118–121.

Cronenwett, L. R. (1995). Molding the future of advanced practice nursing. *Nursing Outlook, 43*(3), 112–118.

Dallek, R. (2003). *An unfinished life: John F. Kennedy, 1917–1963.* London, UK: Brown & Little.

Dock, L. L., & Stewart, I. M. (1938). *A short history of nursing.* New York, NY: G.P. Putnam's Sons, The Knickerbocker Press.

Domino, E. (2005). Nurses are what nurses do—are you where you want to be? *Association of Perioperative Registered Nurses Journal, 81*(1), 187–201.

Donahue, M. P. (1996). *Nursing, the finest art: An illustrated history* (2nd ed.), St. Louis, MO: Mosby.

Donley, R., & Flaherty, M. J. (2008). Revisiting the American Nurses Association's first position on education for nurses: A comparative analysis of the first and second position statements on the education of Nurses. *The Online Journal of Issues in Nursing, 13*(2). Retrieved from http://www.nursingworld.org/MainMenuCategories/ANAMarketplace/ANAPeriodicals/OJIN/TableofContents/vol132008/No2May08/ArticlePreviousTopic/EntryIntoPracticeUpdate.aspx

Dreher, H. M. (2008). Innovation in nursing education: Preparing for the future of nursing practice. *Holistic Nursing Practice, 22*(2), 77–80.

Dreher, H. M. (2009). Education for advanced practice: The question: Is the PhD or DNP the right degree model for future advanced practice nurses? In L. A. Joel (Ed.), *Advanced Practice Nursing: Essentials for Role Development* (2nd ed.), (pp. 58–71). Philadelphia, PA: FA Davis.

Dreher, H. M., Dean, J. L., Moriarty, D., Kaiser, R., Willard, R., O'Donnell, S. et al. (2004). What you need to know about SARS now. *Nursing 2004: The Journal of Clinical Excellence, 34*, 58–63.

Dreher, H. M., Donnelly, G., & Naremore, R. (2005). Reflections on the DNP and an alternate practice doctorate model: The Drexel Dr. N. P. *Online Journal of Issues in Nursing, 11*(1). Retrieved May 6, 2010, from www.nursingworld.org/ojin/topic28/tpc28_7.htm

Dreher, H. M., Lachman, V. D., Smith Glasgow, M. E., & Ward, L. S. (2008). *Educating the global clinical scholar: The first doctoral nursing program to institute a mandatory study abroad program.* Electronic poster presented at the AACN Doctoral Education Conference, Captiva Island, FL, January 2008.

Dunphy, L. M., Smith, N. K., & Youngkin, E. Q. (2009). Advanced practice nursing: Doing what has to be done—radicals, renegades, and rebels. In L. A. Joel (Ed.), *Advanced Practice Nursing: Essentials for Development* (2nd ed.), (pp. 2–22). Philadelphia, PA: F.A. Davis.

Fagin, C. M. (1980). The shortage of nurses in the United States. *Journal of Public Health Policy, 1*(4), 293–311.

Falagas, M. E., Fabritsi, E., Chelvatzoglou, F. C., & Rellos, K. (2005). Penetration of the English language in science: The case of a German national interdisciplinary critical care conference. *Critical Care, 9*(6), 655–656.

Fang, D., Tracy, C., & Bednash, P. (2010). *2009–2010 Enrollment and graduations in baccalaureate and graduate programs in nursing.* Washington, DC: American Association of Colleges of Nursing.

Fawcett, J. (2004). *Contemporary nursing knowledge: Analysis and evaluation of nursing models and theories* (2nd ed.), Philadelphia, PA: FA Davis.

Fitzpatrick, J., Boyle, K. K., & Anderson, R. M. (1986). Evaluation of the doctor of nursing (ND) program: Preliminary findings. *Journal of Professional Nursing, 2*(6), 365–372.

Fontaine, D. K., & Dracup, K. (2007). The accelerated doctoral program in nursing: A university-foundation partnership. *Journal of Nursing Education, 46*(4), 159–164.

Forni, P. R. (1989). Models for doctoral programs: First professional degree of terminal degree? *Nursing Health Care, 10*(8), 429–434.

Friedman, M. (2008). *The great contraction, 1929–1933.* Princeton, NJ: Princeton University Press.

Garfield, G. (1984). Journal citation studies. 44. Citation patterns in nursing journals and their most-cited articles. *Essays of an Information Scientist, 7*, 336–345. Reprinted from *Current Contents, #43*, 3–12, Available at http://www.garfield.library.upenn.edu/essays/v7p336y1984.pdf

Gaspari, K. C., & Wolf, A. G. (1985). Income, public-works, and mortality in early twentieth-century American cities. *Journal of Economic History, 45*(2), 355–361.

Gavin, L. (1997). *American women in World War I: They also served.* Niwot, CO: University Press of Colorado.

Golde, C. M., & Walker, G. E. (2006). *Envisioning the future of doctoral education: Preparing stewards of the discipline.* San Francisco, CA: Jossey-Bass.

Goodrich, A. A. (1936). Modern trends in nursing education. *American Journal of Public Health, 26*, 764–770. (For *American Journal of Public Health* reprint and subscription information, visit www.ajph.org)

Goodwin, D. K. (1995). *No ordinary time: Franklin and Eleanor Roosevelt: The home front in World War II.* New York, NY: Simon & Schuster.

Gortner, S. (1986). Impact of the division of nursing on nursing research development in the U.S.A. In S. M. Stinson, & J. Kerr (Eds.), *International issues in nursing research* (pp. 113–130). Philadelphia, PA: The Charles Press.

Gortner, S. R., & Nahm, H. (1977). An overview of nursing research in the United States. *Nursing Research, 26*(1), 10–33.

Grey, M., & Mitchell, P. (2008). Guest editorial: Nursing and interdisciplinary research. *Nursing Outlook, 56*(3), 95–96.

Hampton, P. (2004). Ethel Byrne. *Encyclopedia of Women's Health* (p. 127). New York, NY: Springer.

Hastings, C. E., Mitchell, S. A., & Loud, J. T. (2010). *Advancing nursing roles in clinical and translational science.* Paper presented at the 2010 Clinical and Translational Research and Education Meeting, sponsored by the Association for Clinical Research Training (ACRT) and the Society for Clinical and Translational Science (SCTS), April 5–7, Washington, DC.

Higonnet, M. R., Jenson, J., Michel, S., & Weitz, M. C. (1987). *Behind the Lines: Gender and the two world wars.* New Haven, CT: Yale University Press.

Hinshaw, A. S., & Holzemer, W. (2000). A national voice for nursing research: Council for the Advancement of Nursing Science. *Nursing Outlook, 48*(5), 240–241.

Hobbs, J. L. (2009). Defining nursing practice: The ANA social policy statement, 1980–1983. *Advances in Nursing Science Issue, 32*(1), 3–18.

Hoekelman, R. (1967). A program to increase health care for children: The pediatric nurse program, by Henry K. Silver, MD, Loretta C. Ford, EdD, and Susan G. Stearly, MS. *Pediatrics, 39,* 756–760.

Honig, J., & Smolowitz, J. (2010). Clinical doctorate at Columbia University School of Nursing. *Clinical Scholars Review, 2*(2), 51–59.

Houldin, A. D., Naylor, M. D., & Haller, D. G. (2004). Physician–nurse collaboration in research in the 21st century. *Journal of Clinical Oncology, 22*(5), 774–776.

Hurd, P. (1995). The national institute of nursing research of the National Institutes of Health. *Nursing Outlook, 43*(2), 89–92.

Irving, F. (2010). *House passes health care legislation.* Retrieved from http://community.advance-web.com/blogs/hx_2/archive/2010/03/22/house-passes-health-care-legislation.aspx

Joel, L. (2002). Education for entry into nursing practice: Revisited for the 21st century. *Online Journal of Issues in Nursing, 7*(2), Manuscript 4. Retrieved from www.nursingworld.org/MainMenuCategories/ANAMarketplace/ANAPeriodicals/OJIN/TableofContents/Volume72002/No2May2002/EntryintoNursingPractice.aspx

Journal of Nursing Scholarship. (2010). Journal information. Retrieved March 24, 2010, from http://www.wiley.com/bw/journal.asp?ref=1527-6546 2010.

Kangas, K. (1997). The great depression: Its causes and cure. *Liberalism Resurgent.* Retrieved April 4, 2010, from http://www.huppi.com/kangaroo/THE_GREAT_DEPRESSION.htm

Karabell, Z. (2010). Our not-so-great recession. *The atlantic.com.* Retrieved from http://davos2010.theatlantic.com/2010/01/taking_stock_of_our_not-so-great_recession.php

Kimmelman, M. (2010). Pardon my French: The globalization of a language. *New York Times,* April 25, 2010, AR1.

Kvarko, J. (2008). *Science is a human right.* Livejournal.com blog. Retrieved March 23, 2010, from http://kvarko.livejournal.com/64285.html

Leininger, M. (1991). *Culture care diversity and universality: A theory of nursing.* Sudbury, MA: Jones & Bartlett.

Li, M., Wei, L., Liu, H., & Tang, L. (2009). Integrative review of international nursing research in Mainland China. *International Nursing Review, 56*(1), 28–33.

Luhby, T. (2009). Americans' wealth drops $1.3 trillion. *CNNMoney.com.* Retrieved from http://money.cnn.com/2009/06/11/news/economy/Americans_wealth_drops/?postversion=2009061113

Lusk, B. (1997). Professional classifications of American nurses, 1910 to 1935. *Western Journal of Nursing Research, 19*(2), 227–242.

Mack, M. (1952). The personal adjustment of chronically ill old people under home care. *Journal of Nursing in Research, 1*(1), 9–30.

Maddox, R. J. (1992). *The United States and World War II.* Westfield, MA: Westfield.

Magyary, D., Whitney, J. D., & Brown, M. A. (2006). Advancing practice inquiry: Research foundations of the practice doctorate in nursing. *Nursing Outlook, 54*(3), 139–151.

Marston, M. V. (1970). Compliance with medical regimens: A review of the literature. *Nursing Research, 14*(19), 312–323.

Mason, D. (1999). Ninety-nine years later. *The American Journal of Nursing, 99*(1), 7.

Meleis, A. (2007). *Theoretical nursing: Development and progress* (4th ed.). Philadelphia, PA: Lippincott, Williams and Wilkins.

Mercer, R. (1981). A theoretical framework for studying factors that impact on the maternal role. *Nursing Research, 30*(2), 73–77.

Mercer, R. (1985). The process of maternal role attainment over the first year. *Nursing Research, 34*(4), 198–204.

Merritt, D. (1987). National center for nursing research is ready for action at NIH. *Public Health Reports, 102*(1), 3–4.

Merton, R. (1964). *Social theory and social structure,* Revised Edition. London, UK: Free Press of Glencoe.

National Institutes of Health. (2005). *Summary of the FY 2006 President's Budget.* Washington, DC: Author.

National Institutes of Health. (2008). *Research teams of the future.* Retrieved March 23, 2010, from http://nihroadmap.nih.gov/researchteams/

National Institute of Nursing Research. (2006). *Changing Practice, Changing Lives: NINR Strategic Plan.* Retrieved September 6, 2010, from http://www.ninr.nih.gov/NR/rdonlyres/9021E5EB-B2BA-47EA-B5DB-1E4DB11B1289/4894/NINR_StrategicPlanWebsite.pdf

Nelson, M. (2002). Education for professional nursing practice: Looking backward into the future. *Online Journal of Issues in Nursing, 7*(3) Manuscript 3. Retrieved from www.nursingworld.org/MainMenuCategories/ANAMarketplace/ANAPeriodicals/OJIN/TableofContents/Volume72002/No2May2002/EducationforProfessionalNursingPractice.aspx

Nichols, E. F., & Chitty, K. K. (2005). Educational patterns in nursing. In K. K. Chitty (Ed.), *Professional nursing: Concepts & challenges* (pp. 31–62). Philadelphia, PA: Elsevier.

Notter, L. E. (1970). Helen L. Bunge, first editor of nursing research. *Nursing Research, 19*(4), 291.

Nutting, M. A. (1925). Greetings. In souvenir programs of the annual convention of the New York State Nurse's Association, the New York State League for Nursing, the New York Organization for Public Health Nursing, Albany, October 27–29, 1925.

Nyquist, J., & Wilff, D. H. (2000). *Recommendations from national studies on doctoral education: Re-envisioning the Ph.D. project.* Retrieved April 4, 2010, from http://www.grad.washington.edu/envision/project_resources/national_recommend.html

O'Sullivan, A. L., Carter, M., Marion, L., Pohl, J. M., & Werner, K. E. (2005). Moving forward together: The practice doctorate in nursing. *The Online Journal of Issues in Nursing, 19*(3), Retrieved May 5, 2010, from http://www.nursingworld.org/MainMenuCategories/ANA-Marketplace/ANAPeriodicals/OJIN/TableofContents/Volume102005/No3Sept05/tpc28_416028.aspx

Pak, V. M., O'Hara, M., & McCauley, L. A. (2008). Health effects following 9/11: Implications for occupational health nurses. *American Association of Occupational Health Nurses Journal, 56*(4), 159–165.

Palmer, S. (1910). The confusion of existing conditions. *American Journal of Nursing, 10*(7), 451–452.

Parietti, E. (1990). The development of doctoral education in nursing: A historical overview. In J. Allen (Ed.), *Consumers guide to doctoral degree programs in nursing* (pp. 15–32). New York, National League for Nursing.

Peplau, H. N. (1952). *Interpersonal relations in nursing.* New York, NY: G. P. Putnam and Sons.

Plohman, J., Cepanec, D., & Heaman, M. (2008). *ISI Journal Impact Factors and Allen (CINAHL) Ratings for Faculty of Nursing Publications 2003–2008. A Report Prepared by the Manitoba Centre for Nursing and Health Research (MCNHR).* Retrieved March 23, 2010, from http:// www.umanitoba.ca/faculties/nursing/collaborative-practice/media/2008_Impact_Factor_ Analysis_of_Faculty_of_Nursing_Pub-Dec22.pdf

Reed, J. (1978). *From private vice to public virtue: The birth control movement and American society since 1830.* New York, NY: Basic Books.

Reed, P. G. (2006). The practice turn in nursing epistemology. *Nursing Science Quarterly, 19*(1), 36–38.

Reed, P. G., & Shearer, N. C. (2007). *Perspectives on nursing theory* (5th ed.), Philadelphia, PA: Lipppincot Williams and Wilkins.

Rotter, A. J. (1999). Introduction. In A. J. Rotter (Ed.), *The light at the end of the tunnel: A Vietnam War anthology* (2nd ed.) (pp. xiii–xxxiv). Wilmington, DE: Scholarly Resources, Inc.

Sanger, M., Katz, E., Hajo, C. M., & Engelman, P. (2002). *The selected papers of Margaret Sanger: The Woman Rebel, 1900–1928,* (Vol. 1). Champaign, IL: University of Illinois Press.

Scannell-Desch, E., & Doherty, M. E. (2010). Experiences of U.S. military nurses in the Iraq and Afghanistan wars, 2003–2009. *Journal of Nursing Scholarship, 42*(1), 3–12.

Schlepp, S. (1987). Hinshaw nominated to direct nursing research center; North Dakota rules on baccalaureate for entry into practice. *Association of Perioperative Registered Nurses, 45*(4), 1016.

Schlesinger, R. (2009). U.S. population, 2010: 308 million and growing. *U.S. World News & Report.com.* Retrieved from http://www.usnews.com/blogs/robert-schlesinger/2009/12/ 30/us-population-2010-308-million-and-growing.html

See, E. M. (1977). The ANA and research in nursing. *Nursing Research, 26*(3), 165–171.

Sheehy, S. (2007). US military nurses in wartime: Reluctant heroes, always there. *Journal of Emergency Nursing, 33*(6), 555–563.

Sherwood, G. D., Brown, M., Fay, V., & Wardell, D. (1997). Defining nurse practitioner scope of practice: Expanding primary care services. *The Internet Journal of Advanced Nursing Practice, 1*(2), 1.

Silver, H., & McAtee, P. R. (1978). The rural health clinic services act of 1977. *The Nurse Practitioner, 3*(5), 30–32.

Smith, S. (2002). *Nursing as social responsibility: Implications for democracy from the life perspective of Lavinia Lloyd Dock (1858–1956).* A dissertation submitted to the Graduate Faculty of the Louisiana State University and Agricultural and Mechanical College, Louisiana.

Stevenson, J. S. (1987). Forging a research discipline. *Nursing Research, 36*(1), 60–63.

Stinson, J. (2004). Reagan did mention AIDS publicly before 1987. *History News Network.* Retrieved March 18, 2010, from http://hnn.us/roundup/entries/5621.html

Sussman, D. (1999). Nursing 1910 style: Camaraderie, housekeeping, and a life of service. *Nurseweek.com.* Retrieved April 5, 2010, from http://www.nurseweek.com/features/99-12/ workhist.html

Ungvarski, P. (2002). 9/11: Redefining the word "normal" in Manhattan. *Journal of the Association of Nurses in AIDS Care, 13*(5), 21–24.

U.S. Bureau of the Census. (1999). *Current population Reports,* Series P-25, Nos. 311, 917, 1095 released on June 4, 1999.

U.S. Census Bureau. (2009). *Census 2000 gateway.* Retrieved March 23, 2010, from http://www. census.gov/main/www/cen2000.html

U.S. Department of Health, Education and Welfare. (1970). *Progress report on nurse training.* Washington, DC: U.S. Government Printing Office.

U.S. Department of Labor Bureau of Labor statistics (2009). Registered Nurses. *Occupational Outlook Handbook, 2010–11 Edition.* Retrieved March 18, 2010, from http://www.bls.gov/oco/ocos083.htm

U.S. Department of Labor Bureau of Labor Statistics. (2010). *Labor Force Statistics from the Current Population Survey.* Retrieved March 18, 2010, from http://data.bls.gov/PDQ/servlet/SurveyOutputServlet?data_tool=latest_numbers&series_id=LNS14000000

Valiga, T. (2004). *The nursing faculty shortage: A national perspective.* Congressional briefing presented by the A.N.S.R. Alliance, Hart Senate Office Building, Washington, DC.

Veteran's Administration. (2010). Vietnam War statistics and exclusive photos. *Veteranshour.com* Retrieved March 18, 2010, from http://www.veteranshour.com/vietnam_war_statistics.htm

Walton, M., & Connolly, C. (2005). A look back: Nursing care of typhoid fever: The pivotal role of nurses at the Children's Hospital of Philadelphia between 1895 and 1910: How the past informs the present. *American Journal of Nursing, 105*(4), 74–78.

Watson, J. (2008). *Assessing and measuring caring in nursing and health science.* New York, NY: Springer.

Wickwire, R. (1937). Forecast for private duty nursing. *The American Journal of Nursing, 37*(3), 244–247.

Williams, D. R. (1945). Present types of collegiate schools of nursing. *American Journal of Nursing, 45*(5), 388–395.

Winnipeg General Hospital/Health Sciences Centre Nursing Alumnae Association Archives. (2001). *Isabel M. Stewart.* Retrieved September 6, 2010, from http://www.umanitoba.ca/nursing/heritage/nurses/stewart/

Wriston, S. (1981). Nurse practitioner reimbursement. *Journal of Health Politics, Policy and Law, 6*(3), 444–462.

World Health Organization. (2004). *WHO guidelines for the global surveillance of severe acute respiratory syndrome (SARS).* Updated recommendations October 2004. Retrieved March 19, 2010, from http://www.who.int/csr/resources/publications/WHO_CDS_CSR_ARO_2004_1/en/index.html

World Health Organization. (2010). *H5N1 avian influenza: Timeline of major events.* Retrieved March 19, 2010, from http://www.who.int/csr/disease/avian_influenza/Timeline_10_01_04.pdf

16

Next Steps Toward Practice Knowledge Development: An Emerging Epistemology in Nursing

What emerges is a more nuanced, more sociologically sensitive, epistemology—which is more resilient than the "hard core" of autonomous self-referential epistemology which scientists have struggled to articulate and to defend. If science is to engage more strongly with the agora[1], its image of impersonal, 'objective', self-organizing structures purged of allegedly subjective elements will need to be complemented and corrected by putting people, human agents, back into science. Our conception of science has to find room for the wide range of people who engage in material scientific activities and are linked in concrete ways to other social spaces in the agora that go far beyond the laboratory. Rather than trying to protect a "hard-core" which turns out to be empty or irrelevant for practical purposes, the many soft layers and clusters need to be strengthened by making their knowledge claims more socially robust.

HELGA NOWOTNY, PETER SCOTT, and MICHAEL GIBBONS

INTRODUCTION

In 1989, Dr. Ada Sue Hinshaw, the Director of the then National Center for Nursing Research wrote "The development of knowledge for nursing poses an exciting, scholarly adventure for the profession's scientists" (p. 161). Just over 20 years later, is it now time for a new cadre of DNP graduates to also assume costewardship of the nursing discipline as *clinical scholars* by developing a new body of *practice-oriented knowledge* too? In this chapter, we present some introductory arguments about what we propose the DNP student and graduate's clinical scholarship, a future

---

[1]*Agora*—"The space in which market and politics meet and mingle, where the articulation of private emotions and meanings encounters the formation of public opinion and political consensus" (Nowotny et al., 2001, p. 183). This definition and this chapter is taken from *Re-thinking Science: Knowledge and the Public in an Age of Uncertainty* which was the follow-up to the ground breaking 1994 book *The New Production of Knowledge: The Dynamics of Science and Research in Contemporary Societies* by Michael Gibbons and colleagues. Both books have had a significant impact on professional doctorate knowledge development, particularly outside the United States.

practice-oriented nursing epistemology, should look like when exiting the DNP degree.[2] We will propose a model of scientific inquiry and stewardship for the nursing discipline through the development of a body of practice-oriented nursing knowledge to improve health. Again, this is a philosophy of science text primarily. Our introductory essays and concluding essays are only designed to better frame the philosophy of science supporting the scientific method for the kinds of formal, clinical inquiry we believe DNP students/graduates should engage in and that DNP faculty should support. We will leave it to other practice scholars and nurse epistemologists to digest these arguments and ideas and begin a journey of discussions about whether DNP graduates should produce nursing knowledge, and if so, what kind? Many of the ideas in this chapter were first fomented in my own teaching of *Nurs 716: The Structure of Scientific Knowledge in Nursing* at Drexel with a classroom full of mostly advanced practice nurses. They discussed at length the very kinds of practical, real, clinical practice knowledge they needed in their practice and which they hoped to create. Finally, in the spirit of doctoral discourse, we present these ideas not to offend, but to sway. We need more debate, dialogue, and critique in the academy, not less.

WHAT KIND OF NURSING KNOWLEDGE SHOULD DNP GRADUATES PRODUCE?

These discussions about the place of philosophy of science and the place of the scientific method in the DNP degree are important questions. In the brief period of its short history, it is not reasonable that absolute conclusions about the nature of knowledge development in this degree should have been already been fully agreed upon, much less codified. In other words, to say so quickly "we thought about it, discussed it, and know what the right course of action is" is folly. Indeed, Reed wrote in 2006, "And during the last decade, scholars within and outside of nursing increasingly acknowledged the role of human practices in knowledge production and critiqued orthodox epistemology with its one path to scientific knowledge" (p. 36). Arriving at some conclusion or set of conclusions about what the final scholarly work product of a DNP degree should ultimately be will not happen if we leave it to national accrediting agencies or specialty organizations to decide. There is already a growing body of literature now criticizing these types of bodies, external to the academy, for thwarting educational innovation through regulation (Dreher, 2008a; Melnyk & Davidson, 2009; Neal, 2008). Though select members of these agencies or organizations may support the mission of knowledge development, it is not the chief function of these entities to which they belong. This mission—extending knowledge development in any discipline—is a responsibility for scholars chiefly *in the academy* (remember discussions in Chapter 2 about "who belongs?" and "who is best prepared to produce this knowledge?"). We predict this will happen, because nursing practice scholars will likely conclude that many past and current DNP students are actually

---

[2]For simplicity, when we refer to the DNP degree we also include the DrNP degree, but fully acknowledge that the DNP degree is overwhelmingly the most predominant degree model. We suggest both can and should aim to embrace practice-oriented nursing knowledge development.

generating evidence for the discipline (yes, including even sometimes empirical evidence) by their current model(s) of clinical or practice inquiry. Others, admittedly, are not. Part of this journey begins with an expansion of the meaning of *evidence* to be addressed in this chapter (Rycroft-Malone et al., 2006)

With half a decade with the new practice doctorate behind us, the kind of inquiry that is taking place in DNP programs toward degree completion needs a label. It needs to be articulated. It will require much more critical reflection and examination on the nature of knowledge development in a practice discipline, however, for us to arrive at a consensus for this label. We provide our own contribution to this discussion in this chapter by asking, is it: (1) *practice knowledge,* (2) *Mode 2 knowledge* (Rolfe & Davies, 2009; Smith Glasgow & Dreher, 2010; Stew, in press), (3) *actionable knowledge* (Coghlan, 2006; Pope, 2007), or (4) *practice inquiry* (Magyary, Whitney, & Brown, 2006)? We will offer some further discussion points about this issue which is beginning to percolate in current academic nursing scholarly circles, particularly as DNP enrollment and number of programs is surpassing the PhD. Moreover, we never want to hear again what some recent graduates[3] at a national DNP conference and at an international conference on the professional doctorate have said, "They wouldn't let me do that" or "They wouldn't let me call it a 'dissertation'" or worse, "The faculty wouldn't let me call it *research.*"

Having also heard the following, we begin the discussion on evidence by asking what does it really mean when a DNP student proclaims "I have to use *existing research* to implement a change that will improve practice?" Figure 16.1 indicates Sackett and colleagues' levels of evidence (Sackett, Strauss, Richardson, Rosenberg, & Haynes, 2000). This highly regarded internationally recognized classification of categories of levels of evidence, though not the only evidence-based classification available, is widely used to classify the scientific health knowledge that is produced en masse around the globe (Rich, 2005; Harbour & Miller, 2001; Petrisor & Bhandari, 2007).

Pearson and colleagues (Pearson, Wiechula, Court, & Lockwood, 2007) nevertheless do challenge this paradigm and write "However, practice discourses across the health professions are characterized by ongoing, vigorous debate on the meaning of evidence when attaching this epithet [evidence] to healthcare practices" (p. 86). Indeed Rycroft-Malone and colleagues (2006) suggest that in the practice domain, the concept of *evidence* is more complex and may mean something different from the traditional, objective, quantitative scientific explanation. The Joanna Briggs Institute model of evidence-based health care proposes four major evidence interests (termed the FAME scale): (1) *evidence of feasibility;* (2) *evidence of appropriateness;* (3) *evidence of meaningfulness;* and (4) *evidence of effectiveness* (Houde, 2009; Murphy, Robinson, & Lin, 2009; Pearson, Borbasi, & Gott, 1997). Further, they report "Any indication that a practice is effective, appropriate, meaningful, or feasible, whether derived from experience or expertise or inference or deduction or the results of rigorous inquiry, is regarded as form of evidence in the model" (Pearson et al., 2007, p. 87). So what does this mean? It sounds like there is a "big tent" for knowledge development in nursing. We suspect

---

[3]In both instances, these two graduates (we have seen others too) were presenting their final DNP projects in peer-reviewed poster sessions.

1a = Systematic Review of Randomized Controlled Trials (RCTs)
1b = RCTs with Narrow Confidence Interval
1c = All or None Case Series
2a = Systematic Review Cohort Studies
2b = Cohort Study/Low Quality RCT
2c = Outcomes Research
3a = Systematic Review of Case-Controlled Studies
3b = Case-controlled Study
4 = Case Series, Poor Cohort Case Controlled
5 = Expert Opinion

While a full explanation of this table is not possible in this text (a simple Internet search will wield a massive amount of information), the table can be summarized as follows for the purpose of our discussion.[1] Primarily used for evaluating studies in clinical care, a [peer reviewed] published paper is first classified according to levels 1 through 5 and sublevels a through c. These are indicated in Table 16.1. The higher the classification of level (1), the higher the likelihood the study is valid, but not necessarily its clinical applicability. The lower the classification of level (5), the lower the likelihood the study is valid, but again, not necessarily its clinical applicability. The sublevel classification is also rated from a (highest) to c (lowest), although in levels 4 and 5 there are not sublevels of classification (Petrisor & Bhandari, 2007). Finally the study is graded A through D as follows: A: consistent level 1 studies; B: consistent level 2 or 3 studies or extrapolations from level 1 studies; C: level 4 studies or extrapolations from level 2 or 3 studies; and D: level 5 evidence *or* troublingly inconsistent or inconclusive studies of any level (Centre for Evidence Based Medicine, 2010). Extrapolations are where data is reinterpreted to some degree in order to help form the recommendation, aside from the original study situation (Harbour & Miller, 2001). One perhaps helpful way to understand the concept of extrapolation similarly occurs in nursing research when investigators use the word "generalizable" when discussing whether the data findings in one study population can be generalized (or extrapolated) to another population. We thus pose the following question: *How will the published work-product of the DNP student be evaluated and classified?* This becomes a critical question if the work is truly designed to be published and disseminated.[2] Whatever the debate, when it comes to working with colleagues from different health professions, Sackett represents the predominant scientific paradigm.

---

[1]David Evans (2003) provides an excellent translation of these evaluative levels for nursing in his article "Hierarchy of evidence: A framework for ranking evidence evaluating healthcare interventions" in the *Journal of Clinical Nursing, 12*, 77–84.

[2]The question here is how will transdisciplinary colleagues evaluate this work product?

FIGURE 16.1
Sackett's levels of evidence

as the DNP degree matures over time, there will be more refinement regarding the nature of practice knowledge development and its place in the wider epistemology of the nursing discipline. So, in the spirit of scholarly discourse among members and future members of the academy, with an aim to advance the nursing discipline, we pose the following questions about DNP clinical scholarship and stewardship.

Is It "Practice Inquiry"?

Practice inquiry has been proposed both by nursing scholars at the University of Washington School of Nursing and by public health and physician scholars affiliated with several medical schools, including the University of California-San Francisco (Magyary et al., 2006; Sommers, Morgan, Johnson, & Yatabe, 2007). In the case of its use in medical schools (first described in Chapter 3), *practice inquiry* is primarily a "set of small-group, practice-based learning and improvement (PBLI) methods designed to help clinicians better manage case-based clinical uncertainty" (p. 246). The aforementioned nursing scholars have introduced the concept practice inquiry differently. For them it is

> an ongoing, systematic investigation of questions about nursing therapeutics and clinical phenomena with the intent to appraise and translate all forms of 'best evidence' to practice, and to evaluate the translational impact on the quality of health and health outcomes
> —*Magyary et al., p. 143*

Magyary and colleagues identify four specific domains of *clinical research* (efficacy research, effectiveness research, service systems research, and practice research) and propose the practice research domain be the particular emphasis for the clinical investigative focus of the DNP.[4] They suggest practice inquiry "portrays clinical research competences that are integral with advanced practice and, thus, relevant to learn during a practice-intensive doctoral program" (p. 143). It does not quite seem logical, however, to equate "educating professionals to primarily engage in practice at the *frontiers of existing knowledge*"[5] (p. 147) with the aims of practice research as outlined by the National Institute of Mental Health (NIMH) (1999).[6] Comparatively a 2006 program announcement by the NIMH (PAR-06-441) described the following as possible research questions within the practice research infrastructure:

- Assess and test methods to more quickly and effectively synthesize and incorporate existing evidence into clinical practice.

---

[4]These four domains are defined in the 1999 NIMH *Bridging Science and Service* report (see footnote 6).

[5]Italics mine.

[6]This report, titled *Bridging Science and Service*, was written by the U.S. National Advisory Mental Health Council's (NAMHC) Clinical Treatment and Services Research Workgroup of the National Institute of Mental Health and outlined what kinds of research paradigms would be most likely to deliver a relevant evidence base for mental health services (NIMH) (1999). Many health researchers, including the University of Washington scholars cited, have indicated these descriptions of "clinical research" could easily apply outside the mental health field as well and be applied broadly to clinical inquiry.

- Determine patient, provider, and contextual factors that may enhance or detract from the effective delivery of interventions.
- Evaluate the effectiveness, safety, and costs of efficacious interventions but not adequately tested in practice settings.
- Evaluate alternative methods of adapting assessment and treatment protocols originally developed in academic settings.
- Determine whether fidelity (by patients and providers) to adapted interventions is related to patient outcomes.
- Test methods to improve the recruitment and retention of patients and providers in community-based intervention studies.
- Determine whether patient and, provider treatment choice is related to positive patient outcomes.
- Determine different stakeholders' perceptions of quality of care and develop instruments to assess the relationship between various definitions of quality and patient/ client outcomes.
- Test the effectiveness of evidence-based care for subsyndromal and comorbid populations.
- Determine how economic factors (e.g., at the patient and community organization levels) affect the provision and receipt of services and pharmaceuticals.
- Test state-of-the-art dissemination and implementation strategies.[7]

Our question is whether these types of practice-oriented, clinical research questions can be answered under the umbrella of nursing practice inquiry in DNP curricula, and whether these questions are at the frontiers of existing knowledge or not (or beyond?)? Magyary and colleagues (2006) and the nursing scholars at the University of Washington School of Nursing should be applauded for one of the very first forays into the context of what is the domain of practice doctorate knowledge development? Nursing scholars at nearby Oregon Health and Science University appear to support this too (Pate & Crabtree, 2009). But we are skeptical that we have carved out the absolute boundaries of the practice inquiry domain yet and even they admit "it is important to be cautious and not prematurely differentiate between the 2 programs [DNP and PhD]" (Magyary et al., p. 147). We conclude the term practice inquiry is a good description of the likely domain of the practice doctorate practitioner/scholar, but we dispute that it properly describes what we should define or call the process or output of practice doctorate scholarship. Practice inquiry is just too oblique a concept (at least at present) for contemporary transdisciplinary usage. We will revisit this argument shortly.

Is It "Actionable Knowledge"?

There is an argument that much of the final scholarly work product in some DNP programs could be termed *action research*, but this method is used by many disciplines. Our purpose here is not to evaluate the contributions of action research-oriented

---

[7]This program announcement is available at: http://grants.nih.gov/grants/guide/pa-files/par-06-441.html.

studies to the body of nursing science. Instead, we are trying to ascertain whether this method is appropriate for the DNP/professional doctoral student, and whether it should be the overriding umbrella over which DNP scholarship should be classified. Coghlan (2006) makes a case for action research in nursing, particularly for students interested in conducting research projects as "insiders in their own organizations" (p. 293). This method is aimed at creating *actionable knowledge* which is designed to be used by both academic and practitioner communities (Adler & Shani, 2001). It is also described as a participatory, democratic, and egalitarian method (Drummond & Themessl-Huber, 2007).

Many DNP students are very interested in addressing problems within their own work environments which can initiate intraorganizational change, including improvements in patient safety, for example (Rapala & Novak, 2007). A significant number of our own DrNP students have chosen to access populations in their work institutions and examined problems critical in their clinical specialty or to the organization. Physicians conduct clinical research on their patients all the time, especially on clinical research units; therefore, this practice should certainly be extended to doctoral nursing students as well. Pope (2007), a reader in health services research in a school of nursing and midwifery in the United Kingdom, describes some of the advantages and disadvantages of action research. Pope, however, promotes its distinctiveness as a method as it dually *enables change while simultaneously conducting the respective research study*. Nogeste's (2008) work is an example of how the action research method has become popular in professional doctorate business programs (DBA, Doctor of Business Administration)[8] and describes how it can be used to both conduct research and solve a real-life problem situation. Certainly this same method could be used by clinical executive DNP students and students who are also examining clinical problems.

Is It "Mode 2 Knowledge"?

There is a strong case to be made that the focus of the professional/practice doctorate ought to be on the generation of Mode 2 knowledge (Rolfe & Davies, 2009; Smith Glasgow & Dreher, 2010; Stew, in press). Internationally, the concept of Mode 1 and Mode 2 knowledge is a lot more prevalent than in the United States where it has barely penetrated the nursing literature. The concept of Mode 1 versus Mode 2 knowledge was first described by Gibbons and colleagues in 1994 in *The New Production of Knowledge: The Dynamics of Science and Research in Contemporary Societies*. Mode 1 knowledge is described as:

> a form of knowledge production—a complex of ideas, methods, values, norms—that has grown up to control the diffusion of the Newtonian model to more and more fields of enquiry and ensure its compliance with what is considered sound scientific practice.
> —*Gibbons, 1994, p. 2*

---

[8]There are lots of DBA programs in the United States and abroad (Neumann, 2005), including at Harvard. The eminent guru of innovation, Dr. Clayton Christensen, who first coined the term "disruptive innovation" and a co-author of *The Innovator's Prescription—A Disruptive Solution for Health Care (2008)*, has a DBA degree from Harvard, not a PhD.

In other words, Mode 1 knowledge is traditional and disciplinary-specific and uses hypotheses that are generated, tested, analyzed, and then disseminated in peer-reviewed, often prestigious journals. Heath (2001) states that it is knowledge based on traditional notions of the objectivity of knowledge, either rational[9] or empirical, but which ultimately depends upon the notion that knowledge must be based in some form of objective reality. Some community health nursing scholars in describing methods of research appropriate for primary care inquiry indicate Mode 1 knowledge is hypothetico-deductive and linear in its orientation (Vydelingum, Smith, & Colliety, 2009). It is a broad generalization, but it is presumed the PhD graduate is supposed to generate original Mode 1 knowledge.

On the contrary, Mode 2 knowledge is generated in the context of application and has an orientation to knowledge that is practical, useful, translatable, and has derivative areas of meaningfulness across disciplines. Gibbons (1994) describes the following:

> Our view is that while Mode 2 may not be replacing Mode 1—Mode 2 is different from Mode 1—in nearly every respect. Mode 2 operates within a context of application in that problems are not set within a disciplinary framework. It is transdisciplinary, rather than mono- or multi disciplinary. It is carried out in non-hierarchical, heterogeneously organized forms which are essentially transient. It is not being institutionalized primarily within university structures. Mode 2 involves the close interaction of many actors, throughout the process of knowledge production and this means that knowledge production is becoming more socially accountable. One consequence of these changes is that Mode 2 makes use of a wider range of criteria in judging quality control. Overall, the process of knowledge production is becoming more reflective and affects at the deepest levels what shall count as "good science."[10]
>
> —*Gibbons, 1994, p. vii*

There is a very strong case to be made that the "good science" evolving from the DNP programs where nursing epistemology and knowledge development is valued is indeed being conducted within the framework of a Mode 2 knowledge production paradigm, even if this is not articulated or clearly realized. Rolfe and Davies (2009) indicate that second-generation professional doctorates will be the primary generators of this kind of knowledge production in the future, and that it will not occur within the confines of a laboratory or the rigid parameters of a traditionalist academic study. They state, "Under Mode 2, the link between theory and practice is more apparent, and because research takes place in the workplace, knowledge-production and diffusion are interlinked" (p. 1268). The emphasis here, however, is that at least from an *internationalist perspective*, the professional doctorate (like the DNP or DrNP) graduate that produces Mode 2 knowledge is engaging in "research" (Dreher & Smith Glasgow, in press). The resistance by the AACN (2006) to eschew any DNP graduate from engaging in the *research enterprise* (beyond translating and disseminating) is therefore

---

[9]Rational knowledge is less discussed in nursing. It is not the kind of knowledge that is experienced. Mathematics and logic, for instance, are examples of rational knowledge.

[10]Gibbons, M. (1994). Preface. In M. Gibbons, C. Lomoges, H. Nowotny, S. Schwartzman, P. Scott, & M. Trow (Eds.), *The new production of knowledge* (pp. vii–ix). London, UK: Sage. Reprinted with permission by Sage.

problematic. The professional doctorate model outside the United States is largely characterized by a de-emphasis on the research enterprise (in comparison to the PhD), but not the absence of it (Dreher, Donnelly, & Naremore, 2005).

We would suggest that the AACN's *Essentials* document may already be largely out of date (AACN, 2006).[11] Produced in 2006 at the beginning of the contemporary DNP degree movement, it was created *before* there was a critical mass of graduates and before anyone could really report any outcome data on what the first graduates' new practice domain would actually look like. And with more DNP programs to be in operation by the end of 2010 than PhD programs, there ought to be a heightened urgency to discuss the future logistics of the production of evidence for our discipline. Isn't any doctoral graduate after all part of the new knowledge economy (Fink, 2006)? Reed does suggest that Mode 2 knowledge may be central to an emerging epistemology and indicates "it seems logical that a nurse–patient practice-centered model rather than a researcher-centered model of knowledge production be employed" (2006, p. 36). Whether or not the language and discourse surrounding Mode 1 and Mode 2 knowledge will ultimately impact the nursing discipline and find its way into our literature more substantively remains to be seen.

Or Is It "Practice Knowledge"?

With a plethora of DNP programs, there is likely going to be a shift or a *practice turn* in our nursing epistemology (a term used by Reed in 2006) away from the overtly theoretical to the practice-focused and directly and expeditiously translational. Our view is that *practice knowledge* by the simplest description, is the by-product of *practice research*. Practice research is characterized by Magyary and colleagues (2006) as "the type of research designs and methods that are relevant and particularly germane to examine clinical questions related to the complexity of everyday clinical situations" (p. 141). Barkham and Mellor-Clark (2003) indicate that the domain practice research, along with the other domains of clinical research described by the NIMH (2006) (efficacy research, effectiveness research, and service systems research) are research areas "placed within the paradigms of evidence-based practice and practice-based evidence" (p. 319). Utilizing the principle of parsimony[12] (all these being equal, the most frugal or simplest explanation is best) and principle of syntactical simplicity, we would subsume each of these four separate domains of clinical research (see page 305) into a singular domain (Bunge, 1961). We believe they can be combined and reframed coherently to represent the expanse of practice knowledge development. In other words, "practice research produces practice knowledge." Extending this analysis, since the nature of practice encompasses inquiry into efficacy, effectiveness

---

[11]The revision to the 2006 *Essentials* document (and we are not aware that any revision is even under discussion at this point) will need more input and be more data driven than the original and be written and vetted in partnership with doctor of nursing practice graduates who are now living out the realities of this new degree.

[12]The theory of parsimony is based on Occam's razor (William of Occam b. 1287, d. 1347) which argues that one should not multiply entities or kinds of entities unnecessarily (Rodriguez-Pereyra, 2008).

and even into health systems inquiry—practice research can be the unifying domain. Another rationale for subsuming these four domains as one (practice research) is also because most current DNP programs emphasize the practitioner *and* clinical executive role under the rubric of a *practice doctorate* (AACN, 2006).

Reed (1996) also offered, a decade earlier, a description of practice knowledge that actually emanated from a revisiting of the works of the renown Hildegard Peplau. Reed has written "Specifically; a closer look at Peplau's theory demonstrates an approach to knowledge development through the scholarship of practice; nursing knowledge is developed in practice as well as for practice" (p. 30). Reed further states, "In this postmodern era, knowledge development is no longer only a concern of theoretical nursing; it is a concern in practice" (p. 30). How prescient Reed was practically a decade before the surge of a new practice doctorate in nursing. Peplau herself later (1988) articulated that nursing practice itself was not a research endeavor, but she did emphasize it is a scientific and scholarly endeavor (or should be). Do we emphasize this characterization of nursing practice today in our baccalaureate programs? In other words, do we talk about *nursing practice* as scholarly? From her classic and heralded *Interpersonal Relations in Nursing* (1952), Pepalu makes a statement that is prophetic and is referenced by Kikuchi in the epigraph that introduced Chapter 3:

> One of the main problems in the observation and study of human behavior and interaction in relations between nurses and patients is the multiplicity of factors to be studied. Some form of organization that will limit the study of unwieldy data to that which can be studied is as necessary in nursing as in any other science that studies human behavior.[13]
>
> *—Pepalu, 1952, p. 276*

One interpretation of this (and of Kikuchi) is that there is a large body of phenomena in nursing that is unique to the nursing discipline, is complex in its manifestation, and is incredibly challenging (perhaps impossible) to explore using traditional empirical methods of inquiry. Interpretative methods offer an alternative, but even those have their own peculiar limitations relative to the study of nursing phenomena. Madeleine Leininger faced this herself in her translation (or adaptation) of very traditional anthropologically oriented enthnographic methods into her creation of the ethnonursing method (1985). As a contemporary example, we offer two scenarios of nursing-sensitive phenomena that challenge our understanding and method of inquiry.

Case 1: *How can some patients who are enduring/experiencing various levels of pain, suffering, discomfort, angst, fear etc. still interact and exhibit behaviors of kindness, selflessness, non-ego-centered, ingratiating, even apologetic gestures <u>toward</u> a new and unknown nurse?* As the nurse co-author of this text, it has bewildered me over my career how so many patients in states of unease and distress can be so *at ease* at the first nurse-patient interaction whether it be in the ER or CCU? My emphasis here is that the exploration of this phenomenon need not be formally explored solely by the PhD nursing student! That is the point. Any prohibition of the DNP student from formal scientific inquiry, even explanation, is

---

[13]Reprinted with permission by Springer Publishing, New York, NY.

ridiculous. Even for an advanced practice nurse like a psychiatric-nurse practitioner student, the nature of this interaction (*practice inquiry*) warrants consideration and begs for a creative mode of inquiry (*practice research*) to explore it further (resulting in *practice knowledge*).

> Case 2: *Question: Is poor weight management a failure of primary care?* In a 2008 publication in *Holistic Nursing Practice* I explored whether physicians and nurse practitioners were accountable for their patients' weight control in the same way as they are being held accountable (and broadcast very proudly in some primary care practices) for the Hb_{1ac} levels in their diabetic patients? I wrote "It appears at least physician primary care providers are as overweight as the general population and this may be interfering with their real ability to credibly encourage aggressive weight loss in their clinic patients" (Dreher, 2008b, p. 316). The question in this article then turned to whether NPs were any better than physicians at encouraging successful weight loss in their primary care patients? After a further review of the literature, I concluded "Nurse practitioners seem positioned to advocate for lifestyle changes in perhaps a little more persuasive way on the basis of their education. However, there is no evidence that nurse practitioners manage weight control better than primary care physicians."
>
> —*Dreher, 2008b, p. 316*

Again, we do not need to wait for the PhD student to answer these questions. If anything, it literally begs inquiry (*practice inquiry*) by the post-master's DNP student who has been treating these kinds of patients for years as an adult, family, or women's health NP? The most appropriate scientific method can be selected from a host of quantitative, qualitative, or mixed-method options (*practice research*) in order to ultimately advance the evidence base of nursing (*practice knowledge*). Further, the findings and implications of this study could have far-reaching immediate implications (translational) for other primary care providers (physicians and physician assistants, certified midwives, etc.), and thus it would be transdisciplinary in application too!

CONCEPTUALIZING PRACTICE KNOWLEDGE

We offer three conceptual diagrams or figures which try to explicate the domain of practice knowledge development within the larger universe of potential nursing scientific inquiry. Figure 16.2 identifies the process of practice knowledge development from inquiry to product (output) that we just outlined in Case 1.

The first and largest arrow represents the possible pool of inquiry by nursing practice scholars. In our definition, *practice inquiry* is *not* a method of inquiry but represents a larger domain of yet analyzed, correlated, explored, tested, hypothesized, and conceptualized (among other modes) data. It is a universal pool of nursing and nursing-related (e.g., health, etc.) phenomena that is poised for inquiry by a practice nursing scholar (**input**). The second arrow represents the chosen scientific method. These methods may be empirical, intermediary/analytical (all the methods that fall between the classic empirical, traditionalist, and quantitative methods, and the interpretive and classically qualitative), or interpretive/classically qualitative methods (*process*).

The last arrow represents *output* or *practice knowledge*. An extremely important point is that this knowledge is *generated* by the doctoral advanced practice student/ practice scholar. It is *not* the everyday practice knowledge often termed personal

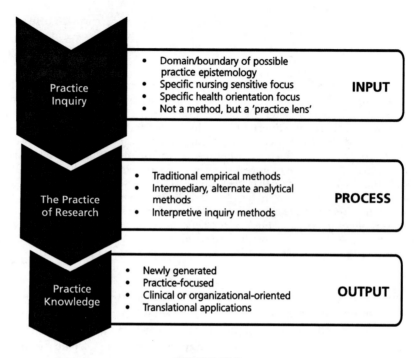

FIGURE 16.2
A model of the path to practice knowledge generation. (Figure 16.2 may be copied/
reprinted only with permission of author H. M. Dreher.)

practice knowledge that is "grasped in a conscious moment of encountering and interacting with a specific patient" and "developed via the dialectical relationship that is created between each patient and nurse" (Mantzoukas & Jasper, 2008, p. 321.) This practice knowledge can have a clinical or organizational orientation and thus would fall within the four domains of clinical research or under the singular rubric of practice research identified earlier. Finally, as described in Case 2, its best representation occurs when this practice knowledge is readily translated through interdisciplinary applications. The two primary care providers working in the same office, but from different disciplines (medicine and nursing), should be looking at their aggregate data on weight for their patients and discussing their disciplinary approach so as to improve overall outcomes (just like the monitoring of Hb_{1ac} levels).

A Proposed Model for Scientific Inquiry in Nursing

First, Figure 16.3 places Figure 16.2 in the context of the larger universe of scientific inquiry in nursing science. Here, the Venn diagram first displays an outer square box which contextually has permeable lines that imperfectly encase the two equivalent circles. Everything inside the box and that which lies outside the permeable lines (representing maybe a future pool of data not yet known) represents the *pool of*

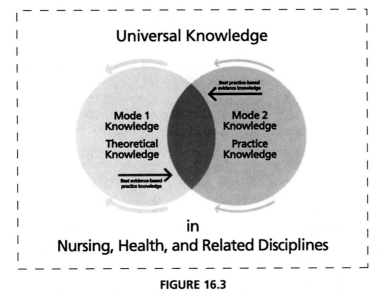

FIGURE 16.3
Model of scientific inquiry in nursing and overlap between competing paradigms.
(Figure 16.3 may be copied/reprinted only with permission of author H. M. Dreher.)

inquiry for nursing science and nursing practice and all the related disciplines and related knowledge that are credible for the theoretical or practice nurse investigator to draw from. For purposes of representation, the Venn diagram (and the square surrounding it) is presented two-dimensionally in this text, but in reality knowledge is multidimensional. By definition, a Venn diagram is a representation of classes or categories and their possible intersection or overlap. In this figure, however, the overlapping area of intersection is far more rich and complex. This will be discussed in detail in this section.

Second, the large left-centric circle represents *Mode 1 knowledge* or *theoretical knowledge. The further to the left* any individual study falls within the circle, as the arrows on the bottom and top of both circles pointing left indicate, the more abstractly theoretical the study. Furthermore, such studies are increasingly less oriented to purely evidence-based practice and have limited translational capacity. These types of studies would likely have a very low classification on Sackett's Level of Evidence, but could still represent serious and rigorous scholarship, just not highly applicable or translatable. Within the same circle, *the further to the right* any study falls, until the overlapping area of intersection, the more it skews toward practice (whether clinical or organizational) and toward the most rigorous *evidence-based practice (EBP) knowledge*. We will address the area of intersection shortly.

Third (and conversely), the large right-centric circle represents *Mode 2 knowledge* or *practice knowledge*. Within this circle, the further to the left any study falls, again until the overlapping or area of intersection, the more it does skew toward practice (whether clinical or organizational) and toward *practice-based evidence (PBE) knowledge*. However, as the arrows on the bottom and top of both circles indicate (they both point to the left), the further to the right any individual study falls, there is an opposing effect. Studies falling more to the right would be classified as *less practice focused* with less emphasis on practice knowledge. They would be moving in the opposite direction away from the overlapping area of intersection and away from a PBE orientation and be less translational. (And perhaps less valid).

Finally, the *overlapping area of intersection* is a very critical area where it might be said the DNP and PhD degree may truly converge, morph or fuse, or be fairly indistinguishable (at least when it comes to the final research product of the doctoral degree or according to the nature of the scientific investigation). Fink (2006) indeed indicates that as the nature of the kinds of directly applicable and translational research changes (what we could call the burden to make research today relevant *now or immediately*), the "scholarly workplace" (p. 38) for the professional doctorate and the academic PhD will also converge and the distinctions between the two degrees may disappear.[14] What does this mean?

The overlapping area of intersection coming from the right (Mode 2/practice-oriented knowledge) signifies the *best PBE*. Barkham and Mellor-Clark (2003) state, "Studies derived from a practice-based paradigm have high external validity because they sample therapy [referring to a specific psychotherapy study] as it is in routine practice" (p. 321). Further, by emphasizing investigation of the practice component in real-time, these types of studies address the applicability of analyzing results *within* a service or clinical setting with a very high likelihood of immediate translational implications. *PBE* has somehow become the contretemps (or the reverse) to the larger EBP movement (Geanellos, 2004; Hellerstein, 2008; McDonald & Viehbeck, 2007). However, even before such terminology (specifically PBE) was being used, there were pioneering clinicians who were creating it. In perhaps the most illustrative case, early HIV clinicians/providers experimented with drug combinations. They discovered that they were highly effective in individual patients (or in select groups of patients) long before the respective clinical trials were conducted to confirm the efficacy of any respective therapeutic regimen. These early HIV specialists (mostly physicians but also a very large cadre of NPs) practiced primary care in very real time and literally "experimented" (Garrett, 1999, p. 1). In Garrett's 1999 article "The Virus at the End of the World," she reports on Dr. Michael Saag, who at the time was supervising the research and care of nearly a thousand patients with HIV/AIDS in Alabama, writing, "In one year, 57 of Saag's patients collectively took 189 different drug formulas, with only three patients taking the same mix of HAART drugs" (p. 1). Like Dr. Saag, they relied on practice evidence to drive their decision-making, because medication adherence studies, drug efficacy studies, especially ones that controlled for the diversity of confounding social, metabolic, and other variables were scarce

---

[14]We would venture to say that the rigor of the nursing research that falls within or near the overlapping area of intersection would mean that in *select* DNP programs the rigor of the respective DNP degree is really *equivalent* to the rigor of *select* PhD programs. Put another way, in *select* DNP programs the Final DNP Project or whatever it is called (see Table 16.1) may be just as rigorous as any (or at least some) PhD dissertation. Pearson and colleagues actually suggest that the professional doctorate and the PhD are "equal but different" (Pearson, Borbasi, & Gott, 1997, p. 366).

(Moitra, 2009). One contemporary argument over the merits of PBE knowledge over EBP knowledge in HIV medicine is stated as follows:

> One driver of recent discussions of "evidence" in HIV prevention is the idea that, rather than ever more tightly defining the conditions under which an intervention might work, prevention research would be better served by a methodology designed to identify those interventions that are robust enough to withstand local variation and implementation. A novel goal of HIV prevention research should be to move beyond the ideal of "best practices" indicated by RCTs and toward a range of good practices, applicable under broader circumstances, and gleaned from multiple ways of knowing.[15]
>
> —*San Francisco Aids Foundation, 2008, p. 2*

The overlapping area of intersection coming from the right also represents crossover into Mode I and theoretical knowledge, and further indicates the amount of rigor and high probability of translational relevance. These are studies that have some semblance of Mode 1 knowledge (and method) and are not devoid of theory or theoretical underpinnings, but again they may likely not be the *prototype type of study* conducted in an average DNP program. Hellerstein (2008), for example, offers the following recommendations for more PBE over EBP in psychiatry:

1. Use real clinical practice environments as laboratories for developing effective treatments.
2. Revive quality improvement (QI) research and scholarship, since QI projects are perfect models for PBE.
3. Develop modular treatments (i.e., medical treatment packages and components with proven efficiency) that can be incorporated into existing protocols of care.
4. Maximize the use of online technologies for: collecting effectiveness data; training providers; disseminating information and health teaching to patients; for testing, monitoring, and rewarding effectiveness.

The overlapping area of intersection coming from the left represents crossover into Mode 2 and practice knowledge, and indicates the study has a very high orientation to practice or to organizational/health systems research with a similar high probability of translational relevance. These studies are likely the PhD dissertations that are very, very clinically based or practice-oriented. Therefore, while movement from the right to the overlapping area of intersection represents movement toward the highest levels of *PBE knowledge*, movement from the left to the overlapping area of intersection represents movement toward the highest levels of *EBP knowledge*. This is a fairly rich interdisciplinary literature, and it is not possible to easily summarize the impact of this movement on nursing knowledge development. But it has had an enormous impact on the practice of medicine (Manser & Walters, 2001; Oxford Centre for Evidence Based Medicine, 2009; Sackett, 1996; Torpy, 2009; White, 2004) and in nursing and general health care delivery.

One of the leaders in evidence-based practice in nursing has been the Dean of the Arizona State University College of Nursing and Healthcare Innovation,

---

[15]Reprinted with permission by the San Francisco AIDS Foundation.

Dr. Bernadette Melnyk. Her work, however, has been primarily concerned with advancing evidence-based care at the bedside by professional nurses (Melnyk & Fineout-Overholt, 2005, 2010). What is needed is *more* evidence-based primary care nursing (and health-related) research, but before NPs and nurse midwives can use this evidence to advance their practice, someone has to create this evidence. Dreher and Gardner (2009) suggest that primary care nursing knowledge development is threatened if it is going to be left to be generated by perhaps PhD-prepared nurse scientists *who are not advanced practice nurses.* It is quite obvious to us in our classroom discussions that it is the seasoned clinician/practitioner in the trenches who knows what questions need most urgently be asked? In the past, PhD programs have relied almost exclusively on masters prepared nurses (very often certified advanced practice nurses) to enter PhD programs, with BSN-to-PhD graduates being a secondary, but very small pool of applicants. With the rise of BSN-to-DNP programs, who will be best positioned to contribute Mode 1/theoretical knowledge for primary care nursing practice? Who will contribute that very highest level of evidence-based practice primary care-oriented knowledge represented by the overlapping area of intersection on the left side of the circle?

We suggest the hybrid professional practice doctorate (the DrNP degree) is best positioned to produce this kind of knowledge (both from the PBE and EBP paradigm), because it falls between the aims of the DNP and PhD degree (see Chapter 2, Figure 2.1). However, the concept of a hybrid doctorate in nursing has not become popular for perhaps various reasons.[16] Similarly, the strongest DNP programs are also well positioned to produce this practice evidence, particularly those very dedicated to practice knowledge development.[17] It is likely that at the beginning of the contemporary DNP movement, it was not hypothesized that in 5 years the DNP degree would overcome the PhD degree in a number of active programs. Therefore, we suggest the importance of nursing knowledge (particularly practice knowledge) and the responsibility of the DNP graduate were absent from the early deliberations. But now, the landscape for doctoral nursing education has changed. The evidence-based knowledge and practice-based knowledge generation/production doctoral nursing educational structures to build this capacity must be re-engineered.

---

[16]The reasons are complex and highly speculative. We understand the AACN in 2004 did not want to revisit the multiple historical and sometimes confusing research degrees (PhD, DNSc, DSN, & DNS) by doing the same with the practice degree and endorsing both the DNP and DrNP (AACN, 2004). However, Physical Therapy and Occupational Therapy have recently had to go back and create a hybrid degree (DScPT, DSc, & DrOT) after their professional doctorates just were not creating (and publishing and disseminating) enough new knowledge for their disciplines. Further, these professions appear to be more receptive to the hybrid doctorate graduate seeking employment in academia, since they do complete a practice or clinical dissertation. We like to think Drexel was ahead of the curve (our nursing school does trace its history back to 1890) and forecast this back in 2004. The jury is still out whether there will be more DrNP degrees in nursing, or whether the DNP will instead become more research-oriented. Since accreditors carry significant influence, the latter scenario seems more likely, but who knows?

[17]We must also be honest in our evaluation of doctoral nursing programs and indicate there are also weak PhD programs (Keithley, 2003), where the mentoring for the research scientist model is not strong. Therefore, it should not be assumed that every PhD nursing dissertation will have an impact on our discipline or on health. The over prevalence of weak PhD programs was also one of the rationales for the *Re-envisioning the PhD Project* (Nyquist, 2002).

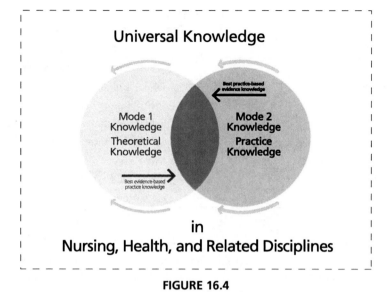

FIGURE 16.4
Conceptual model of practice knowledge development in nursing (Figure 16.4 may be copied/reprinted only with permission of author H. M. Dreher)

We conclude the section of this discussion with Figure 16.4. It places Mode 1/ theoretical knowledge in the background (for de-emphasis) and the large right-centric circle is the focus, with its orientation to Mode 2/practice knowledge. We attest this represents at least a beginning conceptual model of practice knowledge development in nursing. Within the right-centric circle, knowledge to the left (in the area of intersection) would be the most highly developed and practice-based, followed by varying degrees of practice knowledge in the center, and finally including the least developed, lowest contextualized to the extreme right. DNP programs producing Final Projects (or again, whatever the title) here (to the extreme right) would likely be the least valid of all with regard to classification in Sackett's levels of evidence (or perhaps any classification), likely less rigorous, and maybe not even publishable.

HOW TO BEST OPERATIONALIZE PRACTICE KNOWLEDGE IN DNP PROGRAMS

Finally, there is an operational concern for how practice knowledge is made formal within the academy (the university or college setting) before it is then further synthesized, reduced, and disseminated in journal format and oral presentation. Lack of discourse, debate, and clarity of purpose among members of the nursing academy has led us to the current state where Table 16.1 indicates the current diverse types of final projects now used in DNP programs. What is perhaps more astounding is that *this list is not comprehensive!*

There is great confusion and much disagreement about what the final scholarly end product of the DNP degree ought to be (Dreher, 2009a). From the *Essentials of Doctoral Education for Advanced Nursing Practice* (AACN, 2006) it is called the "final DNP product" (p. 19) and the "Final DNP Project" (p. 20) and clarified "Unlike a

TABLE 16.1
Doctor of Nursing Practice End-of-Degree "Final Project" Models

Research Utilization Project	DNP Research Project
Capstone Project	Professional Capstone Project
Leadership Project	Clinical Research Proposal & Implementation
Clinical Dissertation	DNP Thesis or DNP Applied Research Project
DNP Portfolio	Evidence-based Scholarly Project
Capstone Clinical Investigative Project	Scholarly Clinical Inquiry Project
Evidence-based Practice Project	DNP Project
Practice Improvement Project	Practice Dissertation
Practice Inquiry Project	Evidence-based Research Project

dissertation, the work may take a number of forms" (p. 20). However, there is little real discussion or even rationale in this document about *what the proper scholarly end product for a professional or practice doctorate ought to be.* Within the *Essentials* document the following types of *final DNP projects* are suggested:

- Practice portfolio
- Practice change initiative
- Pilot study
- Program evaluation
- Quality improvement project
- Evaluation of a new practice model
- Consulting project
- Integrated critical literature review
- Manuscripts submitted for publication
- Systematic review
- Research utilization project
- Practice topic dissemination
- Substantive involvement in a larger endeavor, or other practice project

Perhaps with more clarity the AACN's (2006) *Essentials* also emphasizes:

> For practice doctorates, requiring a dissertation or other original research is contrary to the intent of the DNP. The DNP primarily involves mastery of an advanced specialty within nursing practice. Therefore, *other methods must be used*[18] to distinguish the achievement of that mastery.
>
> —*AACN, 2006, p. 20*

Our question is: What do you think? Is this a decision for a faculty or an accrediting body? Again with there soon being more DNP programs than PhD programs, the implications for knowledge development are enormous if this dictum is enforced. Further, is a pilot study not permitted to be *original research*? We have found the

---

[18]Italics mine.

pilot study enormously useful in our own DrNP program. Often, it is the seasoned, highly clinically experienced practice doctorate student who has identified a little known phenomenon in nursing that needs initial description and study. A full PhD dissertation on the topic would be premature. Further, access to the population (and recruitment) may be difficult. Here are some examples of clinical dissertation topics from our program (these also could easily be termed practice dissertations too) that are actually pilot studies for the reasons noted above:

Topic A: *The Meaning of Surviving Longer Than Expected and Being Discharged From Hospice: A Phenomenological Study of Elders with Cancer*

Topic B: *Mindfulness-Based Stress Reduction in Kidney Transplant Candidates*

Topic C: *Somatic Awareness and Symptom Attribution in Ischemic Stroke Patients*

In each of these three small pilot studies, the subject recruitment is challenging. In Topic A, the DNP student had seen dozens of patients discharged from inpatient hospice, and she always wondered why some individuals almost seem to thrive when placed in hospice. As an adult NP, also certified in advanced palliative care, she observed improved psychological and physical health status often to the point where the individual outlived their billable hospice length of stay, and were discharged home. She simply wanted to interview a few of them right after discharge and ask them "why do you think you have survived?" Qualitative research guidelines have been published in the prestigious *Journal of the American Medical Association* and physicians do conduct and publish qualitative studies (Giacomini & Cook, 2000a, 2000b; Munday, Petrova, & Dale, 2009). Therefore, it does not seem logical to us that doctoral nursing students would be prohibited from this type of practice inquiry research endeavor (i.e., the generation of *new* practice knowledge), especially when most nursing students (between their BSN, MSN, and doctoral degree) probably have had more exposure to research methods content as any physician who has earned a typical MD degree. There is already a similar body of literature that indicates the average Registered Nurse (with at least a BSN degree) has much more formal coursework in nutrition than the average physician (Dreher, 2009b). In Topic B, the graduate actually studied patients awaiting kidney transplant to determine whether a shorter than standard mindfulness meditation protocol would reduce their pretransplant anxiety. As this was a true pilot study, it was powered at a less rigorous alpha level of 0.10 rather than the more restrictive 0.05. In true pilot studies, this is acceptable statistical practice and permits the student to enroll fewer subjects (Hertzog, 2008). Finally, the student conducting the pilot study in Topic C has hypothesized that some individuals appraise their early symptoms of stroke far differently than if they suspected they were experiencing chest pain or myocardial infarction. She suspects some individuals may thereby wrongly (and often with serious consequences) delay emergency treatment for stroke. This doctoral candidate is also seeking to interview inpatients who are post-CVA (Cerebro Vascular Accident), and with very restrictive enrollment criteria, her faculty mentors believe her study meets the criteria for a small pilot study.

In order that DrNP students indeed do not undertake clinical studies that may be beyond the scope of the degree (with regard to breadth), our faculty does not permit any student to propose a clinical study in which data cannot be collected in 90 days. This does not mean the study *is less rigorous* at all. Collecting data on admission (or 1 day post-op), at discharge (perhaps 3 days later), and at 30-day follow-up, is an enormously popular sequence of three measurement intervals in clinical research. Indeed, the data collected (if the subjects can be adequately accessed) can be exceptionally rich. We also suggest replication studies, however true replication studies are exceedingly rare in nursing for some reason (Beck, 1994; Fahs, Morgan, & Kalman, 2003). Kelder (2005) even describes some of the challenges surrounding the replication of qualitative studies. One reason replication studies may have been discouraged, particularly at the PhD dissertation level, is that some nursing faculty may believe they do not meet the doctoral requirement for original research. However, replication studies could be undertaken by DNP students, or perhaps even downsized and examined with a particular focus (a systematic extension replication) that might be readily translational (Polit & Beck, 2007). What is often overlooked, particularly in nursing, is that it is only after replication that evidence becomes more consistently confirmed. Therefore, with good replication studies, the validity of the research and its use/inclusion in systematic reviews to help change and advance nursing practice is enhanced.

Secondary data analysis also falls in the same category (Aponte, 2010; Magee, Lee, Giuliano, & Munro, 2006). While some PhD students may be prohibited from pure secondary data analysis where they have not actively collected the data (certainly a purist perspective that is thankfully not universal), the DNP student is not so prohibited. How valuable it would be if more DNP students took a fresh look at some already collected data, posed another question, and reanalyzed the data for immediate translation perhaps. Again, two examples from our own DrNP program from two current doctoral candidates[19] who are using secondary data analysis:

Topic A: *Preparedness and Appraisal of Behavior Problems on Role Strain in Family Caregivers of Persons Diagnosed with Alzheimer's Dementia*

Topic B: *The Association Between Underage Drinking, Age of Initiation of Alcohol and Use and Behaviors Contributing to Violence All on School Property*

The doctoral candidate conducting the first study (Topic A) is using secondary data from an NINH/NINR parent study of her supervising professor, and she has also added a small focus group to provide additional original data. The doctoral candidate in the second study (Topic B) is analyzing data solely from a published national database, and she is looking at possible relationships among variables that previously have never been investigated.

Our suggestions for very focused, practical, credible, clinical research methods could almost go on forever (e.g., case method, action research, mixed-method, meta-analysis, and Delphi study). The DNP student doesn't even necessarily need to conduct traditional clinical research. A DNP thesis (or whatever it would be labeled) could be historical, philosophical, advanced policy, or as the *Essentials* suggests, a

---

[19]That is, they have passed their final Comprehensive Exam and are now working on their clinical dissertation proposal or final clinical dissertation.

large, thorough, scholarly systematic review or position paper. We only contend that we ought to call this *final project* something more uniform, scholarly, and titled so that it is immediately understood by other disciplines. For this reason, we prefer "practice dissertation" or "DNP Thesis."[20] By using this approach, a doctoral nursing student, when queried, never has to answer "I didn't do one" when someone learns one is in doctoral study and naturally asks, "So what is your dissertation on?" Practice knowledge generation only needs rigor, proper mentoring, an inquiring mind, and some creativity. *Research* or *creating new knowledge* cannot be words to run away from or avoid in DNP curricula. They need to be embraced. This is doctoral study after all.

Table 16.2 identifies some exemplars of doctor of nursing practice programs that we discern are working toward a practice knowledge development model for

TABLE 16.2
Exemplars of Doctor of Nursing Practice Knowledge Development

Title	Format	University
The Effect of a Multimethod Teaching Strategy of Content Knowledge and Critical Thinking	DNP Thesis	Case Western Reserve University
Sleep Disruption and Interstitial Cystitis Symptoms in Women	Clinical Dissertation	Drexel University
HPV Knowledge and Cervical Cancer Prevention in Older High-Risk Women	Clinical Dissertation	Drexel University
Hospital Room Design and Health Outcomes of the Aging Adult	Clinical Dissertation	Drexel University
Preventing Child Maltreatment in Military Families: Evaluating the Effectiveness of a Web-based Tutorial for Mandated Reporters	Practice Inquiry Project	University of Arizona
Project GENESIS: Community Assessment of a Rural Southeastern Arizona Border Community	Practice Inquiry Project	University of Arizona
Use of Standards of Care by Nurse Practitioners in Providing Care to Adolescents with Asthma at an Academic Nurse Managed Primary Care	Practice Inquiry Project	University of Arizona
Cue based Feeding Protocols May Lead to Fewer Days to Full Oral Feedings and Prevent Oral Aversion Behaviors in Preterm Infants	Capstone Clinical Investigative Project	University of Washington
Translation Research: Bridging the Gap Between Evidence Based Recommendations for Postpartum Depression and the Clinical Setting	Capstone Clinical Investigative Project	University of Washington
Application of the PRECEDE-PROCEED Model of Program Implementation to Development of a Cancer Survivorship Program for Women with Breast Cancer	Capstone Clinical Investigative Project	University of Washington

---

[20]We suggest the term "clinical dissertation" be reserved for hybrid professional practice degrees, since the PsyD degree has already long adopted this "clinical dissertation model" when that degree's founders broke away from the PhD in Clinical Psychology in the 1960s (Murray, 2000; Wheaton College, 2004; Widener University, 2004).

the DNP and DrNP degrees, even if they do not all yet fully embrace practice knowledge development as the epistemological model for this new degree. This is after all partly why this book has been written—to suggest a new paradigm grounded upon philosophy of science inquiry which can provide ongoing discussion among practice faculty, practice students, and practice nursing graduates as we create the future knowledge for one discipline.

DIFFERENTIATING PhD, HYBRID, AND PROFESSIONAL, PRACTICE OR CLINICAL DOCTORATE PROGRAMS

There are many health profession degrees in the United States and around the globe. Table 16.3 first categorizes the three types of health professions doctorates that proliferate in the United States.

Table 16.4 describes some of the important differentiations between the PhD and the professional, practice, or clinical doctorate. The *hybrid professional doctorate* aims would fall somewhere in between each degree model and in some cases the hybrid would look more like the PhD (the DrPH degree for instance) and other times the hybrid would resemble the professional doctorate more if the research project was more modest.

Nursing will have to decide going forward just how much research emphasis the DNP degree is going to have in the future. While nursing may be at a point historically where we are trying to shed an excess of research degrees in particular (with the DNSc degree and others converting to the PhD), the phenomena of degree differentiation is actually moving toward *adding* more types of degrees with more precise missions.

TABLE 16.3
Types of Doctorates for Health Professions Disciplines in the United States. Table modified from Figure 1 in Smith Glasgow & Dreher (2010)

Academic Research Doctorate (Research-Intensive Emphasis)	"Hybrid" Professional Doctorates (Practice/Research-Oriented Emphasis)	Professional Doctorates (Practice/Nonresearch Emphasis)
PhD—doctor of philosophy	**DrPH**—doctor of public health	**MD**—doctor of medicine
ScD—doctor of science	**DSc**—doctor of science	**DPT**—doctor of physical therapy
DNS— doctor of nursing science	**PsyD**—doctor of psychology	**PharmD**—doctor of pharmacy
DSN— doctor of science in nursing	**DSW**—doctor of social work	**DNP**—doctor of nursing practice
DNSc—doctor of nursing science	**DScPT**—doctor of science in physical therapy	**DDS**—doctor of dental science
	DrNP—doctor of nursing practice	**DVM**—doctor of veterinary medicine
	DrOT—doctor of occupational therapy	**DOT**—doctor of occupational therapy
	DCN—doctor of clinical nutrition	

TABLE 16.4
Comparison Between PhD and the Professional/Practice/Clinical Doctorate

Construct	PhD	Professional/Practice/Clinical Doctorate
Orientation	Process-driven	Outcome-driven
	University-driven (rigid)	Student-driven (flexible)
	Fresh researcher (seeking academic training)	Experienced practitioner (or seeking qualification)
	Focus on the aggregate	Focus on the individual(s)
Content	Mode 1 knowledge & Theoretical knowledge	Mode 2 knowledge & Practice knowledge
	Context of discovery	Context of application
	Discipline orientation	Workplace/specialty practice orientation
Outcomes	Traditional	Non-traditional
	Dissertation/Thesis/Published Papers Dissertation	Research Project/Practice Dissertation/Clinical Dissertation
	Seeks explanation & causation	Seeks improvement (doctoral advanced practice)
	Disciplinary scope: vast	Disciplinary scope: focused
	Wide dissemination	Narrow dissemination
Process	Entry through tradition	Entry through experience
	Links with university	Links with industry/workplace
	Complex research training	Practical research training
	Individual	Collaborative

Adapted and modified from Fink (2006, p. 38). The professional doctorate: Its relativity to the PhD and relevance for the knowledge economy. *International Journal of Doctoral Studies, 1*, 35–44.

Table 16.5 indicates how the discipline of occupational therapy has grappled with the very same issues nursing is facing—how to mutually utilize a research doctorate, a professional doctorate, and also embrace a middle-path (a hybrid) that tries to employ the best of both types of degrees (research and practice) (American Occupational Therapy Association, 2007). We have certainly seen a trend for Drexel DrNP graduates to be hired into full-time university positions (even tenure track lines), mostly because prospective employers are excited about hiring a faculty member with a doctorate that included both practice and research.

We suggest the DNP degree needs to be reengineered to embrace at least *formally* and *explicitly (but credibly)* practice knowledge development. We reject any assumption that the DNP degree is not a real doctorate, or is a second class doctorate, or whether it is a watered down PhD (Bollag, 2007; Ellis, 2005; 2007; Toma, 2002). Fink (2006) affirms the professional doctorate (including practice or clinical doctorate) "should not be a watered down version of the PhD but offer a valid alternative in doctoral education" (p. 38). We fully agree. However, the clinging to the proclamation that the DNP graduate will *only* translate and disseminate evidence may be particularly

TABLE 16.5
Types of Graduate Degrees for Occupational Therapy Practice in the U.S.

Masters Entry Level	Professional Doctorate Entry Level (Practice/ Nonresearch Emphasis)	"Hybrid" Professional Doctorates (Practice/ Research-Oriented Emphasis)	Academic Research Doctorate (Research-Intensive Emphasis)
MS—master of science in occupational therapy	**DOT**—doctor of occupational therapy	**DrOT**—doctor of occupational therapy	**PhD**—doctor of philosophy
MOT—master of occupational therapy	**OTD**—occupational therapy doctorate	**DSc**—doctor of science	**ScD**—doctor of science
MSOT—master of science of occupational therapy			

harmful to our discipline if PhD graduations cannot adequately replace faculty retirements. Even despite fairly modest increases in enrollment recently in PhD programs, we worry that there may indeed be a decline in the future. BSN and MSN curricula have long-held evaluation and translation is a degree outcome competency. Surely, doctoral graduates can do more? Doctoral graduates, irrespective of the discipline, ought to be stewards of their discipline and advance knowledge. We portend that the DNP graduate, if utilized properly, can revolutionize nursing knowledge development with an emphasis on practice knowledge and translation. It is certainly not too late for reexamination and a first hard look at outcome data from a first critical mass of graduates.

The 2006 *AACN Essentials* document today, some 4 years plus later, is out of date. It needs revisiting now. Instead of the revision being entirely Dean driven, we suggest the AACN Deans instead appoint a diverse panel of practicing DNP faculty, including outstanding clinical scholar DNP graduates, nursing scholars specifically devoted to practice knowledge development, and scholars who can analyze the outcome data, to spearhead any future revision. The first document was top down. The revision should almost be entirely driven by outcome data, particularly from DNP graduates of all types who are living this degree every day, the academicians who are teaching them, and the employers who have and will hire them.

We envision it will indeed be a journey, perhaps a long one, by scholars in the nursing discipline to eventually provide more clarity to this question of how much research and how much philosophy of science belongs in the DNP degree? It is essential that we do so. Golde and Walker (2006) have boldly called for the preparation of better doctoral educated stewards for their respective disciplines. The Carnegie Foundation in *Educating Nurses: A Call for Radical Transformation* (Benner, Sutphen, Leonard, & Day, 2009) has recently outlined some of the current and future fundamental issues nursing is facing. The authors describe how an ongoing shortage of BSN-prepared nurses (who are needed to care for an emerging major demographic of graying, retiring, baby-boomers) remains under siege by a shortage of nursing faculty to teach them as they can make higher salaries in industry. Further, when they do enter academia, they are poorly prepared to teach. Zungolo's (2009) report that over 30% of new DNPs are entering academia may also worsen this situation (e.g., new faculty without educator skills). For this reason, the National League for Nursing has recently expressed dismay that the production of DNP graduates (unless they are provided additional education and training in teaching pedagogy) are being used as a strategy to allay the nursing faculty shortage (National League for Nursing, 2010). DNP graduates are likely going to continue to enter academia and credible curricular modifications need to be made so that they can do so credibly and skillfully. Does it not make sense that the DNP student be taught by other highly clinically competent DNP graduates? Is this not the ideal type of role modeling in the profession for doctoral advanced practice students "in training" that we aspire to? However, if the DNP graduate is perceived as being poorly equipped to advance knowledge, then the graduate is likely to experience marginalization in the university setting (Gennaro, 2004; McKenna, 2005).

SUMMARY

We predict that where practice knowledge development is weakly contextualized, or where there has been no faculty buy-in that DNP graduates should produce *good practice knowledge* (good science!) sophisticated enough for peer review and dissemination within and outside the nursing literature, there will be great variation in the quality of the DNP graduate. Poorly educated graduates might easily impugn the reputation of graduates from programs that are rigorous, which possess outstanding outcomes. In conclusion, it is worrisome that some doctoral nursing educators, in their honest quest to primarily focus on *practice* within the DNP degree construct, may limit the scope of formal scientific inquiry among inquisitive, eager, and highly clinically seasoned DNP students. Dreher and Gardner (2009) have raised concern particularly over who is going to provide both primary care research and research that will support what is now termed *doctoral advanced practice nursing* and *doctoral nursing practice* (Dreher & Montgomery, 2009). This question is particularly germane as future primary care providers will likely not be MSN prepared (nor later pursue the PhD), but pursue the DNP instead. We are extremely skeptical that the answer here is to encourage the *double doctorate*—DNP/PhD although some have indeed proposed this, and there are already a couple of programs nationally (Mancuso, 2009).[21]

This question poses an urgent reason why DNP scholars ought to be clarifying now what the nature of DNP-generated nursing knowledge is, and what the domain of practice inquiry should be. We are assured that some DNP programs *are engaging* in practice knowledge development in their final projects, but this needs to

---

[21]We are not saying we are opposed to joint DNP/PhD programs much like the MD/PhD. It just seems extreme to propose this degree model to address the relevant knowledge development issues in the profession the DNP degree has presented (or has not resolved). The MD/PhD is a very long, expensive, full-time program of study. We are very skeptical a profession with a shortage of doctoral prepared nurses can generate a critical mass of DNP/PhD graduates.

be more formalized. This also cannot happen if knowledge development is not first supported by sound understanding and grounding in the basic principles of the philosophy of science. Again Nowotny, Scott, and Gibbons write:

> Many of the most powerful scientific techniques—reductionism, normalization, sampling methods, control groups—are based on this presumption of containment or insulation. The laboratory, or wider research arena, has been a sterile space—in a metaphorical as well as physical sense. Good science has been constantly at risk of being contaminated, even overwhelmed, by a surfeit of contexts. Our argument is that this has now been turned on its head . . . . Those [fields] which embrace, willingly or otherwise, a diversity of external factors, and which we have described as strongly contextualized, are not only more 'relevant' (this is an inevitable outcome, whether welcomed or resented), but may also be more successful in terms of both the quantity and the quality of the knowledge they produce.
>
> —*Nowotny, Scott, and Gibbons, 2001, pp. 167–168*

The journey to the recognition of DNP knowledge development in the discipline and in the academy will need real, pragmatic scholarly debate and discussion. In many ways, this journey may very well parallel nursing's journey from a field to a real discipline. A degree mostly five years old is still very young. The stewardship of the DNP graduate to advance the scientific basis of the discipline should be welcomed, but it need not mirror the PhD in order to gain credibility or prestige. Instead its educators/scholars should help create its own identity, rigor, and direction. Rolfe and Davies (2009) indicate that knowledge from a critical mass of contemporary professional doctorate graduates has a great potential to transform nursing practice more than the PhD. We believe there is such a path, but it needs to be paved by tussling among innovators and conformists and by those somewhere in the middle. The path to acknowledging that the DNP graduate *can* and *should* produce *new* knowledge will only occur if the profession revisits the place of instruction and apprenticeship in the conduct of research in the DNP degree. One aspect of instruction well worth revisiting is the question of curricular depth with a grounding of knowledge in the basic principles of science through a philosophical study. The argument should not be whether one degree produces nursing knowledge and one does not, but rather the degree of emphasis on the conduct of research in our *different, but equally valuable doctoral nursing degrees.*

CRITICAL THINKING QUESTIONS

1. Does contemporary knowledge development belong exclusively in a laboratory or in the traditional "ivory tower?" Explain.
2. Do you agree or disagree that the DNP student/graduate might create Mode 2 knowledge that is perhaps more relevant to practice and work quickly translatable?
3. In your own DNP curriculum, how implicit, explicit, or absent is the notion that you will produce *knowledge* that will be useful to the profession? Explain.
4. Describe how theoretical knowledge and practice knowledge are different.
5. The authors indicate a preference for practice knowledge, but acknowledge it may be practice inquiry, actionable knowledge, or Mode 2 knowledge. Divide into groups of four and have each student provide an argument supporting each one.

6. Read more about Sackett's Levels of Evidence. Should DNP graduates be producing *evidence*? Explain.
7. Would you consider a joint DNP/PhD program? Why or why not?
8. Identify a nursing phenomenon that you believe is understudied. Why is it important to study this phenomenon further?
9. If you spent your career in nursing studying about *one specific thing*—about which you, and you alone could become perhaps the leading nurse expert—what would it be?
10. With health care reform and the influx of 33 million new individuals needing primary care, what primary care problem do you think warrants the most investigation and inquiry by a DNP student and why?

Acknowledgement: The authors want to acknowledge Drexel co-op student Joseph Dunphy for his graphical images in this text.

REFERENCES

Adler, N., & Shani, R. (2001). In search of an alternative framework for the creation of actionable knowledge: Table-tennis research at Ericsson. *Research in Organizational Change and Development, 13*, 43–79.

American Association of Colleges of Nursing. (2004). *AACN Position Statement on the Practice Doctorate in Nursing.* Retrieved April 12, 2010, from http://www.aacn.nche.edu/DNP/pdf/DNP.pdf

American Association of Colleges of Nursing. (2006). *Essentials of Doctoral Education for Advanced Nursing Practice.* Retrieved April 10, 2010, from http://www.aacn.nche.edu/DNP/pdf/Essentials.pdf

American Occupational Therapy Association. (2007). A descriptive review of occupational therapy education. *The American Journal of Occupational Therapy, 61*(6), 672–677.

Aponte, J. (2010). Key elements of large survey data sets. *Nursing Economics, 28*(1), 27–36.

Barkham, M., & Mellor-Clark, J. (2003). Bridging evidence-based practice and practice-based evidence: Developing a rigorous and relevant knowledge for the psychological therapies. *Clinical Psychology and Psychotherapy, 10*(6), 319–327.

Beck, C. T. (1994). Replication strategies for nursing research. *Image: The Journal of Nursing Scholarship, 26*(3), 191–194.

Benner, P., Sutphen, M., Leonard, V., & Day, L. (2009). *Educating nurses: A call for radical transformation.* San Francisco, CA: Jossey-Bass.

Bollag, B. (2007). Credential creep. *Chronicle of Higher Education, 53*(42), A10.

Bunge, M. (1961). The weight of simplicity in the construction and assaying of scientific theories. *Philosophy of Science, 28*(2), 120–149.

Christensen, C. M., Grossman, J. H., & Hwang, J. (2008). *Innovator's prescription—A disruptive solution for health care.* New York, NY: McGraw-Hill.

Coghlan, D. (2006). Insider action research doctorates: Generating actionable knowledge. *Higher Education, 54*(2), 293–306.

Dreher, H. M. (2008a). Innovation in nursing education: Preparing for the future of nursing practice. *Holistic Nursing Practice, 22*(2), 77–80.

Dreher, H. M. (2008b). Is poor weight management a failure of primary care? *Holistic Nursing Practice, 22*(6), 312–316.

Dreher, H. M. (2009a, March 24–27). *A novel way to approve DNP projects and clinical dissertation topics.* Paper presented at The 2nd National Conference on The Doctor of Nursing Practice: The Dialogue Continues…, Hilton Head Island, South Carolina, March 24–27, 2009.

Dreher, H. M. (2009b). Obesogenics, nutrition education and the need to deconstruct the concept of a "healthy diet." *Holistic Nursing Practice, 23*(6), 311–314.

Dreher, H. M., Donnelly, G., & Naremore, R. (2005). Reflections on the DNP and an alternate practice doctorate model: The Drexel DrNP. *Online Journal of Issues in Nursing, 11*(1). Retrieved September 6, 2010, from www.nursingworld.org/ojin/topic28/tpc28_7.htm

Dreher, H. M., & Gardner, M. (2009). *With the Rise of the DNP, Who Will Conduct Primary Care Nursing Research?* Drexel University's Second National Conference on The Doctor of Nursing Practice: The Dialogue Continues…, Hilton Head Island, South Carolina, March 24–27, 2009.

Dreher, H. M., & Montgomery, K. E. (2009). Let's call it "doctoral" advanced practice nursing. *The Journal of Continuing Nursing Education, 40*(12), 530–531.

Dreher, H. M., & Smith Glasgow, M. E. (in press). Global perspectives on the professional doctorate. *International Journal of Nursing Studies.*

Drummond, J. S., & Themessl-Huber, M. (2007). The cyclical process of action research. *Action Research, 5*(4), 430–448.

Ellis, L. B. (2005). Professional doctorates for nurses: Mapping provision and perceptions. *Journal of Advanced Nursing, 50*(4), 440–448.

Ellis, L. B. (2007). Academics' perceptions of the professional or clinical doctorate: Findings of a national survey. *Journal of Clinical Nursing, 16*(12), 2272–2279.

Evans, D. (2003). Hierarchy of evidence: A framework for ranking evidence evaluating health-care interventions. *Journal of Clinical Nursing, 12*, 77–84.

Fahs, P. S., Morgan, L. L., & Kalman, M. (2003). A call for replication. *Journal of Nursing Scholarship, 35*(1), 67–72.

Fink, D. (2006). The professional doctorate: Its relativity to the PhD and relevance for the knowledge economy. *International Journal of Doctoral Studies, 1*, 35–44.

Garrett, L. (1999, March). The virus at the end of the world. *Esquire.com*, Retrieved March 28, 2010, from http://www.esquire.com/Virus-End-World-0399?click=main_sr

Geanellos, R. (2004). Nursing based evidence: Moving beyond evidence-based practice in mental health nursing. *Journal of Evaluation Clinical Practice, 10*(2), 177–186.

Gennaro, S. (2004). A rose by any name. *Journal of Professional Nursing, 20*(5), 277–278.

Giacomini, M. K., & Cook, D. J. (2000a). Users' guides to the medical literature XXIII. Qualitative research in health care A. Are the results of the study valid? *Journal of the American Medical Association, 284*(3), 357–362.

Giacomini, M. K., & Cook, D. J. (2000b). Users' guides to the medical literature XXIII. Qualitative research in health care B. What are the results and how do they help me care for my patients? *Journal of the American Medical Association, 284*(4), 478–482.

Gibbons, M. (1994). Preface. In M. Gibbons, C. Lomoges, H. Nowotny, S. Schwartzman, P. Scott, & M. Trow (Eds.), *The new production of knowledge* (pp. vii–ix). London, UK: Sage.

Golde, C. M., & Walker, G. E. (2006). *Envisioning the future of doctoral education: Preparing stewards of the discipline.* Stanford, CA: The Carnegie Foundation for the Advancement of Teaching, Jossey-Bass.

Heath, G. (2001). *Teacher education and the new knowledge environment.* Paper presented to the Australian Association for Educational Research Conference. Retrieved March 28, 2010, from http://www.aare.edu.au/01pap/hea01582.htm

Harbour, R., & Miller, J. (2001). A new system for grading recommendations in evidence based guidelines. *British Medical Journal, 323*, 334–336.

Hellerstein, D. (2008). Practice-based evidence rather than evidence-based practice in psychiatry. *Medscape Journal of Medicine, 10*(6), 141.

Hertzog, M. (2008). Considerations in determining sample size for pilot studies. *Research in Nursing & Health, 31*(2), 180–191.

Hinshaw, A. S. (1989). Nursing science: The challenge to develop knowledge. *Nursing Science Quarterly, 2*(4), 162–171.

Houde, S. C. (2009). Public policy. The systematic review of the literature: A tool for evidence-based policy. *Journal of Gerontological Nursing, 35*(9), 9–12.

Keithley, R. K. (2003). Why Rush will keep the DNSc. *Journal of Professional Nursing, 19*(4), 223–229.

Kelder, J. (2005). Using someone else's data: Problems, pragmatics and provisions. *Forum: Qualitative Social Research, 6*(1), Art. 39. Retrieved September 6, 2010, from http://nbn-resolving.de/urn:nbn:de:0114-fqs0501396

Kikuchi, J. (1999). Clarifying the nature of conceptualizations about nursing. *Canadian Journal of Nursing Research, 30*(4), 115–128.

Leininger, M. (1985). Ethnography and ethnonursing: Models and modes of qualitative data analysis. In M. Leininger (Ed.), *Qualitative Research Methods in Nursing* (pp. 33–72). Orlando, FL: Grune & Stratton.

Magee, T., Lee, S. M., Giuliano, K. K., & Munro, B. (2006). Generating new knowledge from existing data: The use of large data sets for nursing research. *Nursing Research, 55*(2), S50–S56.

Magyary, D., Whitney, J. D., & Brown, M. A. (2006). Advancing practice inquiry: Research foundations of the practice doctorate in nursing, *Nursing Outlook, 54*(3), 139–151.

Mancuso, P. (2009, March 24–27). *The DNP/PHD dual degree option.* Paper presented at the 2nd National Conference on The Doctor of Nursing Practice: The Dialogue Continues. . . , Hilton Head Island, South Carolina.

Manser, R., & Walters, E. H. (2001). What is evidence-based medicine and the role of the systematic review: The revolution coming your way. *Monaldi Archives for Chest Disease, 56*(1), 33–38.

Mantzoukas, S., & Jasper, M. (2008). Types of nursing knowledge used to guide care of hospitalized patients. *Journal of Advanced Nursing, 62*(3), 318–326.

McDonald, P. W., & Viehbeck, S. (2007). From evidence-based practice making to practice-based evidence making: creating communities of (research) and practice. *Health Promotion Practice, 8*(2), 140–144.

McKenna, H. (2005). Doctoral education: Some treasonable thoughts. *International Journal of Nursing Studies, 42*, 245–246.

Melnyk, B., & Davidson, S. (2009). Creating a culture of innovation in nursing education through shared vision, leadership, interdisciplinary partnerships, and positive deviance. *Nursing Administration Quarterly, 33*(4), 288–295.

Melnyk, B., & Fineout-Overholt, E. (2005). *Evidence-based practice in nursing & in healthcare.* Philadelphia, PA: Lippincott Williams & Wilkins.

Melnyk, B., & Fineout-Overholt, E. (2010). *Evidence-based practice in nursing & in healthcare* (2nd ed.). Philadelphia, PA: Lippincott Williams & Wilkins.

Moitra, E. (2009). Acceptance-based intervention to promote HIV medication adherence. PhD dissertation, Drexel University. Retrieved April 4, 2010, from http://idea.library.drexel.edu/bitstream/1860/3035/1/Moitra_Ethan.pdf

Munday, D., Petrova, M., & Dale, J. (2009). Exploring preferences for place of death with terminally ill patients: qualitative study of experiences of general practitioners and community nurses in England. *British Medical Journal, 339*, b2391.

Murphy, S. L., Robinson, J. C., & Lin, S. H. (2009). Conducting systematic reviews to inform occupational therapy practice. *The American Journal of Occupational Therapy, 63*(3), 363–368. Retrieved March 25, 2010, from http://www.thefreelibrary.com/Conducting + systematic + reviews + to + inform + occupational + therapy + practice

Murray, B. (2000). The degree that almost wasn't: The PsyD comes of age. *The Monitor, 31*(1), 52.

National Institute of Mental Health, National Advisory Mental Health Council. (1999). *Bridging science and service: A report by the National Advisory Mental Health Council's Clinical Treatment and Services Research Workshop* (NIH Publication No. 99-4353). Washington, DC: NIH.

Neal, A. (2008). Seeking higher-ed accountability: Ending federal accreditation. *Change: The Magazine of Higher Education Regulation,* Sept–Oct, 25–29.

National League for Nursing. (2010). *Doctor of Nursing Practice (DNP) Addressed by the NLN's New "Reflection & Dialogue" Series.* Retrieved April 9, 2010, from http://haoodnla.com/article/lxy09217160y9j01/363328

National Institutes of Mental Health. (2006). *Interventions and Practice Research Infrastructure Program* (IP-RISP) (R24) (PAR-04-015). Retrieved September 6, 2010, from http://grants.nih.gov/grants/guide/pa-files/par-06-441.html#PartI

Neumann, R. (2005). Doctoral differences: Professional doctorates and PhDs compared. *Journal of Higher Education Policy and Management, 27*(2), 173–188.

Nogeste, K. (2008). Dual cycle action research: A professional doctorate case study. *International Journal of Managing Projects in Business, 1*(4), 566–585.

Nowotny, H., Scott, P., & Gibbons, M. (2001). *Re-thinking science: Knowledge and the public in an age of uncertainty.* Cambridge, UK: Polity Press.

Nyquist, J. (2002). The Ph.D.: A tapestry of change for the 21st century. *Change: The Magazine of Higher Learning, 34*(6), 12–20.

Oxford Centre for Evidence-based Medicine. (2009). *Oxford Centre for Evidence-based Medicine — Levels of Evidence.* Retrieved September 6, 2010, from http://www.cebm.net/index.aspx?o=1025

Pate, M. F. D., & Crabtree, K. (2009, March 24–27). *Practice inquiry in DNP projects: Distinguishing among research, quality improvement, and translation of research into practice.* Paper presented at the 2nd National Conference on The Doctor of Nursing Practice: The Dialogue Continues..., Hilton Head Island, South Carolina.

Pearson, A., Borbasi, S., & Gott, M. (1997). Doctoral education in nursing for practitioner knowledge and for academic knowledge: The University of Adelaide, Australia. *Image—the Journal of Nursing Scholarship, 29*(4), 365–368.

Pearson, A., Wiechula, R., Court, A., & Lockwood, C. (2007). A re-consideration of what constitutes "evidence" in the healthcare professions. *Nursing Science Quarterly, 20*(1), 85–88.

Peplau, H. (1952). *Interpersonal relations in nursing.* New York, NY: G. P. Putnam's Sons.

Peplau, H. (1988). The art and science of nursing: Similarities, differences, and relations. *Nursing Science Quarterly, 1*(1), 8–15.

Petrisor, B. A., & Bhandari, M. (2007). The hierarchy of evidence: Levels and grades of recommendation. *Indian Journal of Orthopedics, 41,* 11–15.

Polit, D., & Beck, C. T. (2007). *Nursing research: Generating and assessing evidence for nursing practice* (8th ed.). Philadelphia, PA: Lippincott, Williams & Wilkins.

Pope, C. (2007). Review: Exploring the effectiveness of action research as a tool for organizational change in health care. *Journal of Research in Nursing, 12*(4), 401–402.

Rapala, K., & Novak, J. (2007). Integrating patient safety in curriculum. *Patient safety and quality healthcare* (pp. 16–23). Retrieved September 6, 2010, from http://docs.lib.purdue.edu/cgi/viewcontent.cgi?article=1014&context=rche_pre

Reed, P. G. (1996). Transforming practice knowledge into nursing knowledge—A revisionist analysis of Peplau. *Image: The Journal of Nursing Scholarship, 28*(1), 29–33.

Reed, P. G. (2006). The practice turn in nursing epistemology. *Nursing Science Quarterly, 19*(1), 36–38.

Rich, N. C. (2005). Levels of evidence. *Journal of Women's Health Physical Therapy, 29*(2), 19–20.

Rodriguez-Pereyra, G. (2008). Nominalism in metaphysics. *Stanford Encyclopedia of Philosophy.* Retrieved March 25, 2010, from http://plato.stanford.edu/entries/nominalism-metaphysics/

Rolfe, G., & Davies, R. (2009). Second generation professional doctorates in nursing. *International Journal of Nursing Studies, 46*(9), 1265–1273.

Rycroft-Malone, J., Harvey, G., Seers, K., Kitson, A., McCormack, B., & Titchen, A. (2006). An exploration of the factors that influence the implementation of evidence into practice. *Journal of Clinical Nursing, 13*, 913–924.

Sackett, D. L. (1996). Evidence based medicine: What it is and what it isn't. *British Medical Journal, 312*, 71–72.

Sackett, D. L., Strauss, S. E., Richardson, W. S, Rosenberg, W., & Haynes, R. B. (2000). *Evidence-based medicine: How to practice and teach EBM.* Philadelphia, PA: Churchill-Livingstone, 2000.

San Francisco AIDS Foundation. (2008). Confronting the "evidence" in evidence-based HIV prevention: Summary report. *HIV Evidence-Based Prevention.* Retrieved April 4, 2010, from http://www.sfaf.org/files/site1/asset/sfaf-confronting-evidence-summary.pdf

Smith Glasgow, M. E., & Dreher, H. M. (2010). The future of oncology nursing science: Who will generate the knowledge? *Oncology Nursing Forum, 37*(4), 393–396.

Sommers, L. S., Morgan, L., Johnson, L., & Yatabe, K. (2007). Practice inquiry: Clinical uncertainty as a focus for small-group learning and practice improvement. *Society of General Internal Medicine, 22*, 246–252.

Stew, G. (in press). Enhancing the doctoral advanced practice role with reflective practice. In H. M. Dreher & M. E. Smith Glasgow (Eds.), *Role development in doctoral advanced nursing practice.* New York, NY: Springer Publishing Company.

Toma, J. D. (2002). *Legitimacy, differentiation, and the promise of the Ed.D. in higher education.* A paper prepared for the Annual Meeting of the Association for the Study of Higher Education, Sacramento, CA.

Torpy, J. M. (2009). Evidence-based medicine. *Journal of the American Medical Association, 301*(8), 900.

Vydelingum, V., Smith, P., & Colliety, P. (2009). Research perspectives applied to primary health care. In D. Sines, M. Saunders, & J. Forbes-Burford (Eds.), *Community Health Nursing* (4th ed.) (pp. 74–79). San Francisco, CA: Wiley & Sons.

Wheaton College. (2004). *Clinical dissertation manual for the doctor of psychology degree (Psy.D).* Wheaton College Psychology Department, Wheaton, IL: Author.

White, B. (2004). Making evidence-based medicine doable in everyday practice. *Family Practice Management, 11*(2), 51–58.

Widener University. (2004). *Manual for the clinical dissertation for the doctor of psychology degree (PsyD).* Widener University Institute of Graduate Clinical Psychology. Chester, PA: Author.

Zungolo, E. (2009, March 24–27). *The DNP and the faculty role: Issues and challenges.* Paper presented at 2nd National Conference on the Doctor of Nursing Practice: The Dialogue Continues..., Hilton Head Island, South Carolina.

Appendix A

Sample Philosophy of Science Syllabus: Drexel University 2005–2009

Drexel University
College of Nursing and Health Professions,
Doctor of Nursing Practice Program (DrNP)

Nurs 700: Philosophy of Natural & Social Science: Foundations for Inquiry into the Discipline of Nursing
Term: Fall 2009
Prerequisites: None
Credit Hours: 3
Class Hours: Wednesday, 5:40–8:30
Office Hours: Wednesday, Thursday, 4–5 P.M.
Faculty: Michael D. Dahnke, PhD

Office: 12th Floor, Bellet Building
Phone: 8937
E-mail: mdd23@drexel.edu
Fax: 215-762-8429

Required Textbooks/Supplies

Rosenberg, A. (2000). *Philosophy of science: A contemporary introduction*. London: Routledge.
Rosenberg, A. (2008). *Philosophy of social science*. Boulder, CO: Westview Press.
Woodhouse, M. B. (2006). *A preface to philosophy*. Belmont, CA: Wadsworth Publishing.

Course Description

This introductory course will focus on the logic of inquiry in the natural and social sciences. Concepts for discussion include cause, determination, measurement, error, prediction, reduction, and the roles of theory and experiment. In addition to these central issues of scientific inquiry, the broader question of values in science will be discussed. Also, the distinction between natural and social science—laws, theory, methodology, confirmation and acceptance—will be explored. The course will conclude with introductory discussions on how nursing as an applied science discipline connects to these intellectual developments.

Course Objectives

The successful student will

- Critically investigate the foundations of science and scientific inquiry.
- Learn the epistemological and ontological bases and presuppositions for scientific methodology, theory, explanation, and knowledge.
- Appreciate philosophical challenges to these bases and presuppositions.
- Understand the role science has within culture and society, and the effect of culture, society, and values on science.
- Learn and appreciate the addition of feminist perspectives on science in the realms of epistemology, values, and methodology.
- Learn the traditional distinctions between natural and social science, and the philosophical challenges to these distinctions.
- Be able to apply the insights and knowledge gained in class to nursing science.

Attendance/Participation

Being a graduate course, attendance and participation will not be calculated directly into the final grade. At this level, the importance of these should be apparent and taken for granted. Thus, both will be expected and may indirectly affect grade if gross deficiencies occur. This is primarily a seminar course that depends on the participation of all students in class discussion.

Methods of Evaluation

1. Response Papers   30%
2. Group Project   30%
3. Term Paper   40%

Assignments

Response Papers

During weeks 2 through 9 each student should submit a response paper based on the handouts assigned for that week with about a single typed, double-spaced page of thoughtful reflection and interpretation. Summarize the main points and issues or problems addressed, explicate new concepts introduced and present any questions you have regarding the content of the chapter. Utilize the assigned textbook readings in analyzing and interpreting the text with some clear reference to the assigned textbook reading assignment. This should be submitted as a hard copy document and brought to class. I may ask you to read your response, as we will use these as the basis of class discussion.

Group Project

In the last module of the course we will be applying what we've learned to some recent examples of nursing science. The class will be divided into three groups and assigned one of three articles from a nursing science journal in order to apply the inquiry learned throughout the course to this example of nursing science. The purpose of the assignment is to engage class discussion, particularly toward the question as to whether and in what way "nursing" is a science. Length: 3–5 pages in APA style, abstract unnecessary.

Term Paper

Each student will write a 10–12 page term paper on one of the questions listed below. The class readings should be viewed as only a jumping off point for this paper. Research into the many sides and complexities of this question should be done. You should identify and explicate the various standard views regarding the question with a critical analysis of each and a thesis that argues in favor of some considered answer to the question. Standard APA style and formatting should be followed, including abstract. Due date: December 8.

1. How do we distinguish science and nonscience?
2. What is a scientific explanation?
3. What is a scientific theory?
4. Is the distinction between natural and social science a real distinction?
5. What is the logical structure underlying scientific claims?
6. Is science masculine? Can there be a feminine science? What would that be like?
7. Do faith (religion) and reason (science) conflict or can they be reconciled without contradiction?

Journals

Hahnemann library subscribes to a number of excellent philosophy of science journals. These can be helpful in providing insight for the article analysis, case study, and reading presentation assignments. And of course they can be invaluable sources of research for the term paper.

Philosophy of science journals
Journal for General Philosophy of Science
The British Journal for the Philosophy of Science

Philosophy of Science
Studies in History and Philosophy of Science
Isis
Synthese

Grading Scale

Letter Grade	Numerical Grade
A+ = 4.0	96–100
A = 4.0	92–95
A– = 3.7	90–91
B+ = 3.3	87–89
B = 3.0	84–86
B– = 2.7	82–83
C+ = 2.3	79–81
C = 2.0	76–78
C– = 1.7	74–75
D+ = 1.3	71–73
D = 1.0	68–70
F = 0.0	below 68

Class Topical Outline

Module One

The Scientific Revolution and Introduction to the Philosophy of Science Lecture: The Essence and Influence of the Inception of Modern Science in the 17th Century. What is Philosophy of Science? One Hundred Years of the Philosophy of Science

Module Two

Readings: Woodhouse, Chapters 1 and 2; Rosenberg (2000), Chapters 1 and 2; Carl G. Hempel, "Laws and Their Role in Scientific Explanations"; Wesley Salmon, "Why Ask, 'Why?'?"

Module Three

Readings: Rosenberg (2000), Chapters 3 and 4; Bas van Fraassen, "The Pragmatics of Explanation; Philip Kitcher, "Explanatory Unification."

Module Four

Readings: Rosenberg (2000), Chapters 5 and 6; Thomas Kuhn, "Introduction: A Role for History"; Thomas Kuhn, "The Route to Normal Science."

Module Five

Readings: Rosenberg (2000), Chapter 7; Bruno Latour and Steve Woolgar, "The Social Construction of Scientific Facts."

Module Six

Readings: Rosenberg (2008), Chapters 1 and 2; Michael Scriven, "A Possible Distinction Between Traditional Scientific Disciplines and the Study of Human Behavior."

Module Seven

Readings: Rosenberg (2008), Chapters 3 and 4; Charles Taylor, "Interpretation and the Sciences of Man."

Module Eight

Readings: Rosenberg (2008), Chapters 5 and 6; Jon Elster, "Functional Explanation: In Social Science."

Module Nine

Readings

Rosenberg (2008), Chapters 7 and 8; Alison Wylie, "Reasoning About Ourselves: Feminist Methodology in the Social Sciences."

Module Ten

The Philosophy of Nursing Science—Guest Facilitator: H. Michael Dreher, PhD, RN, Department Chair, Doctoral Nursing Department Readings: Jacobs, B. B. (2001). Respect for human dignity: A central phenomenon to philosophically unite nursing theory and practice through consilience of knowledge. *ANS, Advances in Nursing Science, 24*(1), 17–35; Morse, J. M. (2001). Toward a praxis theory of suffering. *ANS, Advances in Nursing Science, 24*(1), 47–59; Dixon, J. (2002). An integrative model for environmental health research. *ANS, Advances in Nursing Science, 24*(30), 43–57.

Disability Statement

Student with disabilities requesting accommodations and services at Drexel University need to present a current accommodation verification letter ("AVL") to the faculty before accommodations can be made. AVL's are issued by the Office of Disability Services ("ODS"). For additional information, contact the ODS at www.drexel.edu/edt/disability, 3201 Arch St., Ste. 210, Philadelphia, PA 19104, V 215.895.1401, or TTY 215.895.2299.

Academic Integrity

Students are responsible for complying with academic integrity standards as set forth in the *Nursing Student Handbook* and the *Drexel University Student Handbook*. Cheating, plagiarism, forgery, or other forms of academic misconduct are not tolerated at this institution, nor are they consistent with professional nursing. Plagiarism is a serious offense and will not be tolerated. Please see http://www.drexel.edu/cchc/studentlife/Judicial/code/acadintegrity.html

N.B. All cell phones, beepers and other noise emitting electronic devices should be turned off or otherwise silenced during class. This is merely electronic age courtesy.

The instructor reserves the right to make changes to this syllabus if circumstances warrant such change.

Appendix B

Suggestions for Syllabi Using Philosophy of Science for Nursing Practice

This text is intended for the education of students of doctoral nursing practice; however, PhD nursing programs which have a strong grounding in practice may also find it very appropriate. It includes information and arguments regarding the state of nursing and advanced nursing education today, the history of science and the problems of science as raised by the philosophy of science. A coherent schedule can be designed with these various, related elements in mind. Alternatively, the text could be used with a central focus on the philosophy of science if the contentious issues regarding advanced nursing practice and knowledge development are less of a concern in a particular program; or the nursing chapters could be easily used later in a course on nursing epistemology or doctor of nursing practice professional issues. We actually plan to use this text at Drexel in two courses. Below are suggestions for scheduling in both a 14-week semester and a 10-week quarter curricula.

Semester Schedule

Week 1

Chapter 1: What is a Practice Discipline?

Week 2

Chapter 2: Nursing as a Practice Discipline

Week 3

Chapter 3: Philosophy of Science in a Practice Discipline
Chapter 4: Philosophy and Philosophizing

Week 4

Chapter 5: The Scientific Revolution
Chapter 6: One Hundred Years of the Philosophy of Science

Week 5

Chapter 7: What is Science? The Problem of Demarcation

Week 6

Chapter 8: Scientific Methodology

Week 7

Chapter 9: Observation: The Scientific Gaze

Week 8

Chapter 10: Theory and Reality

Week 9

Chapter 11: Explanation and Laws

Week 10

Chapter 12: The Feminist Critique of Science

Week 11

Chapter 13: Philosophy of Social Science

Week 12

Chapter 14: *Philosophies* of Social Science

Week 13

Chapter 15: The Path to Nursing Science Today, 1910–2010

Week 14

Chapter 16: Next Steps Toward Practice Knowledge Development: An Emerging Epistemology of Nursing

Quarter Schedule

Week 1

Chapter 1: What is a Practice Discipline?
Chapter 2: Nursing as a Practice Discipline

Week 2

Chapter 3: Philosophy of Science in a Practice Discipline
Chapter 4: Philosophy and Philosophizing

Week 3

Chapter 5: The Scientific Revolution
Chapter 6: One Hundred Years of the Philosophy of Science

Week 4

Chapter 7: What is Science? The Problem of Demarcation

Week 5

Chapter 8: Scientific Methodology

Week 6

Chapter 9: Observation: The Scientific Gaze

Week 7

Chapter 10: Theory and Reality
Chapter 11: Explanation and Laws

Week 8

Chapter 12: The Feminist Critique of Science

Week 9

Chapter 13: Philosophy of Social Science
Chapter 14: *Philosophies* of Social Science

Week 10

Chapter 15: The Path to Nursing Science Today, 1910–2010
Chapter 16: Next Steps Toward Practice Knowledge Development: An Emerging
   Epistemology of Nursing

Appendix C

Glossary of Philosophical Terms

Abduction: Also called abductive logic, abductive reasoning, or abductive inference. Identified and defined by American philosopher Charles Sanders Peirce (1839–1914) as a third type of logical reasoning (in addition to deduction and induction) in which one reasons to the best explanation of a phenomenon. Like induction and unlike deduction, such inferences are not certain or absolute. Like deduction and unlike induction, the number of cases involved in the premises (the sample) is usually irrelevant to the quality of the inference. A classic example is "When you hear hoof beats think horses not zebras." The best explanation for the sound of hoof beats in this part of the world is horses. It is not impossible that the explanation for the hoof beats you here is zebras, but that is not the most plausible explanation. In Africa, zebras might be a more plausible explanation, but again not a certain one.

Peirce meant this form of logic as descriptive of the type of reasoning employed in reaching a scientific hypothesis. He did not believe deduction or induction properly characterized this mode or reasoning. Abductive logic, however, has not achieved widespread acceptance as a distinct form of logical reasoning independent of deduction and induction. Many philosophers and logicians recognize it simply as a form of induction.

Analytic Truth: A statement is an analytic truth if it is necessarily true or true by definition. For example, "All bachelors are married."

Androcentric: Presuming, favoring, oriented toward male views and values.

A posteriori: After experience. *A posteriori* typically refers to knowledge gained from sensory experience.

A priori: Prior to experience. *A priori* typically refers to knowledge (especially knowledge of logic and mathematics) that is not due to experience.

Ceteris Paribus: Latin for "all things being equal." A qualification invoked in order to mentally strip away uncontrollable variables.

Cogency: The quality of a good inductive argument such that (a) it is strong and (b) all its premises are true.

Conclusion: The statement of an argument that premises are meant to provide reasons or evidence for belief.

Contingency: Logically, the quality of two statements such that there is no logical relationship between them. Epistemologically, the term can refer to statements which are true or false dependent upon actual states of the world. Metaphysically, the term may refer to an object which does not exist of necessity.

Critical Theory: A movement in philosophy and social science, influenced largely by the works of Marx and Freud, that asserts that philosophy and social science should work to free people from political and other forms of oppression.

Deductivism: Also called deduction, deductive logic, deductive reasoning, or deductive inference. A form of logic in which one claims to argue to a certainty. Take this classic argument from Aristotle (the first person in Western philosophy to formalize and systematize deductive logic) as an example:

1. All men are mortal.
2. Socrates is a man.
3. Therefore, Socrates is moral.

Not only is this argument deductive, but it is a "good" (valid) deductive argument, because not only does the arguer *claim* to argue to a certainty, but with this argument, they *do* **argue to a certainty**. Another way of saying that this argument reaches a certainty (is valid) is that *if* **the premises** (statements 1 and 2) **are true, then the conclusion** (statement 3) *must* **be true**. Try to hold in your mind that statements 1 and 2 are true but statement 3 is false. You should find this to be an impossible task. This is because **the truth of 1 and 2 (the premises) guarantees the truth of 3 (the conclusion)**. We say that this argument is "good" in a particular way: it is valid.

Dogmatic: The acceptance of beliefs without critical thought. The irrational, absolutist commitment to a belief system.

Dualism: A metaphysical position which holds that there are two basic, irreducible substances in the universe, of which everything is composed. The most well-known form of dualism is mind/body dualism, particularly that of Descartes. According to the theory of mind/body dualism, everything is made of immaterial (nonphysical) mind or spirit (souls/minds, ideas, mental states, etc.) or material (physical) body (human bodies, trees, stars, rocks, mountains, etc.) or some combination of the two (persons).

Elenchus: A method of inquiry associated with Socrates in which discussants of various views test one another's claims through critical questioning.

Empiricism: An epistemological position in which knowledge claims are based on and confirmed by sensory experience, usually posed against rationalism. "Empiricism" is sometimes used to refer generally to any epistemological position or theory that focuses on or affirms the authority of sensory experience. In this way, empiricism could be used to describe the theories of philosophers dating back to Aristotle. Sometimes, though, it is used to describe more narrowly the empiricism of a group of modern philosophers known as British Empiricists (sometimes Classical Empiricists) and later 19th- and 20th-century philosophers who were influenced by their specific approach to empiricism. The three primary British Empiricists were John Locke (1632–1704), George Berkeley (1685–1753), and David Hume (1711–1776). The school of philosophy most influenced by this approach to empiricism was logical positivism.

Entelechy: In Aristotelian philosophy a force within objects (both living and inanimate) that leads them to their proper, natural place.

Epistemology: The branch of philosophy that studies the source, nature, scope, and confirmation of knowledge and knowledge claims.

Explanandum: Latin term for a phenomenon to be explained.

Explanans: Latin term for the explanation given for an *explanandum*.

Functionalism: An approach to social science which presumes understanding can be attained by searching for manifest and latent functions of human and social action.

Gynocentric: Presuming, favoring, oriented toward female views and values.

Hermeneutics: Relating to interpretation. Originally "hermeneutic" referred to the study of Biblical interpretation. Later it was expanded to refer to the study of interpretation in general. It also refers to a philosophical and social scientific approach that focuses on the interpretation of human action in the context of social rules.

Holism: The view that understanding can only be attained from a perspective of wholes. Things are more than the sum of their parts.

Idea: A common philosophical meaning of the word "idea" is any content of the mind, including thoughts, perceptions, doubts, wishes, etc.

Idealism: A metaphysical position in which it is held that everything is composed of immaterial or spiritual substance. According to idealists, matter does not in fact exist. This does not mean that the table in front of you is not real. It is real as an "idea" (a mental object) but not as a physical object.

Implication: Logically, the quality of a statement (or statements) that its truth guarantees the truth of an implied statement.

Incompatibility: Logically, the quality of a statement (or statements) that its truth guarantees the falsity of the incompatible statement.

Inductivism: Also called induction, inductive reasoning, inductive logic, or inductive inference. A form of logic in which one claims to argue to a probability. There are three common types of inductive argumentation: generalization, analogies, and causal arguments. Generalizations are instance of arguing from a claim which predicates a property to a sample and infer the likelihood that the population to which the sample belongs also holds that property. The primary criteria for an argument of this type are that the sample be of sufficient size and representative of the diversity of the population. Statistics is a sophisticated form of this type of reasoning. An analogy is a comparison between two or more things. In the premises of an analogical argument it is asserted that the things being compared have certain properties or qualities in common. From the similarity of these qualities it is inferred in the conclusion that they are similar in some further, relevantly similar manner. The main criteria for this type of argumentation are that the items being compared are not only similar in some respect but in enough respects that are relevant to the inferred quality to support the conclusion, and that they are not relevantly dissimilar in a way that would weaken the inference. A causal argument merely maintains that some event A brings about a second event B. The difficulty of causal arguments can be seen in the difficulty of research into the etiology of certain diseases like AIDS.

Since in induction we are only arguing to a probability, inductive inferences can be judged as a matter of degree. This is different from deductive reasoning which an argument is either valid or invalid, a very black and white standard. Inductive arguments are judged as strong or weak (with a variety of degrees of strength or weakness) depending on the degree of probability that the conclusion does indeed follow from the premises.

Inference: Also, inferential reasoning. The mental act of starting with knowledge claims that are known or assumed to be true and drawing further knowledge claims from those. A very simple example is Aristotle's famous syllogism:

1. All men are mortal.
2. Socrates is a man.
3. Therefore, Socrates is mortal.

From the first two statements (the premises), we can infer the third statement (the conclusion).

Instrumentalism: The view that cognitive tools such as mathematics or scientific theories are just tools (instruments) for achieving specific goals like predicting phenomena and are not necessarily reflective of reality.

Intentional: Referring to elements, perceptions, and beliefs of the mind, that which is subject to interpretation.

Invalidity: The quality of a bad deductive argument, such that the premises do not guarantee the truth of the conclusion. It is possible to have all true premises but a false conclusion.

Logic: The branch of philosophy that studies inferential reasoning. Logic is traditionally divided into deductive logic and inductive logic, though the American philosopher Charles Sanders Peirce (1839–1914) introduced a third type, abductive logic. The first philosopher in the West to systematize logic was Aristotle, whose system dominated logic and logical studies until the development of propositional logic in the late 19th century.

Logical Positivism: A school of philosophical thought that grew out of the intellectual movement known as the Vienna Circle. Logical positivists were especially interested in the philosophical study of science. They saw science as merely empirical study structured and justified logically.

Materialism: The metaphysical position which holds that all that exists is made of matter or physical substance. Souls, spirits, and immaterial objects in general do not exist. Minds are explained as part of or processes of the physical, organic brain.

Metaphysics: That branch of philosophy which studies ultimate reality, what the nature and essence of existence is, what things and types of things actually exist, and in what nature they exist.

Monism: The metaphysical position which holds that only one type of irreducible substance exists. Everything in the universe is in fact made of this one substance. Many of the earliest philosophers expressed a monist view, asserting the underlying reality to be water (Thales), air (Anaximenes), or fire (Heraclitus). The modern world generally recognizes two forms of monism: materialism and idealism— although there are numerous varieties of both of those views.

Naive Realism: The view that our common sense beliefs and perceptions accurately reflect the world.

Nomological: Law-like, pertaining to laws and values, prescriptive as opposed to descriptive. From the Ancient Greek *nomos* which means law or custom.

Objective: Relating to knowledge of independent reality; distinct from and unaffected by specific, personal, invested views.

Paradigm: A term used by Thomas Kuhn to refer to the broad conceptual frameworks that shape and inform the beliefs, views, and research of scientists.

Paradigm Shift: A fundamental change in worldview that amounts to possibly a change in reality.

Phenomenalism: An empirical view in which the reality of physical objects is reduced to their perceptual existence.

Phenomenology: A movement in philosophy and social science which focuses on inner subjective experience to attain understanding.

Positivism: A philosophical position on science attributed to French philosopher Auguste Comte (1798–1857). Positivism emphasized empirical study as the only means of acquiring knowledge. Comte particularly advocated this approach for the social sciences. Comte's use of this term was adopted later by the Logical Positivists of the 20th century.

Postmodernism: A broad philosophical, literary, artistic, and cultural movement in which the presumptions of modernism are powerfully criticized and questioned.

Pragmatism: A philosophical school originally associated with the American philosophers Charles Sanders Peirce (1839–1914), William James (1842–1910), and John Dewey (1859–1952). Later pragmatists include W.V.O. Quine (1908–2000), Richard Rorty (1931–2007), Hilary Putnam (1926–), and Ian Hacking (1936–). Pragmatists generally eschew metaphysical flights and attempt to connect our philosophical beliefs and inquiries to practical life.

Premise: Sometimes premiss. A statement in an argument intended to provide evidence or a reason to believe that the conclusion of the argument is true.

Rationalism: An epistemological position in which knowledge claims are based on and confirmed by the mind and the mental processes of the mind, usually posed against empiricism. "Rationalism" is sometimes used to refer generally to any epistemological position or theory that focuses on or affirms the authority of the mind. In this way, "rationalism" could be used to describe the theories of philosophers dating back to Plato. Sometimes it is used to describe any philosophical position with an emphasis on the employment of reason, especially as opposed to recognition of nonrational (especially emotional) elements of human nature and thought. Sometimes, though, it is used to describe more narrowly the rationalism of a group of modern philosophers known as Continental Rationalists. The three primary Continental Rationalists were René Descartes (1596–1650), Gottfried Leibniz (1646–1716), and Baruch Spinoza (1632–1677). Rationalists tend to hold a very high standard of knowledge, usually with models of epistemic certainty being logic (deductive) and mathematics. Strictly speaking no one has ever had sensory experience of the kinds of geometric figures that Euclid defined: squares, circles, etc. Every attempt at one of these in the sensory world will always be imperfect and not live up the exacting standards of the Euclidean definition. Ironically, irrational numbers like π, $\sqrt{2}$, or 1.222..., are good examples of nonempirical knowledge because they can only be known through the rational minds not through sensory experience. Rationalists tend to point to the uncertainty of empirical knowledge (due to the limitations of the sensory organs, illusions, etc.) to argue that empirical knowledge is not really knowledge as it lacks certainty. Empiricists admit the uncertain nature of empirical knowledge but argue for a lower standard regarding legitimate knowledge.

Rational Choice Theory: An approach to social science in which it is presumed that humans are essentially rational and will generally make rational, self-interested decisions.

Reductio ad absurdum: A type of argument in which another's claim or argument is criticized by showing that it logically leads to an absurd or otherwise untenable conclusion.

Reductionism: The view that understanding comes from breaking entities down to their constituent parts. Things are no more than the sum of their parts.

Scientific Realism: The metaphysical view that science accurately informs us about the state of the world.

Soundness: A quality of a good deductive argument such that (a) it is valid, and (b) all the premises are true. Logically, then the conclusion must also be true. This means that it is possible for an argument to be valid but not sound, but not possible for an argument to be sound but not valid.

Statement: Also, proposition. A declarative sentence, the kind of sentence that can be true or false. More technically, "statement" refers to the thought behind the declarative sentence. For example:

1. "The moon is made of green cheese."
2. "The Earth revolves around the sun."
3. "The Louvre is in Paris."
4. "The location of the Louvre is Paris."

Numbers 3 and 4 are in fact the same statement expressed in different sentences.

Strength/Weakness: Qualitative assessments of inductive arguments. Strong arguments are ones in which the premises provide good support for the conclusion. Weak arguments are ones in which the premises provide poor or little support for the conclusion.

Subjective: Relating to the internal workings of the mind; affected by specific, personal, sometimes invested views.

Synthetic Statement: A statement that is not analytically true or analytically false. Its truth is dependent upon contingent states of the world as it brings together (synthesizes) separate, distinct concepts.

Teleology: From the Ancient Greek *telos* which means end, purpose, or goal. This is the ancient and medieval worldview that all things in the world have an inherent purpose. Rain falls not due to meteorological laws, but in order to nourish plants and animals.

Validity: Colloquially, people use "valid" in a nebulous manner as a general synonym for good. In deductive logic, it is a technical term which refers to the quality of a deductive argument such that *if* **the premises are true, then the conclusion** *must* **be true.** Another way of saying this is that **the truth of the premises guarantees the truth of the conclusion.** Note the conditional nature of the definition. Validity is not about the actual truth of the statements that comprise the argument. Validity is a quality of the form of the argument, a structure that guarantees that if you start with true premises you will generate (infer) a true conclusion. The question of actual truth is covered by the concept of soundness.

Index

Note: n = footnote